Customers and Patrons
of the Mad-Trade

MEDICINE AND SOCIETY
Andrew Scull, Editor

This series examines the development of medical knowledge and psychiatric practice from historical and sociological perspectives. The books contribute to a scholarly and critical reflection on the nature and role of medicine and psychiatry in modern societies.

1. *The Regulation of Madness: Origins of Incarceration in France,* by Robert Castel, translated by W. D. Halls.

2. *Stubborn Children: Controlling Delinquency in the United States, 1640–1981,* by John R. Sutton.

3. *Social Order/Mental Disorder: Anglo-American Psychiatry in Historical Perspective,* by Andrew Scull.

4. *Inheriting Madness: Professionalization and Psychiatric Knowledge in Nineteenth-Century France,* by Ian R. Dowbiggin.

5. *Madness and Social Representations,* by Denise Jodelet, translated by Tim Pownall, edited by Gerard Duveen.

6. *Inventing the Feeble Mind: A History of Mental Retardation in the United States,* by James W. Trent, Jr.

7. *Impure Science: AIDS, Activism, and the Politics of Knowledge,* by Steven G. Epstein.

8. *Mental Ills and Bodily Cures: Psychiatric Treatment in the First Half of the Twentieth Century,* by Joel Braslow.

9. *Medicalizing the Mind: The Invention of Modern Psychotherapy,* by Eric Caplan.

10. *Imperial Bedlam: Institutions of Madness in Colonial Southwest Nigeria,* by Jonathan Sadowsky.

11. *Undertaker of the Mind: John Monro and Mad-Doctoring in Eighteenth-Century England,* by Jonathan Andrews and Andrew Scull.

12. *Customers and Patrons of the Mad-Trade: The Management of Lunacy in Eighteenth-Century London,* by Jonathan Andrews and Andrew Scull.

Customers and Patrons of the Mad-Trade

The Management of Lunacy
in Eighteenth-Century London

With the Complete Text of John Monro's
1766 Case Book

Jonathan Andrews
and Andrew Scull

UNIVERSITY OF CALIFORNIA PRESS
Berkeley · Los Angeles · London

Publication of the illustrations in this book has been made possible by grants from the Scouloudi Foundation in association with the Institute of Historical Research, and from the Marc Fitch Trust.

University of California Press
Berkeley and Los Angeles, California

University of California Press, Ltd.
London, England

Library of Congress Cataloging-in-Publication Data

Andrews, Jonathan, [date]–.
    Customers and patrons of the mad-trade :
the management of lunacy in eighteenth-century
London : with the complete text of John Monro's
1766 case book / Jonathan Andrews and Andrew
Scull.
        p.   cm.—(Medicine and society ; 12)
    Includes bibliographical references and index.
    ISBN 0-520-22660-7 (alk. paper)
    1. Monro, John, 1715–1791.
2. Psychiatrists—England—Biography.
3. Psychiatry—England—History—18th century.
4. Mentally ill—England—Case studies.
I. Scull, Andrew T.   II. Title.   III. Series.

RC450.G7 .A645 2003
616.89'0092—dc21   2002067881
[B]

Manufactured in the United States of America

12   11   10   09   08   07   06   05   04   03

10   9   8   7   6   5   4   3   2   1

The paper used in this publication meets the mini-
mum requirements of ANSI/NISO Z39.48-1992
(R 1997) *(Permanence of Paper).*♾

To the memory of the late Roy Porter

Contents

List of Illustrations   ix

Preface   xi

Acknowledgments   xv

PART I · *Managing Lunacy in Eighteenth-Century London*   1

  1. Customers, Patrons, and Their Mad-Doctor   5

  2. A Rare Resource: John Monro's Case Book   13

  3. Profiling Patients and Patterns of Practice   28

  4. The Craft of Consultation: Managing Patients and Their Problems   45

  5. Diagnosing the Mad   58

  6. Religion, Madness, and the Case Book   82

  7. Treating Patients and Getting Paid   92

  8. Being Mad in Eighteenth-Century England: Patients' Views of Their Own Illnesses   107

PART II · *John Monro's 1766 Case Book*   117

Notes   119

Bibliography   177

Index   203

Illustrations

1. Portrait of Dr. John Monro by Nathaniel Dance (1769)   7

2. The White House, Bethnal Green (1794)   10

3. Scene viii from William Hogarth's *A Rake's Progress* (1735)   38

4. Caius Gabriel Cibber's "Raving and Melancholy Madness," as engraved by William Sharp (1783)   39

5. Thomas Rowlandson's caricature of John Monro and Charles James Fox (1784)   40

6. "The Fatal Effects of Despair" (1789)   72

7. "The Distressed Mother" (1788)   73

8. "The Suicide" (1788)   74

Preface

This is the second of two books we have devoted to the examination of John Monro, his patients, and the world of eighteenth-century madness and mad-doctoring. Once again, as with its predecessor *(Undertaker of the Mind)*, *Customers and Patrons of the Mad-Trade* is the product of a close and continuing collaboration that has been facilitated by (indeed, in many ways, made possible by) the wonders of email and the internet, which have allowed us to work together closely, even in the face of the almost six thousand miles that physically separate La Jolla and Oxford. Both of us have worked and reworked the text and exchanged ideas about the meaning of the case book that forms the core of the analyses we present here, pooling our intellectual talents and resources (such as they are) to what we hope is good effect. Once more (as with our work on *Undertaker of the Mind*), though our internal debates and exchanges have often been spirited, we have readily reached an interpretative consensus, and the process of working together has been a remarkably smooth and enjoyable one for both of us. Needless to add, perhaps, it follows that we are jointly and equally responsible for whatever errors of omission and commission others detect in our text, just as we have shared equally in its production.

The present volume had its origins in a serendipitous discovery made during the late 1980s by one of the authors while he was doing post-graduate work on the history of the first and most famous asylum in the English-speaking world, Bethl(eh)em Hospital, or Bedlam. Alerted by the hospital's current archivist to the fact that some distant relations of the Monro family, the dynasty who served as physicians to the hospital from 1728 to 1853,[1] might have in their possession some of their ancestors' papers, Jonathan Andrews made contact with a St. Mary's Hospital and Harley Street practitioner, Dr. F. J. G. Jefferiss (d. 1998), and found that such a cache had indeed survived. Among the extant papers, Dr. Jefferiss drew particular attention to the existence of a small, nondescript, leather-bound volume. Its unimpressive exterior, he enthusiastically pointed out, concealed a case book kept by the second member of the dynasty to serve as Bethlem's physician, John Monro (1715–91). Here was a rich and fascinating, if also frustrating, document that would eventually provide a unique window into the practice of mad-doctoring in Augustan England.

Dr. Jefferiss generously provided a photocopy of the case book for Jonathan's use during the course of his research. Although the case book was not central to Jonathan's dissertation or subsequent publications, he did not forget it in the ensuing years, thinking that he might produce an annotated edition and commentary and append it to a short overview of its author's career. This long-gestating idea began to take concrete form when the two of us first discussed this rare and remarkable find some years later, at a springtime conference of the Society for the Social History of Medicine at the University of Exeter. During the course of a long conversation on an organized bus trip around some of Devon's nineteenth-century asylums, we agreed that the case book could present us with an interesting opportunity for collaborative research. Certainly, we were both convinced, it was too precious a resource to leave hidden away in a private archive.

With the approval of Dr. Jefferiss and others among Monro's descendants, we therefore began work on a modern, annotated edition of the case book. Dr. Jefferiss was kind enough to permit another copy to be made and to sanction access to the original text, as he was keen to see the case book in print. Dr. Jefferiss also obtained the consent of his cousin, James Mackenzie (the owner of the case book), for its publication, and since Dr. Jefferiss's death the family has continued to be very supportive of our efforts to produce this edition. Neither of us actually saw the original manuscript until 1999, when the present manuscript was very far advanced and not long after Dr. Jefferiss had unfortunately passed away. Even a perusal of the facsimile of this extraordinary document, however, was sufficient to inspire us to write this book together. Precisely because the original manuscript was intended purely for Monro's private purposes and was never expected to see the light of day, it provided a direct and unmediated insight into the practice of Augustan England's most eminent mad-doctor. For the same reason, however, its contents were often elliptical and in need of further explication for a modern readership.

The publication of Monro's case book occurs at a time of renewed interest in the history of the public institution that was central to his career and reputation—Bethlem having celebrated its 750th anniversary in 1997. The oldest and most famous/infamous psychiatric establishment in the English-speaking world, Monro's hospital has long occupied a singularly powerful place in our collective (un)consciousness. Not least, it has served as the mythical and mystical Bedlam of our imaginings: the scene of riot, turmoil, and tumult—a veritable (or perhaps not so veritable) theater of folly, where Reason wrestled with the demons of Unreason in a continuing drama of brutal beatings, callous cruelties, and the massive maltreatment of the mad. Given that historians have recently sought to replace the legend and mystery that swirled about in earlier Gothic fantasies with a more prosaic portrait of Bethlem as it really was,[2] we feel that it is also time to reexamine the beliefs and practices of a man who long served as its physician—someone whom historians have stigmatized, not always fairly or on the basis of much direct acquaintance with his clinical endeavors, as a bastion of conservatism and reaction, the epitome of the supine and neglectful *ancien régime* mad-doctor.[3]

John Monro's eighteenth-century case book, a rare if not unique document, offers us a chronicle, in his own unself-conscious and unguarded words, of the medical practice of one of the most famous English mad-doctors of the period. Though its counterparts for other years have been lost, presumably forever, this surviving volume reveals an unmatched array of information about the customers of the mad-business. We have sought here to provide an extensive analysis of these materials, placing them in a wider historiographic context and seeking to explore how much we can learn through a thorough interrogation of such an invaluable resource.

Some readers may prefer to first undertake their own reading of Monro's text (reprinted in part 2 of this volume), "uncontaminated" by the suggestions made in our commentary in part 1, and only subsequently compare what they made of his jottings with the analysis we ourselves present. Others may choose instead to digest our readings before tackling and trying to make sense of the elusive and allusive shorthand in which this particular mad-doctor recorded his impressions of his patients and those who brought them to his attention. Both of these strike us as viable approaches to these rich materials, and each mode of reading has its own virtues and limitations. Whichever route an individual reader takes, however, he or she will encounter a disturbed and disturbing world, one filled with anecdote and gossip, humor and sadness, travail and tragedy—the world in which John Monro plied his trade, sought his patrons, treated his patients, and made his fortune. We have found it a fascinating one, and we suspect (and hope) that our readers will, too.

Acknowledgments

Naturally, we are especially grateful to the late Dr. F. J. G. Jefferiss; his widow, Phyllis Jefferiss; his son, Jeremy James Jefferiss; and his cousin, James Mackenzie, for agreeing to permit the publication of the case book that forms the basis of the analysis of the patrons and customers of the mad-trade that we present in part 1, and that we reprint in its entirety (with annotations) in part 2. We would both like to thank them for their support, courtesy, and encouragement during the period in which we have worked on this project. Without them, obviously, we could never have produced this book, and we hope they will be pleased with the volume that their generosity has made possible.

It would be remiss of us not to thank colleagues and friends who have given us extremely valuable suggestions and feedback on matters associated with this study. A number of people have gone further, and have read and commented on drafts of our discussion of the issues raised by Monro's case notes, and on the annotations we have made to the case book itself. In these contexts, we should particularly like to acknowledge the assistance of Joel Braslow, William Bynum, Matthew Craske, Stephen Cox, Liz Foyster, Elaine Murphy, Steven Shapin, and Trevor Turner, and the constant prodding and enthusiastic support we have received from Howard Boyer. Our thanks, finally, to Helen Coward for a great job with the transcription (and for patience over getting paid!), and to Lynnette Turner for her support and encouragement. For sterling assistance with the copyediting and production of this book, we would like to thank Laura Harger and Sue Carter of the University of California Press. Thanks, too, to Stan Holwitz, and to Brian Southam.

As this book went to press, we learned with shock and dismay of the death of Roy Porter. A man of boundless energy, wit, generosity, and kindness, he will be deeply missed by all who knew him, and by the thousands of people who were acquainted with him only through his prodigious scholarly output. Roy was a friend and an immensely supportive colleague to both of us for many years (and the former doctoral supervisor of one of us). While his eloquent scholarship has graced a dizzying array of fields in social, cultural, medical, and scientific history, Roy was most at home in the eighteenth century. His pioneering history of madness in this period, *Mind Forg'd Manacles,* led many, including ourselves, to re-examine the place of insanity in Enlightenment England, and it is no exaggeration to say that, but for him, this book would never have been written.

PART ONE

Managing Lunacy in Eighteenth-Century London

Goodwife Jackson, aged 39, of a burnt high-coloured
sanguine Complexion, black Hair, 12 Years since fell mad,
ran up and down the Streets, bare footed, Cloaths torn, Hair
loose, was ready to lye down and pull up her Cloaths to
every one, pretended Love to one Mr Holland her Master,
then a Prisoner in the King's Bench; at last she tore all things,
and struck every one, and was raving mad; being poor, I have
her a Glass of Antimony a Scruple in Beer, each other
Morning for 14 Days . . . sometimes of Scamony in Beer or
Ale . . . not omitting Bleeding and Sleepers; and . . . Broth
and Posset-Drink, with much Plantaine boiled in it, and thus
cured her, and she is well to this Day, having been half a Year
mad to a high Degree.

Daniel Oxenbridge, *General Observations of the
Practice of Physick* (1715; quoted in Roy Porter
[ed.]), *The Faber Book of Madness*, p. 241)

I was desired to visit a woman who resided at no great distance from the man whose case has just been described [that
of a respectable farmer, in the country]. I found her sitting up
in the bed—she was wrapped about the head, neck and
shoulders with cloaks and flannels—she received me with
a smiling countenance, and when I enquired into her
complaints, she laughed, and enumerated a great variety of
symptoms; but I could not really discover that she had any
bodily indisposition, except what was occasioned by laying in
bed. In a chair at the bed-side, were, Wesley's Journal, Watt's
Hymns, the Pilgrim's Progress, and the Fiery Furnace of
Affliction. I prescribed according to the usual form, but could
do her no good; and I was afterwards informed, that she
became so mad as to require confinement. I was told by her
husband, that there was not the least pre-disposition to
Madness before this attack [but] . . . a Methodist preacher,
who had much infested the parish, was frequently in her
company, and they were perpetually conversing on religious
topics.

Reverend William Pargeter, *Observations
on Maniacal Disorders* (1792, pp. 32–33)

. . . should every one who displayed the smallest symptoms of insanity be immediately deprived of his liberty, and treated as a madman, nobody can tell where the spirit of confinement might end. . . . If it be true, as some Moralists have ventured to assert, that every person is to be considered insane who submits his reason to the dominion of any ruling passion . . . it would be difficult, perhaps, to fix upon any one person who ought to be indulged with the privilege of walking through the world without a keeper.

Thomas Monro [of Magdalen College], "Vicious and Foolish People Considered Insane," *Essays on Various Subjects* (1790, p. 69)

CHAPTER I

Customers, Patrons, and Their Mad-Doctor

The history of psychiatry, as David Ingleby wittily remarked some years ago, once resembled "the histories of colonial wars[: it told] us more about the relations between the imperial powers than about the 'third world' of the mental patients themselves."[1] In recent years, his gibe has lost some of its sting, as historians belatedly have begun to make efforts to uncover the fates and the experiences of patients and their families.[2] Still, it is remarkable how much less we know of these customers and patrons of the mad-trade than we do of those who managed, cared for, and confined the (putatively) insane. Nor, until recently, have we learned much about the nuts and bolts of psychiatric practice and therapeutics[3]—about what the alienist and the madhouse-keeper actually did to and for their patients—a neglect equally manifest in the history of medicine more broadly construed.[4] The difficulties presented by each of these enterprises are manifest and major. They are not insurmountable, however, and the distortions of understanding that flow from avoiding these tasks are at least as apparent and as significant.

This book is centrally about patients and their families and their inter-action with the mad-doctor who managed their troubles and who pro-vided for their care and (in some instances) confinement. Concerned, nonetheless, to offer a balanced, multifaceted account, it also explores in some depth the reactions of the physician to the stories he heard from and about the insane, and the nature of the interventions he recommended and employed in the course of his daily practice. The patients and families whose lives and travails we explore here were all attended by the same mad-doctor, John Monro (1715–91), Physician to London's Bethlem (or, as it was popularly known, "Bedlam") Hospital for most of his profes-sional career. Monro was perhaps the most prominent of the emerging coterie of medical men specializing in the management of the mad in Augustan England. With only rare exceptions, however, the patients we deal with here were not among the ranks of Bedlam's mad-folk. Rather, they constituted a sample of those Monro treated in his private practice, which was far more financially rewarding and consumed far more of his time, energies, and talents than did his more visible involvement with the inmates of what for centuries has been the most celebrated (and anathematized) hospital for the insane in the English-speaking world.

It was, of course, John Monro's family connections and his long association with Bethlem that accounted, in substantial measure, for his standing at the very head of a newly emerging eighteenth-century profession. Monro was the second of a veritable family dynasty who continuously presided over London's Bedlam from 1728 to 1853. His tenure as the hospital's physician began in June 1751, barely a year before the death of his father and predecessor, James, and extended over four decades, to within a few months of his own demise. On the foundation provided by the limited income but extraordinary visibility his hospital appointment generated for him, and building upon his father's reputation and contacts among the aristocracy and well-to-do, John created a remarkably extensive and extremely lucrative practice ministering to the mad. He acquired madhouses of his own, obtained substantial retainers and consulting fees from his contacts with a range of establishments owned and operated by others, and provided advice and treatment to a wide array of nervous and distracted patients in more domestic settings. The wealth and property he accumulated secured the family's fortunes, and his professional prominence made the Monro name virtually synonymous with the specialty that he did much to create and consolidate.

Bethlem itself was a monastic foundation dating from as early as 1247, and it had been involved with the care of the lunatic since at least the early fifteenth century, early acquiring and never losing an identity almost isomorphic with the institutional treatment of the insane. In its corrupted form, "Bedlam," the institution's very name became identified in the English-speaking world with chaos, tumult, danger, and disorder. In John Monro's day, the institution was one of the sights of London, visited regularly and in substantial numbers by metropolitan sophisticates and country bumpkins alike. A staple of the stage at least since the age of Shakespeare (1564–1616) and Ben Johnson (1573[?]–1637), it surfaced as a cliché in Grub Street novellas, as a satirical weapon in the poetry and prose of men such as Swift and Pope, in the paintings and prints of Hogarth and Rowlandson, and in repeated (if often throwaway) references among the diaries and letters of the English elite.

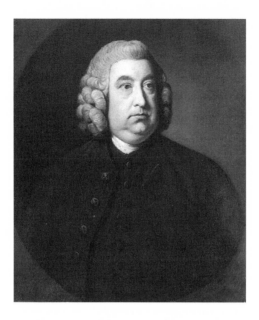

FIGURE I. Portrait in oils on canvas of John Monro, M.D., in his younger days, painted in 1769 by one of the leading portrait artists of the day, Nathaniel Dance (1735–1811). This picture was donated to the College of Physicians by the mad-doctor's great-grandson, Dr. Henry Monro, in 1857 and is currently on loan to the Bethlem Royal Hospital Museum. Reproduced by kind permission of the Royal College of Physicians, London.

The inmates of Bedlam—both literally, in the eyes of those who came to gawp at them, and metaphorically, in a variety of literary renditions of insanity—gave seeming substance to long-standing cultural stereotypes of mad behavior. They stood (or squatted) as an indictment of the lunatic, seen variously as the embodiment of extravagance, incoherence, incomprehensibility, melancholia, menace, and ungovernable rage. The cells and galleries of the ancient foundation—ironically, the smallest, most specialized, and least affluent of the great London hospitals of the Georgian age—were emblematic of Unreason, their occupants both unwilling and performing actors in a theater where the throngs of visitors might inspect the product (and price) of immorality, the wreck of the human intellect, the dolor of the downcast, and the rages of the raving. Once housed in the modest accommodations provided by an old monastic building at Bishopsgate that Henry VIII had granted to the City of

London at the time of the dissolution of the monasteries that formed part of the English Reformation, Bethlem had grown dilapidated and boxed in by the encroaching city by the early seventeenth century. It moved, however, to its Moorfields location in 1676, occupying an externally ornate edifice designed by Robert Hook and constructed (with little regard for the long-run integrity of the building itself, but with symbolic appropriateness) on the liminal space just beyond the City of London wall, built upon the uncompacted accretion of discarded rubbish and effluvia that had filled up the old moat. Here was a spectacular new palace designed to display the benevolence and solicitude of the capital's citizens and to symbolize the Restoration of royal and civic unity and to connect it to the restoration of reason. Its architecture was conceived pre-eminently as fund-raising rhetoric rather than for its present and future inmates, whose interests took distinctly second place. As late as the mid-seventeenth century, there were between thirty and fifty madmen (and madwomen) at the old Bishopsgate site. However, with the 120 cells that comprised new Bethlem soon fully occupied, and a series of further extensions from the late 1720s onward (when provision was made for more than 100 "incurable" patients in newly constructed wings), the hospital's population multiplied many-fold. In the new building, both internal and external arrangements were manipulated and compromised to achieve the higher goals of impressing upon both the institution's patrons and the public at large the virtues of civic pride and Restoration renewal. Contemporaries could be relied upon to point out the ironic contrast between the sober splendor of the hospital's exterior and the impoverishment and chaos that lurked within. Yet—and again the qualification makes salient another important facet of the ambivalent place occupied by madness and the mad in early modern England—notwithstanding all its contradictions between inner and outer, ditch and palace, deprivation and ornament, as Christine Stevenson has shown, new Bethlem was still planned with a firm (if subordinate) attention to "therapeutic efficacy." In terms of air, light, and space, it was fundamentally designed for the restitution of its inmates' health and to exploit the advantages of its bright and airy Moorfields location. And, undoubtedly, new Bethlem represented a rather impressive and grandiose application of resources by its governors to the creation of a new lunatic hospital, bringing it "a new dignity among London's charitable institutions and international renown."[5]

By the time John Monro succeeded his father, James, as Bethlem's physician, however, the hospital had long since lost its distinction as the sole specialized establishment for the confinement of the mad in the metropolis. When Thomas Guy left his fortune to endow one of the rapidly proliferating new charitable hospitals that graced the capital,[6] one of the stipulations of his will was the setting aside of a sum of money to endow a ward in his new institution for the chronically ill, including the insane. And in the very year that John succeeded to "the throne of folly," St. Luke's Hospital, another charity asylum dedicated entirely to the care of the insane, was founded in London, partly at the initiative of one of Bedlam's governors (and one of Monro's major rivals in the mad-business), William Battie.[7] Moreover, these were only the most visible manifestations of a transformation in the management of madness that had been gathering steam in England since the Restoration.

For the growing affluence of London and its hinterland was fueling an expanding marketplace for all manner of goods and services, as the rich found ever more extensive (and expensive) ways of expending their surplus, and the middling sort hurried to ape and emulate their "betters."[8] The entrepreneurially inclined soon realized that a lucrative living could be derived from the provision of all manner of novelties, not least finding ways to relieve the well-to-do of the burdens of life's (and even death's) unpleasantnesses. If undertakers could make death the occasion for profit, helping to invent and then satisfy a whole array of new wants, so too were there fresh prospects to earn lucre from the care of lunatics, and a thriving business speculating in this variety of human misery had begun to establish itself several generations before John Monro appeared on the scene.[9] A growing demand on the part of the upper classes for some system of private care that would relieve them of the burden of their troublesome and unmanageable relations and sequestrate them from public view, together with the ability of the rich to provide substantial rewards for those who obliged them in this way, was a crucial catalyst for the development of an expanding array of "madhouses." To an increasing extent parish authorities also got in on the act, paying small sums to those willing to provide places of confinement for difficult characters of a meaner sort. In Bethnal Green, in Hoxton, and in Hackney, men such as Matthew Wright took leases on large old houses and converted them into places to which one could consign the most disturbed and disturbing.[10] And west of the city, in the village of Chelsea, still another cluster of madhouses now emerged, including Michael Duffield's madhouse, a handsome building erected by a Mr. Mart that was located between Lord Shaftesbury's house and Lord Wharton's park.

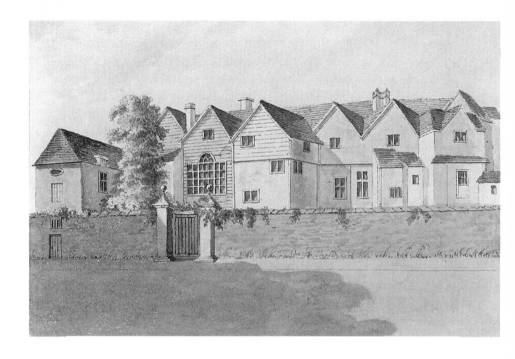

FIGURE 2. The White House, Bethnal Green. Bethnal House was built in 1570 for John Kirby immediately adjacent to the Poor's Land or Green. It appears to have acquired the nickname "Kirby's Castle" after its owner virtually bankrupted himself getting it built, and its folly was satirically linked with that of Fisher in John Snow's *Survey of London:* "Kirby's Castle, Fisher's Folly." This illustration, by an unknown artist and executed in pen, ink, and wash, dates from 1794 and shows the whitewashed exterior for which the building was subsequently renamed. Leased by Matthew Wright and transformed into a madhouse in 1727, it remained a receptacle for lunatics for nearly two centuries. After Wright's death, his widow ran the establishment for a year till the lease was taken up by a George Potter, one of whose patients between 1759 and 1763 was the poet Christopher Smart. (Smart wrote his master work, *Jubilate Agno*, while confined here.) Subsequently the enterprise passed into the hands of the venal Thomas Warburton, who used the White House and the adjacent "Red House" primarily for paupers, well over three hundred of them at a time. For the early-nineteenth-century lunacy reformers, the White House became a byword for cruelty and neglect. As Lord Robert Seymour testified before the 1815 Select Committee on Madhouses, "the house having been built for the use of a private family, as houses of a like nature have generally been, is very unfit for the great number of persons it now contains; the ceilings are extremely low, the beds are so closely stowed as to be nearly in contact with each other, and the airing or exercise yards are most inconveniently small." Two or three patients were squeezed into a single bed when space grew tight, and many slept naked in unheated rooms, amid the stench of their own excrement and on soiled straw infested with vermin. Most were chained at night to their bedsteads and were mopped down in the yard in the morning, whatever the weather. Information kindly supplied by the Tower Hamlets local history archivist, Malcolm Barr-Hamilton, and by the historian of Bethnal Green's madhouses, Elaine Murphy. Illustration reproduced by kind permission of Tower Hamlets Local History Library and Archives, London.

Nor was the "trade in lunacy" confined to the institutional care of the seriously disturbed. If madhouses provided one mechanism for drawing a discreet veil over the madman's very existence, families often recoiled from taking advantage of such sinister silences (for the reputation of these places was dire almost from the outset). Demonstrably, most preferred to seek other solutions to the problems their mad relations posed, and, if affluent, they possessed the wherewithal to do so. Hence, those who sought to minister to minds diseased often found themselves treating the mad in family or community settings.

Not that the mad-doctors of the age reacted purely passively to the demands of their customers and patrons. Many of them, on the contrary, actively sought to expand their practices to encompass all sorts of "nervous" troubles and distress. Here were protean disorders of uncertain provenance and even more uncertain extent, diseases whose very existence the doctors helped to establish and legitimize—the fashionable hyp (or hypochondria), hysteria, the spleen, and the vapors proving at least as rewarding and attractive an arena for the display of their professional talents as the more alarming and urgent manifestations of Bedlam madness. The fashionable Scottish physician George Cheyne's lucubrations about "the English Malady"[11] were but one especially visible manifestation of a far wider marketplace for the services of the specialist in mental disorders than a traditional historiographic emphasis on the growth of an institutional sector would lead us to expect. And John Monro, as one of the leading actors in this particular morality play, provides us with a revealing and intimate set of insights into the multifaceted clinical realities of the age.

CHAPTER 2

A Rare Resource

John Monro's Case Book

THE ORIGIN, FORMAT, FUNCTION, AND INTENT OF MONRO'S CASE BOOK

In common with at least some other physicians of his generation, John Monro kept careful notes of the cases he treated—more particularly of those he encountered in his private practice. Like the records kept by his colleagues, most of his case notes have long since disappeared. Abandoned in obscure places and left to endure the gnawing criticism of mice, or effaced by the simple ravages of time and circumstance, they have vanished without trace, taking with them our chance to recover the intimate secrets of a deliberately obscured corner of the medical marketplace.

Carefully preserved by one of his descendants, however, a single volume of John Monro's case notes has fortunately (and fortuitously) survived. This rare and quite possibly unique document offers us a fascinating window into Monro's private practice, and permits us a privileged peek into a subterranean world where secrecy and discretion were the very essence of becoming a successful practitioner. Consisting of Monro's record of his private attendance on one hundred cases of nervous and mental disorder among the moneyed classes during a single year (1766), the case book provides immediate and telling access to the diagnosis and treatment of a whole range of mental afflictions by a specialist practitioner. It also tells us a great deal about the sociocultural milieu in which medicine was practiced and how ordinary people evaluated and responded to the often bizarre and distressing appearance, behavior, speech, and thought-worlds of the deranged. The expectations and the experiences, the coping strategies and the crises, the behaviors and the beliefs of both patients and their families emerge vividly in Monro's jottings. Although such phenomena are recorded, to be sure, at one remove, and filtered through the lens of the mad-doctor's perceptions and pen, nevertheless, they are preserved for posterity, as all too often they were not, in the pages of what turns out to be a remarkably rich and revealing document. Finally, and not the least of its value, the case book provides ample material to highlight and further explore some of the traditional historical evaluations of psychiatry as "mad-doctoring," providing special insight into the day-to-day practice of a leading contemporary physician, and into the networks and internal markets that constituted the eighteenth-century "mad-trade."

The case entries are written in a style and form that, while requiring the degree of explication that an annotated edition provides, tell a coherent narrative story about each patient. Moreover, the text is, for the most part, both comprehensible and engaging. The records testify to the enormous scope of Monro's private practice dealing with the insane, quite beyond the demands of his duties at Bethlem and Bridewell (the house of correction with which Bethlem had been amalgamated under the same Court of Governors since ca. 1574). In the 1730s, Alexander Cruden (the famous compiler of a Biblical concordance, who was to be one of the Monros' most troublesome and vociferous patients) queried whether the numbers of patients being tended by John's father, James Monro, might be "too many to be well minded by one man" and whether he might "better have minded his Patients in the several Madhouses."[1] This question seems even more telling for John, who had evidently substantially enlarged the family business. Cruden, unwilling patient of both father and son, sardonically suggested that if a mad College of Physicians was set up between Bethlem and St. Luke's, it might be filled up with "but a third of John Monro's practise."[2]

The past three decades have witnessed a veritable explosion in historical, sociological, and other academic analyses of medicine, psychiatry, and allied sciences. The recent growth of the history of psychiatry as a subdiscipline has led to the establishment of the first specialist journals and of European and national societies for the study of psychiatry's past.[3] The same period has also been marked by considerable growth in postgraduate and undergraduate university courses in the history of medicine and science, including those in the history of psychiatry, aimed at an audience of both arts and science students. Yet this intellectual development and ferment have been only partially matched by a comparable expansion in the range of readily available primary source materials essential to the study and teaching of such disciplines. For all these reasons, the case book should appeal to a wide readership among a range of academics interested in the history of medicine, and to those seeking to teach or to study the history of medical and psychiatric practice. Although they were "meant only as a mnemonic device for himself, Monro's jottings about his consultations have an unmediated simplicity" that renders the case book "a particularly compelling document."[4] As no secondary account does or could, Monro's cases provide us with a series of snapshots, from a variety of angles, of the intricate sociomedical context of mad-doctoring in the mid-eighteenth century, taken and reproduced for us by one of its leading exponents in England. Here we are given a striking and unretouched series of pictures of the very underbelly of the mad-trade, less its public face than its most private parts, all left relatively undoctored by the mad-doctor. Clinicians also will discover in Monro's notations a riveting chronicle of a medical world not so radically divorced as might be presumed from the set of social relations that currently subsist among doctors, patients, and their families, a world that has often tended to remain hidden or underrepresented in previous accounts of psychiatric practice. Perhaps to their surprise, we suspect that contemporary psychiatrists will agree with Trevor Turner in finding that "the case book has a delightful immediacy [and that] the patient vignettes, from the more detailed to the brief, are extremely recognisable":

> Roughly speaking, it seems [as though] one is reading one's own diary, slightly transcribed by eighteenth-century language and beliefs. The people being poisoned, punished, bewitched, starved, etc., and their families in two minds, and decisions whether to confine or not to confine, are what we mad-doctors are still doing today.[5]

On still another level, the material presented here is of more than just academic and clinical interest, in the narrow sense of those terms. The stories and observations Monro recorded for his private use turn out to be just as fascinating and illuminating for the general reader. They offer access into an intimate underworld of personal griefs, anxieties, fears, ambitions, and psychological distress that are by turns familiar, disturbingly alien, enthralling, diverting, bizarre, anguished, and even poignant.

We have already explained at some length in the Preface how John Monro's case book (reproduced as part 2 of this book) first came to the attention of one of us and led to our decision to collaborate on this project. There is no need to repeat that account here. However, we believe that it *is* worth commenting, at this juncture, on some aspects of the form, function, and intent of the case book. Not only can we thereby provide some assistance in navigating its text and in comprehending the nature and meaning of Monro's sometimes confusing style of annotation, but we can also help the reader to form a more concrete picture of the case book as a physical entity. Last, but not least, our discussion here aims to help the reader to understand Monro's text as a particular product of its time, and of the specific branch and form of practice in which its author was engaged.

It was not until the summer of 1999 that one of the authors first saw the original, when he was able to take advantage of the generous hospitality of Dr. Jefferiss's widow and son. The case book, in its extant manuscript form, is written on 124 small pages, generally of between 13 and 14 lines each, with between 5 and 7 words on each line, and is around 10,200 words in length. It is bound in leather, with a brass clip fastener, and it is 12 centimeters (5 inches) wide, 19 centimeters (8 inches) long, and 1.5 centimeters (half an inch) thick. The case book is thus of a handy pocket size, which would have made it easily transportable for the mad-doctor as he went about his daily business during the year. Monro records his entries in a neat hand, in what now appears as brown ink (though its current color may, of course, be an effect of the aging process). Dated 1766 on its cover and inscribed with Monro's name on its first page, the book's format suggests that Monro had for some time been accustomed to discreetly keeping track of his private patients in separate case books compiled for each year. More likely than not, therefore, Monro originally kept a whole series of case books extending over the many years of his private practice, and it is regrettable that the record of only one year of his cases appears to survive. The pagination and overall form of the case book are more or less faithfully reproduced in this modern edition, including Monro's original abbreviations, annotations, deletions, and corrections, which have been preserved for the extra insights they offer into the idiosyncratic ways in which an eighteenth-century physician kept tabs on his patients. Problems with the legibility of the original counseled against the production of a facsimile version.

The specific notations and properties of Monro's case book to some extent correspond to those found in other contemporary medical case books. In other respects, however, they are peculiar to this particular book's form and format. Potentially they have a great deal to tell us about the intentions and function of keeping such a record, as well as the wider context of medical practice in this period. Significantly, Monro employs three basic but rather informative types of marginalia: two number notations and a textual description. The latter is quite patently and straightforwardly used to record the outcome of a case, if known, and is normally rendered succinctly in one or a few words and in a smaller hand (replicated here, in our transcribed edition of the text, by a smaller type). These marginal outcome references are a form of notation that tails off as this particular year of Monro's practice proceeds and are a subject that we discuss in more detail in chapter 7 of our commentary.

The number notations in the margins, on the other hand, are continued throughout the case book and signify respectively, in order of appearance: (1) the day of the month on which the patient was seen or the day on which Monro was consulted in a case (the doctor recorded the name of the month above the first case entry on a particular page for that month); and (2) the case number that the mad-doctor assigned to each case over the course of the year. The marginal date tends to be recorded not only first, but also in a larger hand, than the case number (and once again we have been careful to replicate this subtle distinction throughout the transcription via distinctive font sizes). This suggests that Monro tended to conceive of and account for his attendance on private cases on a monthly and annual basis, in conformity with a typical calendar or diary-like format.

These latter forms of notation reflect a real concern on Monro's part with keeping an accurate and thorough record, which he might easily consult or look back on in the future if he felt this to be necessary. Perhaps Monro copied this approach from his father, or else he may have derived it from his training at medical school. It seems likely that Monro, like many other contemporary physicians, also derived some of his methods for keeping a faithful record of his business as a physician from the necessary, everyday practice of ordinary household accounting. The doctor's precise rationale for numbering each case is open to debate. Possibly, Monro was keen to quantify the growth and success of his practice on a yearly basis, and in some small measure this form of notation does seem to reflect the "quantifying spirit" of the eighteenth century.[6] It may also be that these case numbers were intended to facilitate tracing the history of a particular case, not merely during that year but over Monro's entire period of practice. However, the absence of any sort of index or index page casts doubt on this theory. Monro's failure to refer back in detail, let alone with reflexivity, to any previous case book in any of the entries he made about a patient in 1766 implies a rather limited commitment to follow-up. In fact, Monro's way of recording case numbers in the margins signifies that, rather than ascribing unique numbers to every case he saw, he preferred to start afresh each year, numbering cases from 1 upward, and merely to cross-reference back in a textual form to cases he remembered seeing in previous years. On the other hand, if the same case was seen or advised on more than once on different dates in the same year, no new case number was assigned; only the date of the new consultation was recorded. This manifests a meticulous and careful form of note-taking but does not suggest a physician who was striving for an especially innovative or scientific enumeration or classification of cases.

Most other contemporary physicians seem to have followed this or a kindred practice. Indeed, since Monro practiced in a period long before the keeping of medical records and case-taking or the compilation of statistics was seen as relevant to any sort of scientific or clinical understanding, one should scarcely expect him to have done otherwise. Even after 1815, when asylums in the public sector became almost universally accustomed (indeed, were statutorily required) to keep case notes, an approach similar to the one Monro made use of was evidently adopted. Every separate asylum admission tended to be accorded a different case number, and patients' notes were recorded as continuous records, often across a series of volumes of chronologically maintained case books. It was not until well into the twentieth century that patients normally were assigned unique case numbers or unique files and their records kept individually, in separate folders.

The most likely explanation for the assignment of case numbers is that Monro was seeking an easy means of keeping his financial accounts in order, and that these numbers corresponded with those in an accompanying (but no longer extant) receipt book for that year.[7] A name-index clearly would not have worked as effectively for this purpose because a number of the cases he consulted on remained anonymous (for reasons we shall elaborate on later). These notations also reveal how the patient was already medicalized and objectified to some extent, or was seen as "a case," even if in a pre-Foucauldian "clinical" or "arithmetic of cases" sense.[8] The case book also must have been seen by Monro as an important means of recording his own diagnostic, prognostic, or even therapeutic insights and, to some extent, of following up and applying what he had gleaned during former consultations. Monro's approach to case-taking presents a stark contrast to that of general provincial physicians such as Richard Loxham of Poulton, Lancashire. Loxham chronicled his practice in a large and plainly nonportable ledger measuring about 40 centimeters (15.75 inches) by 16 centimeters (6.25 inches), which served

the dual purpose of an account book and case book, in which he fastid-
iously recorded the costs of treatments and the very processes of getting
his clients to pay up. Monro's portable case book, on the other hand,
concentrated more or less exclusively on patients' histories, symptoms,
and treatment and made no mention at all of bills, receipts, and debts.[9]
In this sense, Monro's case book is clearly a more medicalized document
than Loxham's, although the latter doctor devoted much more space to
registering the nature and efficacy of his medical treatments than did
Monro.

Monro clearly saw a number of cases more than once and was careful to record when he recalled seeing a patient before or treated a patient
his father had seen. On pages C-45–46 of the case book, for example, he
notes that a patient had "rec.d benefit from my father's advice, many
years ago," a characteristic marker of his filial engagement with the
memory and former practice of James Monro. Such cross-references
may even be a way of reminding himself to look back over James's own
notes (presuming that this practice of case-taking was something that,
like much of John's style and craft of practice, had been passed down
from father to son). Despite the patently private nature of Monro's
pocket-size notebook, his neat handwriting indicates that it was very
much intended to be read and re-read by the doctor himself and possibly
by intimates in his business. It seems likely that Monro adopted the
same approach to note-taking in other case books completed over the
years of his practice. However, the extent to which this was so, and the
degree to which Monro adapted his craft as time went on, must remain
a matter of conjecture in the absence of any other surviving case books.

Monro may have had other specific purposes in mind in his method of
case-taking. His notes could have proved valuable if he sought to share
information with other doctors, and they likewise could have constituted
an information resource and insurance in the event of his involvement in
contested confinements, habeas corpus, and prosecutions, or of other
courtroom appearances. We know from the case book itself and a variety of other sources that Monro was certainly named, summoned, and
required to give evidence in a number of false-confinement cases in this
period. It was relatively standard practice for eighteenth-century physicians to number cases in their publications, as did George Cheyne,
Nicholas Robinson, and a number of other specialists in nervous disorders, and it is conceivable that Monro had a similar use in mind for his
own cases. On the other hand, Monro's courtroom appearances were
still comparatively rare, and the case book seems a profoundly private

document, not designed or destined for publication or public use. There is little evidence that Monro was especially concerned to keep or exploit the case book in ways that would come to characterize the case-taking of most nineteenth- and a few eighteenth-century mad-doctors: for the active communication of medical knowledge or as a rich pathological reservoir in which to dip for the purposes of publication and career promotion, let alone as a set of cases with which to educate students. This is a set of aims that, as his earlier published exchanges with Battie had clarified, conflicted with Monro's gentlemanly taste and physicianly *modus operandi.* Monro can hardly be distinguished in his career for the enthusiasm with which he sought to share the fruits of his knowledge of cases of insanity with other practitioners—at least those outside his family. Furthermore, there are actually relatively few instances of Monro recalling the details of previous attendances in much more than a curious or incidental fashion, and none of him overtly adjusting his practice in 1766 in the light of a previous year's case book jottings. The forms of notation he adopted may well, therefore, have had more to do with the fact that Monro had the longevity and transmission of the family business very much in mind, and in this connection conceived of the case book as, at least in part, a means of keeping tabs on and retaining a clientele. Monro was probably concerned to pass on an accurate and useful record to the son(s) and grandson(s) who were to follow in his mad-doctoring footsteps.

Of course, the anonymity of some patients and the common recording of very little identifying information about others, beyond (at most) their surnames, occupations, and street names, also reflect the strong patronage and class-determined context of early modern medicine. It was clearly important for Monro to sustain a discreet, private practice in which clients were known to the doctor and the practice but were somewhat protected from public exposure, whether through careless gossip or the mislaying or theft of the case book. The use of ellipses was a common contemporary literary convention and is found again and again in eighteenth-century literature and also (though less often) in private correspondence. It was a standard ruse to avoid offense and libel prosecutions, and Monro may have adopted this strategy for not dissimilar reasons. However, some of his customers and patrons were quite evidently treated more confidentially than others, no doubt because of their more elevated social status or at their own explicit request (and it is notable that most, if not all, of Monro's anonymous patients were those who had personally consulted the mad-doctor). In some cases, Monro simply may have forgotten or neglected to record a patient's identity (and may have planned to fill in details later). Yet, in most instances he was almost certainly exercising discretion or had been deliberately kept in the dark by the patient/family because the details of a case were peculiarly sensitive (as in the case of a gentleman onanist) or because of especially strong fears about the potential stigma (and outcome) of a consultation with such a well-known mad-doctor (as in the case of a lady friend of Mrs. Blinkhorn).[10] Other contemporary doctors, who treated the ordinary sick and drew their clientele from more lowly social circles, such as the Lancashire physician Richard Loxham, always named their patients, even when the patients were suffering from sexually transmitted diseases or other potentially stigmatizing ailments.

Assuredly, too, it was not unusual for contemporary mad-doctors to attend and observe a patient anonymously, or secretly, in order to obviate anticipated opposition to such a (potentially humiliating) consultation. Occasionally, ellipses were employed in Monro's case book for patients' friends and acquaintances rather than for the patient, as in the case of Miss Gilchrist, a woman of "small fortune" and disappointed betrothals whose suitors were only partially named. These patterns indicate once again how large a part class played in the discretionary content of the mad business.[11]

On a few rare occasions, Monro utilized underlining in order to emphasize certain passages in the notes he recorded, and these emphases may be of some interest to the historian and other readers. For example, his underlining on page C-45, where he discusses a case whose eyes "seem'd fix'd as if regarding the object they were directed towards," apparently reflects the prevailing diagnostic weight placed on the eyes by contemporary mad-doctors, as well as the influence of sensational theories of mind that ascribed mental functioning to the strength and nature of sensory impressions made upon the mind or "sensorium." It seems unsurprising that an orthodox eighteenth-century mad-doctor such as Monro would have drawn attention to such symptoms, and the pathological processes they revealed, especially in a case that clearly seemed classic or archetypal to him—a man who "had the true mad stare." In accordance with sensationalist theory, after all, mad-doctors often stressed the need for their patients to be removed from the "objects" that were deemed to have disturbed their senses.[12]

In some places in the case book, Monro sometimes also struck out words or brief passages of text and/or added words and phrases (usually above existing text), evidently because he had changed his mind as to what he wanted to record or had decided to correct an inaccurate entry. Most, if not all, of these corrections evidently were applied at the time of writing, and their presence seems to indicate that Monro normally wrote directly into the case book as he went about his business, rather than waiting to write up his entries on each case at a substantially later stage, either from loose sheets of notes or from another rough pocket book. And yet the overall neatness of the case book and the small number of such corrections may, to the contrary, imply some sort of delay and space for reflection in the compositional process. It seems quite likely that Monro may have habitually written up the case book at the end of the day, and occasionally a little later. The brief notes Monro often added at the conclusion of an entry, in a smaller hand (once again rendered here in a reduced type), sometimes recorded after a few days and sometimes after a considerably longer time period, do nonetheless suggest a regularly maintained, if very sketchy, record. They argue that he was accustomed to come back to the case book record, usually to record the outcome of the case but also to add anything substantive he had heard later about a patient's symptoms or progress.[13] This is a clear reflection of the mad-doctor's preparedness to consistently follow up cases to their denouements, even if the content and brevity of these entries suggest his rather limited practical role in the ultimate outcome of many cases after an initial consultation and prescription had been provided.

The sorts of presentational features we have discussed are all retained in this edition of Monro's text. We have done so not merely in order to maintain the accuracy and originality of the case book in its transcribed form and to preserve the historical source record in as intact and authentic a form as seems feasible, but also, and more importantly, because of the light these features throw on the doctor's compositional and thinking processes and on his wider relations with his patrons and clients. For some of the same reasons (and also on other grounds), all other ellipses and abbreviations, as well as superscripts and unusual punctuation—including dashes after periods to highlight ends of sentences and colons or equals signs (rather than hyphens, as in modern usage) to signal word divisions—are also retained, even when sentences or punctuation marks are clearly, or seemingly, ungrammatical. Most of these latter features, however eccentric they may appear to modern eyes, should be understood as eighteenth-century English usage or contemporary note-taking conventions and were regularly employed not only by Monro but by many of his contemporaries. Only where abbreviations are not obvious to readers are words filled in (and the addendum placed in square brackets) in the case book text. And only where the case book is quoted in our commentary are original notations altered in other ways—for the sake of clarity in the exposition and in accordance with our publisher's conventions.

HISTORIOGRAPHICAL BACKGROUND

The use of case book material, as a number of historians from Ackerknecht and Sigerist to Porter and Weindling have pointed out,[14] is an important means by which the patient may be brought more centrally into an account of the history of medicine. Analysis of case books may also reveal much about the changing nature of relations between patients and practitioners, about the way in which, in their day-to-day practice, medical practitioners diagnosed and treated their patients, and the manner by which patients negotiated their "sick roles."[15] With the exception of patients' own writings and oral testimonies, case books provide us with our best available purchase on patients' actual experience of insanity and of their treatment at the hands of doctors and their own friends and relations. Much recent work in the history of medicine has addressed itself to these latter issues, allowing for a closer exploration not only of "disease" as defined by the medical profession, but of "sickness" as defined (in part, at least) by patients.[16] Studies of medicine in early modern England by Porter, Beier,[17] and others have exploited case books and writings by patients themselves to restore balance to a historiography that had previously tended to pay excessive attention to elite and professional standpoints, and such trends have also begun to manifest themselves in the history of twentieth-century psychiatry.[18]

More recently still, medical historians have begun to focus on the history of the case history itself. Work in this vein by scholars such as Trevor Turner, Akihito Suzuki, Günter Risse, and Robert Jütte testifies to a resurgence of interest on the part of leading medical historians in case history material.[19] In substantial measure, this heightened attention to a previously neglected set of records reflects a new-found appreciation of the importance of these materials to the development of a behaviorist, narrative, and experiential, rather than purely intellectual, history of medicine. Case histories also help us to reach a balanced assessment of the nature and development of clinical medicine in different national, regional, and historical contexts. Research in this field has tended to concentrate on how the case history has evolved and what purposes it served, what its ideological and paradigmatical bases were, what it tells us about the complicated relationships between medical ideas and medical practice, and (less directly, perhaps) what it may reveal about patients themselves and their relations with medicine and its practitioners. Porter and other historians of psychiatry, informed in part by the importance of the case history for modern psychologists and psychoanalysts, and in part by the imperative of "doing medical history from below,"[20] have accorded the case book, the case history, and the patient narrative[21] a central place in historical accounts of the changing meaning of mental illness and of psychiatric care and treatment.

Some notable recent asylum histories and histories of lunacy administration have also begun to accord more substantial space to the variety of insights derivable from a close examination of the case book and the case note.[22] On the one hand, these sources allow, if in variable and inconsistent fashion, some assessment of the dominant and changing preoccupations of medical men in constructing the medical record, of the consonance and contrasts between lay and medical judgments of illness, and of the ways in which official oversight and wider sociocultural and political agendas also shaped the medical record. On the other hand, the case book and the case history commonly furnish detailed information about the types of behavior on which the identification of illness and the medical intervention were based. They demonstrate, too, how such behavior/illness impinged upon (and beyond) the domestic sphere. Such materials present the historian with vital information about the socioeconomic background and illness history of individuals. Simultaneously, they chart the subsequent behavior and symptoms of patients, and they provide a record of the responses and attitudes provoked by or mediating such behavior. Naturally, by the nineteenth century the surviving record tends to provide a more comprehensive history of an individual patient when it is generated out of an institutional context than when, as here, it records the perhaps more infrequent and casual visits of a private practitioner. In early modern times, however, before detailed record keeping and case notes, let alone patient-centered records, became the norm, asylums and other medical institutions relied heavily on medical case books and correspondence in the reconstruction of specific doctor-patient relations and of patients' illness histories.

Despite a growing appreciation of the need to address individual cases[23] in historical research on mental illness, historians (and their publishers) have sometimes been unwilling to reproduce case book and case history material as resources for historical study. Understandably, but, we believe, sometimes mistakenly, publishers have anticipated a rather narrow demand among readers, while some medical historians have tended to see the work of preparing critical editions of such texts as a laborious and rather thankless task. There is still another difficulty, of course: in contrast with, for example, the case books of lawyers and legal advocates, few medical case books have actually survived. Certainly, until we are well into the nineteenth century, with its heightened emphasis on the importance of statistics and record keeping, case books are rather like the nearly extinct California condor. Without question, those seeking to write the history of psychiatry (and those attempting to teach it) have been handicapped by the lack of availability of such texts.

There are a few significant exceptions to the above account. Most notable, perhaps, are the voluminous *Case Books of John Hunter* (1728–92), F.R.S. (Fellow of the Royal Society), reproduced in their five-volume entirety in 1993.[24] The records of the Glasgow-born, London-based Hunter do include a number of mental and nervous cases, although, because he was a surgeon and anatomist, the bulk of his practice was—as one would expect—devoted to surgery, morbid dissection, and general medicine. However, on the basis of our review of the current literature, we are convinced that no British psychiatric case book from the period before 1800 has ever been published.[25] Nor does any mad-doctor's case book of comparable importance appear to exist for eighteenth-century England. There have been, we acknowledge, a few modern editions of general medical case books from the early modern period,[26] and a handful of these, including the Hunter case book and Joan Lane's superb edition of John Hall's case book,[27] contain a number of mentally afflicted cases, though patients of this sort were marginal to the main thrust of these men's practices. More pertinently, Michael MacDonald's superb study, *Mystical Bedlam* (1981), was largely based on the seventeenth-century case books of Richard Napier. However, these case books have never been published in their own right.[28]

During the 1980s and early 1990s, a number of historians combined with Tavistock and Routledge to produce a series of facsimile classic texts in the history of psychiatry. These included William Pargeter's *Observations on Maniacal Disorders* (1792), a work that, like many other contemporary treatises on insanity, gave considerable space to the case histories of individual patients. Pargeter's text must have been based substantially on case books that he had kept.[29] Also published in this series was an excellent edition by Roy Porter of John Haslam's *Illustrations of Madness* (1810).[30] Haslam, the Bethlem apothecary and a colleague of Thomas Monro (John's son and successor as Bethlem physician), used his book to present a single case history of the Bethlem patient James Tilly Matthews, drawn from the hospital records. His main objects were simply, as his title suggests, to illustrate Matthews's insanity, while also vindicating his own management of Matthews's case, and he selected from the available manuscript materials accordingly.

Still another volume in the Tavistock/Routledge series was George Cheyne's *English Malady* (1733), again in an edition annotated and introduced by Porter.[31] This was a treatise in which the Scottish physician dramatized his own case history, alongside other cases he had attended (presumably composed from his bedside scribblings), to confirm the reality of nervous disorders and their peculiar national characteristics. Concurrently, Cheyne's book served to promote his own approach to such conditions, which blended dietetic, Newtonian, naturopathic, and humoral medicine.

None of these works, however, despite their origins in medical observations, fully reproduces the case book record. None of them, in consequence, allows the sort of privileged insight into the everyday private world and activities of a contemporary medical practitioner that the material presented here does. As we shall see, Monro's case book is particularly revealing about the customers of the mad-business. It documents a hitherto hidden network of referrals and cross-referrals that underpinned the emerging "trade in lunacy" in England's metropolis. Simultaneously, it illuminates in unparalleled fashion the relatively fluid, reciprocal, and negotiable relations that existed among perhaps the most famous English mad-doctor of his era and his patients, their families, and other practitioners.

If read carefully, Monro's text provides us with a whole series of revealing glimpses of the mad-doctor's attitudes and activities—and those of his clientele. The very form in which medical men chose to record the mundane aspects of their day-to-day encounters with their customers potentially reveals a great deal about their assumptions and worldview. The treatment of patients' narratives in the Monro case book should thus be of particular interest and value to those historians, sociologists, and psychiatrists who have sought to investigate and analyze the construction of the medical narrative during the early modern period.

The tone of Monro's case book is sometimes obtrusively evaluative, serving to legitimate and valorize his own particular views of and approaches to the patients he saw, as well as occasionally to cast aspersions on those of others. By and large, however, its language is rather detached. In contrast to some other early modern case books, such as that of John Hall (which is almost exclusively confined to cases with successful outcomes),[32] there is little evidence of selectivity in the cases described and presented by Monro. The nonrecovery or death of a substantial number of patients (as well as the restitution of others) is faithfully recorded, even if for some the outcome remains unrecorded and hence a mystery. Monro is at times critical and dismissive of the information that patients and their friends provide to him, but at others is rather noncommittal or nonjudgmental in the observations he makes, displaying a concern to report accurately what he heard and saw.

Here, then, is a document of considerable historiographic interest, one that is quite possibly unique in the English-speaking world, and very likely beyond. We now turn to an examination of the conclusions that can be drawn from a systematic review of the contents of this remarkable manuscript.

CHAPTER 3

Profiling Patients and Patterns of Practice

WHO WERE THE CUSTOMERS?
PATIENTS' SOCIOECONOMIC AND DEMOGRAPHIC PROFILES

Possibly the most interesting details provided in Monro's case book are those that give us clues about the identity of the customers of the mad-doctor, an aspect of the mad-business that historians, thus far, barely have begun to investigate.[1] On the one hand, Monro's case book reveals, as one might expect, that a significant number of his clients came from the "respectable," moneyed classes, including merchants, lawyers, journalists, and established tradesmen. Monro was called to attend, for example, on prominent city politicians and tradesmen, including Alderman Richard Peers and the wife of Alderman Barlow Trecothick (both men were also prominent governors of Bethlem).[2] At still higher levels of the social hierarchy, his services were sought by members of the aristocracy. Besides being consulted in the cases of Earls Orford and Ferrers, for instance (interventions we have discussed in our first volume, *Undertaker of the Mind*),[3] the case book records that he was also called in to deal with the case of Sir Francis Chester by the latter's relation through marriage, Sir George Robinson, baronet.[4]

Such cases indicate the substantial reliance of eighteenth-century medical practitioners on familial links between their clients in order to spread the word and market their services, patterns of practice also discernible in other early modern case books.[5] Not surprisingly, there is no evidence that Monro ever felt the need to advertise his services, something that was disdained as the method of quacks, itinerants, and tradesmen. Such overtly mercenary behavior unquestionably would have compromised the appeal of elite physicians to the types of social circles they primarily sought to cultivate and with whom they sought to associate themselves.

However, to assume that the aristocracy and the merchant elite were Monro's primary clientele would be mistaken. The case book suggests, on the contrary, that the majority of Monro's clients were from either the middling and lower ranks of society—the shopkeepers, smaller tradesmen, and craftsmen who comprised the city's modestly heeled bourgeoisie—or else from the ranks of the *nouveaux riches*. Patients such as a Shoreditch distiller; the cooper to the brewer, Samuel Whitbread; a Fleet Market grocer; and bakers' wives and sisters from Wood Street, Turnstile, Cow Cross, and Crown Court were hardly the elite of London life, but were far more typical of Monro's customers than were baronets, knights of the realm, aldermen, and their ladies. As for patients drawn from the ranks of the major professions, it was captains, not admirals (but also not common sailors!), whom Monro saw, and country parsons and city clergy, not bishops and deacons.

Monro's attendance on eminent lawyers such as Dr. William Macham of Doctors Commons, on merchants' families, and on various individuals styled "ladies," "maiden ladies," or "gentlemen" suggests that the higher-ranking professionals, wealthier tradesmen, and the gentry constituted a significant portion of his clientele. Among city tradesmen, he attended the Swiss merchant Mr. Rosat, but only after the latter's trading fortunes and mental health had declined and forced his return from Turkey to England, while he also attended Mr. Bevan, a well-traveled clerk to the established and reputable London merchant company Messrs. Drake and Long. Some of his customers, though, were from distinctly humble backgrounds, including servants and even slaves. Among the sizable number referred to as "poor," at least some must have been in the service of relatively well-off families who presumably paid for their treatment, while a number of others in distressed circumstances appear to have suffered rather dramatic reversals in their fortunes, either precipitated by or precipitating their mental troubles. One can identify similar cases in other surviving contemporary sources, such as a patient Monro attended in consort with William Pargeter: a "Mr Wood, who formerly kept the Assembly-House at Kentish-Town, was tried at the Old Bailey for a highway-robbery, and was acquitted," but who was allegedly so badly affected by these circumstances "that he became *epileptic mad,* and died."[6]

All in all, Monro's socially heterogeneous patient population seems to suggest that, however lucrative and successful his practice became, he was never (or not, at least by 1766) able to attain the kind of social status enjoyed by fashionable physicians from superior family backgrounds—those who became court physicians and who were regularly called upon by the uppermost echelons of society. Monro's social aspirations were compromised, perhaps, by his somewhat unorthodox family roots and by the ambiguous aura of respectability with which the specialist mad-doctor and physician of Bethlem was almost automatically endowed. Too close an association with him brought obvious perils in its wake, while the commerce the mad-doctor made out of madness left an indelible stain on his social pretensions.

Female patients were disproportionately represented in the single year's sample of patients chronicled in Monro's case book. Sixty-five of the cases recorded were women, as against forty-five men (in one case the sex was unrecorded).[7] Possibly, this reflects a gender bias in the identification of mental troubles among privately treated patients. What we cannot determine from the surviving evidence is whether this discrepancy indicates a greater liability on women's part to present or acknowledge their mental afflictions in this period, or a greater propensity for women to be perceived as mentally deranged by a society and medical profession dominated by men. Certainly, this gender discrepancy among his private patients is at odds with what we know of Monro's public practice at Bethlem, where poor male patients predominated. Although some studies have argued for the prevalence of single, unmarried women among the mentally deranged, at least forty-three (69 percent) of Monro's female customers were married or widowed, as against just eighteen cases who are identifiable as unmarried (the marital status of other cases is unspecified).

The age range of the patients Monro treated or was consulted about is impossible to chart accurately from the case book, as age is seldom registered explicitly. Nevertheless, many appear to have been young "maiden women" and young gentlemen in the prime of life. Only a few were recorded as elderly;[8] the mental problems of most of these latter cases probably arose in part as a result of the aging process. Yet, even if some of Monro's private clients are identifiable as in their dotage (and a few of these were clearly close to death), it seems unlikely that the attentions of the mad-doctor were directed very often to the problems of senile decay and deterioration. These, after all, were predicaments that tended to be more easily containable and manageable in the home.

In rather exceptional circumstances, if symptoms were especially severe, the mad-doctor might be called to attend on the cases of children. The youngest patient mentioned in the case book was Bella Tuten, a nine-year-old girl whom Monro seems to have adjudged mentally disabled rather than insane. Bella "had been from birth in the state I saw her," namely "incoherent" and incontinent. Monro also acknowledges in the case book that he attended a Mr. Fletcher "while a boy."[9]

THE MAD-DOCTOR IN BUSINESS: INHERITING AND BUILDING A PRACTICE

The record of just one year's attendance can allow only limited insight into the degree of follow-up on cases. However, as we have already indicated (see chapter 2), Monro was careful to cross-reference cases by assigning them marginal numbers, and to remark on those occasions when he made further visits to a patient (as in the cases of Mr. Bevan, whom he saw four times in 1766, Mr. Griffin, who had been his patient "3 or 4 times," and Mrs. Harris, who "had been my patient twice before in the time of her first husband").[10] Notations of this sort imply a degree of relatively personalized attention, as do entries indicating that he had previously seen some cases not just months but years before. This impression is strengthened by recorded instances of attendance on other family members and by references to some of the patients also having been treated by his father. John takes the trouble to indicate that he first attended Mrs. Shoreland "before she was married," and Mr. Moore "once before." He attended two brothers called Whitehead, and noted that a sister was also mentally afflicted; Mrs. Webb was sister to Mr. Fletcher, who "was my patient while a boy, & again about 2 years since at Highgate where he died after an illness of 10 days"; Miss Sutton was sister to a baker Monro had "attended the last year in the same way"; Mrs. van Hock's mother had been attended by Monro "about 4 years ago in Glocester street in the same complaint," and Mr. Inge's father had been in Bethlem "near 40 years ago." Mrs. Godwin "received benefit from my father's advice, many years ago"; Mr. Coltman's uncle "informed me he had a near relation under my father's care," and Captain Knackstone "was a patient of my father's once or twice, and likewise of mine, for a short time."[11]

Apart from attesting to Monro's interest in the hereditary nature of insanity, such cases seem an indication of some of the advantages that flowed from a continuous family practice when one faced the problem of "making a medical living." Generational succession offered advantages not just in terms of building up a practice or preserving one's professional patch, but also in enabling one to offer an intimate service to clients across generations.[12] The numerous references to patients John had gleaned from his father's practice nicely illustrate the importance of nepotistic connections in medical careers in early modern Britain. The prevalence of endogamy was perhaps nowhere more marked than in the mad-doctoring trade, where we can point to multigenerational practitioners besides the Monro dynasty, such as the Mason-Cox family, associated with Fishponds Asylum and Cox's swinging chair;[13] the Fox family, who owned Brislington House throughout the nineteenth century and into the twentieth;[14] the Willises, headed by the infamous "Dr. Duplicate," Francis Willis, the provincial mountebank who "cured" the mad King George;[15] and the Newingtons of Ticehurst, proprietors for more than a century of the English aristocracy's favorite madhouse[16]— to cite only some prominent examples. Some houses were run by a mixture of lay and medical proprietors within a family spanning a number of generations. These included Laverstock House, in Wiltshire, which was in the hands of the Finch family—William and his medically qualified grandson and namesake—from at least the 1770s until 1854;[17] Hook Norton House in Oxfordshire, managed by the Harris family from ca. 1725, who continued as licensees through 1825;[18] and Spring Vale Private Asylum in Staffordshire, run by the Bakewells from 1808 to 1840.[19]

Nor were the Monros the only contemporary practitioners who combined public service at a hospital or asylum with involvement in the private mad-business: like William Battie, for example, Thomas Arnold (1742–1816) also wore both hats, as a founding father and the first physician to Leicester Lunatic Asylum from 1794, as well as proprietor of Belle Grove Private Asylum, Leicester.[20] Similarly, most contemporary physicians who held posts at general hospitals, from Richard Mead to William Cullen, also kept up a vigorous private practice alongside their not always demanding hospital duties.

Normally, Monro appears to have made house calls, attending patients at their own homes or at the houses and madhouses to which they had been removed. However, he was also prepared to offer consultations to a few of his patients at his own residence, as in the case of one woman who "came to me at home to ask my advice." Some relatives also called on him directly, such as a Mrs. Theobald, who "call'd on me about her daughter," and Mr. Kinder, who "consulted me about his wife."[21] While Monro was summoned to attend many cases by patients' relatives and other associates, quite a number of his visits were made at the request of the patients themselves. Cases such as Mrs. Gordon, whom Monro records as having "sent for me to consult me" after being bitten by a cat she supposed "mad" (or rabid),[22] emphasize the limits of overly simplistic social control interpretations of medical care for the insane in this period and the significance of patient demand for the specialist services of the mad-doctor.

Monro's practice was plainly focused in the metropolitan regions. Most of his patients whose addresses are mentioned were residents of the city and the surrounding communities, and other evidence suggests that the vast majority of his clients hailed, as one might expect, from the City of London and from Westminster and neighboring parishes. Nevertheless, Monro also traveled further afield in pursuit of custom, venturing into the home counties and even into rural districts at a further remove from the metropolis. Some of the patients whose treatment is recorded here had addresses in Hertfordshire, Sussex, and Kent, and Monro also saw a fair number of foreigners working or living in the City and its environs.[23]

Again, the pattern we see in Monro's case book seems to coincide with what we generally know about patterns of practice among well-established metropolitan doctors in the medical mainstream.[24] A relatively wide theater of operations might be readily anticipated by such physicians. Clearly, Monro enjoyed rich pickings from his custom in the capital alone, where he faced limited competition from other practitioners. Like most of his prosperous colleagues, however, Monro sought to strike a genteel balance as a man of the city and the country, maintaining a residence in both environments. Physicians, in this respect, imitated the lifestyle adopted by most of the better-heeled families of the city, who divided their time in this way for reasons of health, pleasure, and social decorum. In Monro's case, this meant that the family enjoyed a country seat in Barnet.

The specialist nature of much of Monro's medical attendance probably contributed to his need to extend his catchment area beyond that of the typical city general practitioner. Most of his patients who came from further afield, though, were probably already residing temporarily or permanently in the London area. Some (such as Mr. Stanfield of Huntingdonshire)[25] had more than likely been brought up specially to see Monro, or some other metropolitan practitioner, and others had friends in London and Middlesex, such as an anonymous Chichester woman who was an acquaintance of a Mr. Richardson of Mount Pleasant, Barnet.[26] Their willingness to travel considerable distances to see him underlines the advantages of city practice but also implies that there was a genuine and relatively widespread recognition of Monro's special area of expertise among clients, patrons, and his medical colleagues.

A number of his patients, indeed, were seen on referrals from other practitioners. Besides this source of business, Monro also seems to have attended a substantial number of Scottish patients residing or sojourning in the city.[27] Here his own Scottish origins, and the social connections of his family north of the border, doubtless did much to recommend him to his compatriots. John's father's attendance on patients such as a Mr. MacCune suggests that this pattern of referrals probably had been established in the previous generation. John's library, which must itself have been partially handed down to him by his father, was certainly full of medical, historical, lexicographical, topographical, and travel literature relating to Scotland.[28] A strong, if not growing, awareness of English prejudice toward the Scots may also have encouraged some of them to seek out the Monros.[29] Monro's case book thus allows substantial access not only to the identities of the mad-doctor's customers, but also to the various avenues of referral and patronage by which the mad-doctor went about acquiring his patients.

THE MONROS AND THE
CONTEMPORARY ART WORLD

One of Monro's sources of patients is at first sight somewhat unusual and surprising. A fair number of those Monro saw had interesting connections with the eighteenth-century art world, a reflection, as we shall see, of an interest in the fine arts that the aspiring mad-doctor had begun to cultivate while a student at Oxford, and of the extent to which John (and subsequently, to an even greater extent, his son Thomas) cultivated ties with members of London's artistic community. One of John's patients in 1766, for example, was "Mrs [Elizabeth] Moreati, the wife of an Italian employ'd in designing for the king by Mr Dalton,"[30] who had evidently been brought over by Richard Dalton (1715[?]–91), the librarian and antiquary to George III.

Dalton was also responsible for collecting works of art and commissioning artwork for the king, particularly works from foreign shores, and he had brought a number of Italian artists and craftsmen over to England in the 1750s and 1760s, provoking considerable resentment from less well-connected British artists such as [Sir] Robert Strange (1721–92). The most famous of the Italians imported by Dalton was Francesco Bartolozzi (1727–1815), regarded as perhaps the best European engraver of his generation. Bartolozzi came over from Milan in 1764 and worked for Dalton for three years, ultimately becoming one of the main figures in the establishment of an Italian school of engraving in England. However, so far as we can tell, Moreati was not part of the Bartolozzi school, or even an engraver. In all probability, he was a more minor craftsman who worked instead on some aspect of the interior design of royal properties. Also in contrast with Bartolozzi, who left his wife behind in Italy, never to visit her again, Moreati brought his wife with him. Apparently, though, Elizabeth found adapting to London a considerable strain on her health and nerves.[31]

The connection with Dalton, who was also one of the securities[32] for the admission of Moreati's wife to Bethlem, underlines the fact that we are dealing with one of these Italian artists and craftsmen. Dalton's patronage was evidently considerable, extending to making Mrs. Moreati his maid and taking responsibility for her care when she became ill. Possibly with the benefit of Monro's advice, however, he evidently preferred the cheaper care available in Bethlem to any private arrangement for the disturbed woman.

Besides the Moreatis, Monro was called in to attend someone else connected to a famous artist — a Mrs. Walker, a servant in the household of Joseph Goupy (1689–1769), a well-known London-born watercolorist and etcher of Huguenot extraction who served as drawing-master to George I, the young George III, and other royal family members. Mrs. Walker was in Inskip's Chelsea madhouse in 1766 when Monro attended her, ca. 7 January. She was, he noted, "mad enough," with many "paralytic" symptoms. Marginalia indicate that she was (subsequently) "brought to the hospital," and the implied Bethlem admission would reflect her humble social status. However, attempts to identify her in Bethlem's admission registers have been inconclusive.[33]

Monro probably already knew Goupy's work, and it was commonly reported that Goupy had since his youth supported a "mistress," a woman who "became mad" in later life. According to an acquaintance, the artist had taken his mistress "into his own house" in Kensington, as "he could not bear to see in her old age the object of his love and pleasure confined in Bedlam," but "the expense of attendance, etc., was so great that he lived and died in very indigent circumstances."[34] Goupy's will (dated 16 February 1769) makes detailed provision for her future well-being, calling her "Sarah Wright Spinster." Goupy confesses to "have a great regard for" this woman, "she having Lived with me many years and is now so unhappy as to be deprived of her reason," and cared so deeply for her that he left virtually all his (somewhat modest) real and personal estate in trust to her sister, Elizabeth Williams, to be sold and then invested (if sufficient) for Sarah's "Maintenance and benefit."[35] Perhaps Sarah Wright and Mrs. Walker were the same woman. It was standard practice for contemporaries, to sustain a socially necessary illusion of moral respectability, to maintain mistresses under the guise of domestic servants, and perhaps Monro was intentionally misinformed about his patient's real identity.[36] Yet the different names and marital status of Sarah Wright and Mrs. Walker, and the fact that a private madhouse and Bethlem were plainly thought fit for one and domiciliary-based care for the other, make this conclusion unlikely.

The interest of the Monros in contemporary art and the family's long-standing association with some of the leading artists of the eighteenth and early nineteenth centuries are matters of record and have been alluded to in a limited way by a number of historians.[37] The case book clearly adds a few more pieces to the jigsaw of what is already known about their connections with the art world. John Monro had evidently acquired his taste for the arts at Oxford. In a (1735) diary account of a tour of England he conducted when he was a student at the university, Monro shows a particular concern with noting down the works of art he saw, detailing at some length the names of artists and sculptors and remarking on those works he found particularly striking (or valuable) in the churches and country houses he visited.[38] His interest was probably furthered while he was traveling on the continent as a Radcliffe scholar, a much-coveted appointment allowing him a stipend to tour the medical schools of Europe that he owed to his father's connections to the Walpole family.[39] Surviving evidence demonstrates that he was particularly interested in and knowledgeable about not only art and antiquities, but more especially about engraving and its history, and that he gathered a substantial collection of books, drawings, and engravings.[40]

John Monro senior's consultation in the insanity of John Bennett, the business partner of the famous print and mapseller Robert Sayer (whose firm established a deserved reputation for superlative engraving and employed a whole team of engravers), may well have been the result of acquaintances he had already made through his artistic interests.[41] We know that John's broad grasp of the subject enabled him to assist the engraver Joseph Strutt (1749–1802) in the preparation of his biographical dictionary of engravers.[42] On still another occasion, his cultivated taste for classical and more modern literary works, from Horace to Shakespeare, and his research into the latter, allowed him to be of considerable assistance to George Steevens (1736–1800), who was then jointly working with Samuel Johnson (1709–84) on an edition of Shakespeare's works.[43]

Although there is little evidence that James Monro was as much of a connoisseur as his son became, both he and John evidently knew William Hogarth (1679–1764). Indeed, it may well have been one of the Monros who recommended Hogarth for a governorship of the hospital in 1752.[44] Significantly, it was John, along with another governor of Bethlem and Bridewell, Moses Mendez, who in 1751 was requested by the Court of Governors "to Ask Mr Hogarth what Painting he thinks wou'd be proper for the Altar in the Chappell" at Bridewell.[45] There is no further record in the hospitals' minutes of what Hogarth advised or what was decided, but it was almost certainly this artistic consultation with Monro and Mendez that helped to secure Hogarth his governorship, conferred on him almost exactly a year later.[46] Monro's extensive library included a number of works by and about Hogarth.[47] Furthermore, James may well have had some role in granting Hogarth the opportunity to make his studies for the famous Bethlem scene (viii) in his (1735 and 1763) *Rake's Progress* series. This scene (figure 3), which was set in the hospital's new incurables wards, displays a be-wigged physician (sporting a bright red coat in the oil version) who bears more than a passing resemblance to the young James. The Bethlem physician is depicted stooping in a concerned fashion over the prone, semi-naked, and shaven-headed Tom Rakewell, possibly taking his pulse, while an attendant is manacling his leg.[48]

As well as his role in procuring Hogarth's services for Bridewell and Bethlem, three decades later John Monro was one of six governors on a 1783 Bethlem subcommittee that was asked to negotiate terms with artists "for Drawing and Engraving" Cibber's statues of raving and melancholy madness (figure 4). The picture that resulted formed the frontispiece of Thomas Bowen's celebratory book, *An Historical Account of the Origin, Progress and Present State of Bethlehem Hospital*, the first official history of that institution.[49]

James's and even John's somewhat adventitious connections with the art world scarcely compare, however, with the extensive encouragement given in subsequent years by John's son Thomas Monro to a number of famous young water-colorists at the beginning of their careers. Notable among the younger Monro's protégés were William Turner ([Joseph Mallord] 1775–1851) and Thomas Girtin (1775–1802). Monro junior's efforts extended to setting up a studio for them in his own home at Adelphi Terrace and have led some historians to regard him as one of the founders of the British school of water-colorists. Nor was Thomas just a passive patron: he was no mean water-colorist himself, and his work continues to attract collectors.

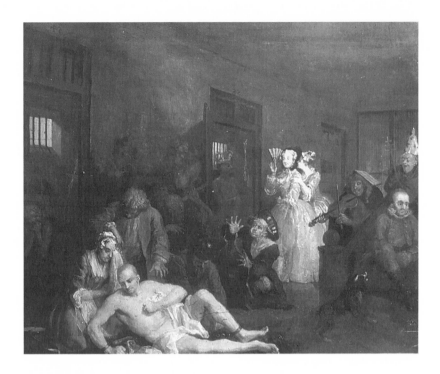

FIGURE 3. Scene viii from William Hogarth's   Reproduced by courtesy of the Trustees of Sir
A Rake's Progress, oil on canvas, painted in 1735.   John Soane's Museum, London.

It was partly this background that led another of the leading eighteenth-century water-colorists, John Robert Cozens, to be placed under
Thomas's care when he became deranged circa 1794. Other aspects of
Thomas's links with artists can easily be traced in numerous references to
him in Joseph Farington's diary, as well as in the manuscript diary of his
son (and successor as physician to Bethlem), Edward Thomas Monro.[50]
It seems, however, that Thomas may well have followed his father's lead
in his artistic endeavors, as he did in so much else. We know, for example, that John passed on a portion of his picture collection to Thomas
(the rest was auctioned off after his death).[51] Surviving catalogues of
Monro's drawings and collection of watercolors and engravings include
quite a number of items that had been collected by John,[52] and
Farington reported Thomas as confessing that "he inherited from his
Father an inclination for drawings."[53]

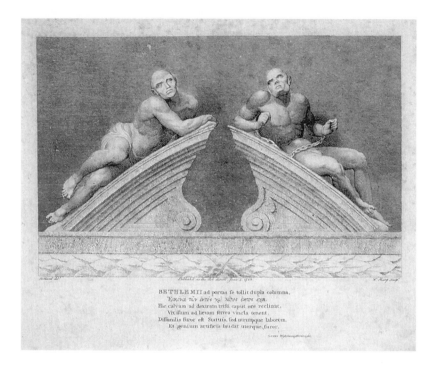

Although much is known about Thomas Monro's artistic pursuits, rather less has been written about John's. The exception is William Schupbach's 1983 study of the Rowlandson caricature of John Monro and Charles James Fox (figure 5).[54] As Schupbach points out, Rowlandson portrays Monro in the guise of both mad-doctor and connoisseur, examining Fox, his patently lunatic patient, with a quizzing glass, as if he were one of the valuable works of art Monro clearly spent much of his spare time inspecting and treasuring. The caricature is far from flattering to either of Rowlandson's subjects. Fox is shown in a mad rage, disheveled and with straw in his hair, and under restraint in a straitjacket, after losing the elec-

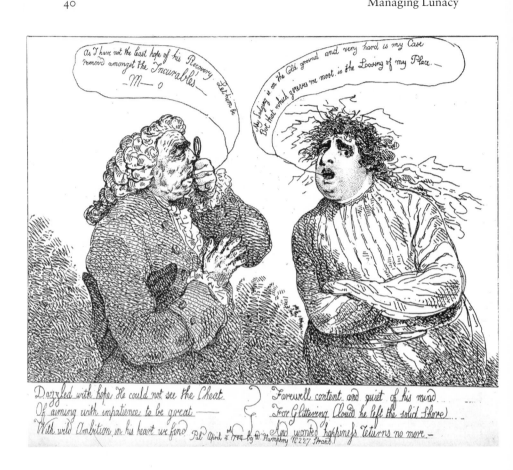

FIGURE 5. Thomas Rowlandson's caricature of John Monro and Charles James Fox. A caricature designed to skewer the Whig leader, who had just lost the 1784 election and had (as Rowlandson represents it) been driven mad by his loss of office and power, the picture equally pokes fun at the corpulent Dr. Monro (see figure 1), who is seen inspecting his prize patient through a quizzing glass and ordering him to be carted off to the ward for incurables. Reproduced by kind permission of the Wellcome Institute Library, London. © Copyright the British Museum.

tion of 1784 to Pitt and his followers, which brought an end to the previous years of coalition government. (Many contemporaries liked to depict Fox thereafter as a furious and frantic leader of the opposition.) Monro, on the other hand, is depicted pronouncing authoritatively on Fox and ordering his removal to Bethlem's incurables ward, the blend of mad-doctor and connoisseur casting both of Monro's pursuits in a somewhat ridiculous and dubious light. Monro's corpulence was already evident, although to a lesser degree, in the earlier, more dignified portrait of him (figure 1, page 7) in his younger days that was painted in 1769 by one of the leading contemporary portrait artists, Nathaniel Dance (1735–1811), and subsequently donated to the College of Physicians by his great-grandson, Dr. Henry Monro. But in Rowlandson's rendition, the girth of this connoisseur of madness, and his wrinkled ugliness (Monro was about seventy years old when the caricature was done), are magnificently exaggerated to savage comic effect. It was not uncommon for mad-doctors and other physicians to be represented in caricature with grotesque and forbidding features, such as would be apt to strike up aversion and fear in their patients, and a number genuinely had features to match and inspire such responses. For example, many contemporary accounts dwelled on the "frightening" appearance of Thomas Warburton, proprietor of Bethnal Green madhouse. Warburton's height (at six feet plus), heavy build, "knock-knees," and "long nose" (which some estimated at three inches) created a fearsome look, and contemporaries noted that when he attended George III, the king "could not bear to look at him."[55] John Mitford was among those to report the shockingly protuberant size of the mad-doctor's "proboscis," as well as his sovereign's characteristically reiterated reaction to it: "I heard the King said 'Take away that fellow with the long nose—take him away-away-away.' "[56]

Nathaniel Dance's connection with Monro may have arisen through the work of his grandfather George Dance the Elder (1695–1768), architect of the first St. Luke's building in Upper Moorfields, and his father, George Dance the Younger (1741–1825), portrait painter, City Surveyor of London, and perhaps the leading architect of the day, a man who was regularly employed in works on the city's hospitals.[57] Dance the Younger had been the architect responsible for the second St. Luke's building at Old Street (ca. 1782–89). He continued to be involved in other work there, designing, for example, a covered seat for the airing ground ca. 1790.[58] He was also the architect of Mansion House and Newgate Gaol, and employed some of his spare time in making caricatures and humorous sketches.[59] His role as city surveyor had brought him into close contact with governors and officers at Bethlem Hospital. In the 1760s and 1790s, for example, Dance drew up detailed plans of parts of Bethlem adjoining London Wall, and of other premises abutting Bethlem.[60] He refused to contribute to the subscription raised for Cozens when he went mad and came under the care of Thomas Monro in 1797, but he was a regular visitor at Thomas Monro's houses at Adelphi Terrace and Merry Hill, Bushey.[61]

Apart from their genuine appreciation of fine arts, the Monros must also have seen their artistic and literary pursuits as genteel accoutrements wholly befitting men of superior social standing, learning, culture, and income. Their role as patrons and connoisseurs provided them with vivid, material means of displaying such gentlemanly accomplishments. Yet, as the Rowlandson print demonstrates so well, the stigmatizing effects of their involvement with the mad-business were a perpetual source of status instability and strain. For the inevitable consequences of their links to this disreputable trade threatened to overthrow at any moment their best efforts to sustain their preferred identity as cultured and well bred, and made them an easy target for satirical attacks on their social pretensions.

MONRO AND THE MADHOUSE TRADE

If the mad-business flourished as never before in the entrepreneurial climate of the eighteenth century, so too did social fears and fantasies about those who practiced its dark arts. For all the efforts of some society physicians to transform nervous complaints into fashionable disorders, mental disorders remained a potent source of shame and scandal, especially in more extreme cases of distress and disturbance. Although most of Monro's patients consulted him on a discreet, out-patient basis and coped with their troubles in a domestic setting, others found themselves consigned to a madhouse, an environment that provided both secrecy and physical isolation. However, what were distinct virtues, from one point of view, simultaneously gave birth to fearful imaginings about what transpired in those hidden places—fears that were by no means always misplaced.

A substantial minority of Monro's patients, almost a quarter of those recorded in the 1766 case book, found themselves consigned to such establishments. Monro's case notes record the close ties that existed between him and the proprietors of many metropolitan madhouses, and the numerous visits he paid to those held in confinement. Monro, for example, saw patients in more than one of the madhouses in the Hoxton area, east of the city, most frequently attending patients at the sizable establishment run by John Miles. In 1763, when parliament briefly inquired into the mad-business, Miles was accused of falsely confining sane people on his premises, but the unsavory aroma that attached to the keeper's activities obviously did not deter Monro from maintaining and building upon the intimate and financially rewarding relationship that his father, James, had first developed, for at least sixteen of the patients mentioned in the case book found their way into Miles's hands.

West of London, in the village of Chelsea, still another cluster of madhouses had developed, and Monro sent at least four of his patients to one of these establishments, Michael Duffield's, and still another to a house run by Duffield's nephew, Peter Inskip. Small, ephemeral businesses of this sort had begun to emerge in a number of neighborhoods, and Monro's private patients also could be found in madhouses in Bloomsbury, in Paddington, and at Bethnal Green. In all these places, Monro appeared on the scene as an outside consultant, often providing medical services that the keeper was not qualified to provide, and seldom interfering in the broader management of the individual case.

The more successful madhouse-keepers often made considerable sums of money from their businesses. The Miles family, for instance, acquired a considerable fortune from the trade, and in the provinces, Anthony Addington's madhouse at Reading provided the financial wherewithal to launch Addington's own career as a court physician and to underpin the political career of his son, a future prime minister. To operate such a business directly was, however, to court scandal, and many physicians preferred to share in the wealth as visiting consultants, rather than to traffic more directly in such an unpleasant and stigmatizing endeavor. As "professionals" they could thus collect fees for the disinterested provision of their skills and advice, rather than overtly relying upon the profits of a tradesman, those that derived from charging for the lodging and confinement of the afflicted.

Status concerns thus played an important part in shaping the structure of the emerging trade in lunacy, and at least partially explain the numbers of lay proprietors of madhouses in this period. Yet, on occasion, as Monro's own situation makes plain, appearances could be deceptive, for some physicians were not averse to participating more directly and profiting from speculation in this species of human misery, and a number appear to have lurked as silent partners behind the public pretense that an establishment rested in other, lay hands. Besides his role as a consultant to a number of madhouses, John put the family fortunes on a solid footing by developing his own establishment, Brooke House in Hackney, nominally set up and run by William Clarke in the late 1750s but almost certainly an operation with which Monro was connected from the very outset. Significantly, once the 1774 Act for Regulating Madhouses instituted a requirement that the proprietor obtain a license from the College of Physicians, it was John who became the licensee, and there are a number of patients in the 1766 case book who appear to have been treated there by him—the print- and mapseller John Bennett quite certainly, and probably several more. Like other madhouses where his involvement was more limited and indirect, Brooke House was not a purpose-built establishment especially designed as a receptacle for the insane, but a decayed old mansion patched and adapted to fulfill its new role. For almost a century and three quarters it remained at the core of the family's involvement in the mad-business, though generally the grubby task of day-to-day management was left in other hands.[62]

CHAPTER 4

The Craft of Consultation

Managing Patients and Their Problems

A significant proportion of Monro's patients were plainly regarded as serious cases of madness. He refers to these cases with such terms as "violent," "raving," "furious," "lunatic," "mad," and so forth. Many more among those Monro encountered, however, were observed to be merely "bewildered," "nervous," "hysterical," "dull," or "low/high in spirits," or were fearful and anxious about being harmed themselves, rather than being inclined to hurt others. This suggests that although the special expertise of the mad-doctor was naturally thought to be necessary in cases of full-blown raving madness, Monro was more often summoned to deal with patients with milder mental problems. Cases of the latter sort were, after all, considerably more common. If Monro's clients were in any sense typical of those mad-doctors were called upon to treat in this period, then it would seem that much of the existing historiography of eighteenth-century psychiatry has had a misplaced focus, being overly concerned with the extreme case of the violent maniac or the suicidal melancholic and with the growth of the tougher machinery of confinement and restraint.

The case book evidence likewise implies that, although he was often called on as something of a last resort, after the mentally afflicted had been ill for a considerable length of time, Monro's attendance was not infrequently summoned in incipient cases, too, as a preventive or early curative measure by families keen to ward off a worse mental explosion or to avoid more serious consequences. For all that, families seem to have been generally more prone to downplay rather than to exaggerate the mental oddities of their members, to contain the distracted and the frantic within the confines of the domestic sphere, and to persuade themselves that they could cope at home.[1]

Monro employed a multiplicity of terms to describe the mental afflictions he encountered. On one level, the variety of conditions these cate-

gories purport to identify serves to highlight the adaptability and flexi-
bility of medical definitions at this time, particularly for those cases that
fell short of a definitive diagnosis of madness. Yet, in many cases, the
terms of reference Monro used reflected the preferences and choices of
patients' families and friends. Besides, like Purcell, Cheyne, Blackmore,
and other contemporary specialists in fashionable "nervous" disorders
such as the vapors, the spleen, and hypochondria, Monro had good
social, commercial, and professional reasons for blurring the boundaries
between full-blown madness and a whole series of milder nervous ailments. Families themselves, keen to eschew the social taint that the
insanity of one of their members brought with it, were often at pains to
encourage a less damning diagnosis.

In one case Monro detailed, it was the patient who wanted to accept
her affliction for what it was. By contrast, the family appears to have
come to the mad-doctor only when the patient insisted on it, and with
great hesitation and circumspection.[2] Brought to the mad-doctor "rather
to see her than any thing else [that is, to humor her, with no expectation
that matters would proceed further]," this young Chichester woman
"was herself more willing to call her unhappy complaint by its true
name, than her friends seem'd to be." Although Monro also tactfully
avoided attaching an explicit label to his patient's condition, not even
specifying it in his case book, he was plainly in little doubt as to the seri-
ousness of her mental derangement. The patient herself obliged by presenting Monro with "a very regular good account of herself without the
least inconsistency"—something that he evidently did not invariably
see as a contraindicator of insanity. The young woman had been ill for
six years by the time Monro saw her, half of which time she had spent
"continually in bed," and throughout this lengthy disturbance her family apparently had resisted facing up to the nature of her malady. These
and other symptoms Monro was apprised of would have struck him as
a quite familiar account of nervous illness. "She felt no joy, seem'd a burthensome creature in the world, & if she attempted to amuse herself,
seem'd much the worse for it afterwards complain'd of great tightness
round her head. . . ."[3] Indeed, this is a representation that is closely mir-
rored in writings throughout the early and middle decades of the century
by physicians specializing in nervous disorders.[4]

The aversion that many families appear to have felt toward the ministrations of the mad-doctor and toward confinement outside of the
home are unambiguously present here. Calling in a mad-doctor and,
even more so, placing a relation in a madhouse threatened to rupture

the intimacy of familial ties and implied an inevitable loss of control over a family member's fate. When one adds to these factors the social stigma and scandal that an open avowal of madness in one's domestic circle unavoidably entailed, it becomes easy to understand a pattern of prevarication over seeking out specialist treatment. Here, as well, is certainly one explanation for the slow pace at which the machinery of confinement developed in this period. A century and more later, such considerations were still at work, often prompting the well-to-do to go to great lengths to circumvent or postpone the disgrace of incarcerating one of their nearest and dearest in an asylum.[5] Possessing the financial wherewithal to cope with the unproductive, the ability to employ large numbers of servants to manage their troubled relatives, and the capacity to remove them to a quiet and secluded part of the country or, if all else failed, to pack them off abroad if need be, upper- and upper-middle-class families—even in the age of the asylum—still exhibited a strong preference for extra-institutional solutions.[6] For at least some patients themselves, however, as the case of the young lady from Chichester shows, home "care" could in practice prove a far from attractive alternative. Indeed, given that this woman had, as Monro discovered, spent three of the previous six years confined "continually in bed," it may come as no surprise that she felt so depressed and seemed to welcome his intervention.[7]

Other cases show us a Monro who was at pains to exercise his professional acumen, expending considerable effort in an attempt to identify the distinctive features of a variety of conditions. Tailoring specific diagnoses to specific cases would have had obvious appeal to many clients in search of a personal form of medical attention. Moreover, such an approach was well supported by traditional classically and humorally founded medical theories, which had long stressed the individuality of patients' temperaments and the specificity of their disorders.

A number of early modern treatises on madness, from that of Cheyne to that of Pargeter, underline how important individual case histories were for mad-doctors: they provided a means to assert the possession of medical knowledge and simultaneously to communicate aspects of that knowledge to professional colleagues and potential customers. Such sources demonstrate, furthermore, how much the practices of early modern mad-doctoring involved one-to-one negotiation with clients and accommodation to their perceived needs, and yet also demonstrate that it was more often patients' families, rather than patients themselves, who predominated in this bargaining process. This is a pattern that lends support to Jewson's influential argument that early modern medicine was highly dependent on its patrons (and customers) and that medical knowledge was itself heavily conditioned by this dependent relationship.[8]

Jewson has also stressed how much eighteenth-century medical practice was formed by the manifold demands of patronage, and Monro's case book—despite (or because of) its private nature and function and its relative lack of concern with knowledge transmission or assertion—provides a number of illustrations of this dynamic at work. Some patients clearly put up more resistance to their families and friends than they did to the mad-doctor, whose intervention might (in principle at least) appeal to them as promising relief of their symptoms. The therapeutic encounter might also provide some patients with the hope—or, if nothing else, the illusion—that they were once more in a position to give voice to their own preferences. Sir Francis Chester, for example, was described as "not caring to do anything without the advice of a Physician to which he very readily submitted."[9] Others who had grown suspicious of their families clearly had high, if not unrealistic, expectations about Monro's arrival on the scene and intervention in their treatment. Captain Prowsett was recorded as being "very apprehensive . . . of the people round him [and] wanted to go out of the house with me tho not able to walk." He indicated that he was "apprehensive that poison & improper things were given him . . . & seem'd to have more confidence in me than his own brother & sister."[10]

The somewhat detached tone Monro generally adopts when making observations on such cases makes his underlying attitude difficult to decipher. He probably regarded disaffection toward relatives such as that cited above as delusional and irrational. One suspects, too, that he would not have made any record of patients' behavior and speech in the case book if he did not consider his observations to consist of likely signs and symptoms of derangement. Part of his clinical acumen, and almost certainly not the least of the services he provided to the families who consulted him, was surely his capacity to draw upon his experience in order to render clear judgments about what was irrational or delusional and what was understandable—and his authoritative pronouncements on such matters undoubtedly in themselves provided a measure of relief for relations confused and uncertain of how to react to disturbances of behavior, emotion, and cognition.[11] Nevertheless, the nonjudgmental nature of many of the entries he records suggests a degree of professional caution and an unwillingness to make hasty or highly interventionist decisions about cases and how to cope with them.

For all the evidence of negotiations between doctor and customer, it must also be noted that the sort of argument Jewson makes can easily be pushed too far. As a number of historians have recently pointed out, far from being invariably deferential to their clients, eighteenth-century physicians were often prepared to contradict their patients' desires and whims, and doctor-patient relationships in this period had their fair share of conflicts. George Cheyne's surviving correspondence with Samuel Richardson and with Selina, countess of Huntingdon (1707–91), provides a fascinating and instructive set of contrasts in this regard.[12] Samuel Richardson achieved public fame with the publication of *Pamela* in 1740; but novels were his avocation, printing his trade, and his correspondence with Cheyne began in 1733, long before he achieved fame as a writer. Cheyne sprinkled his correspondence with tirades against booksellers and printers, convinced—like many an author—that the publishing trades were filled with fools and rogues. He made an exception for Richardson, however, with whom he had long and friendly relations: "I have a sincere Regard for you and am convinced you are a Man of Probity and Worth beyond what I have met with among Tradesmen."

But a "tradesman" Richardson remained in his eyes, and one suffering from a series of maladies Cheyne did not hesitate to diagnose at a distance: "All your complaints are vapourish and nervous, of no manner of Danger, but extremely frightful and lowering."[13] Cheyne offered his advice freely and at length, his tone often peremptory and his prescriptions firm and unyielding.[14] He criticized Richardson for concealing his symptoms ("I wish you had imparted [your Complaints] frankly to me") and cast doubt on the courses of treatment others had prescribed:

> As to your sweating Machine for the Head, I own I can see little Use it will be to you in your Case. Your Giddiness is from the Stomach and Fumes rising from the Prima Viae, from a Thickness of Blood and Want of Perspiration. Not only a temperate but an abstemious Diet, Exercise, and gentle Evacuation must relieve you most effectually. . . .[15]

And on another occasion, he was scathingly dismissive of his rivals: "Get rid of Doctors and all the quacking Trade as soon as you can. I find few of them that understands your case."[16]

With the countess, however, daughter of one earl and wife of another, Cheyne's tone was very different. Flattery was laid on with a trowel, and anything likely to offend her ladyship's sensibilities or to suggest that her physician was disposed to trespass above his station was avoided at all costs. His patient's judgment and good sense were repeatedly celebrated

("I much admire your ladyship's courage and firmness. . . . Your low living was wonderfully judged";[17] "I think you did right in taking a vomit and will do well, if you can, daily to chew a little rhubarb. . . . As to your diet, I can add nothing"[18]); and unctuous "advice" and tactful suggestions were the order of the day:

> This (if I can have credit enough with your ladyship to be believed) I most sacredly assure you—that the regimen and medicines I have advised your ladyship never yet failed me. . . . Therefore I earnestly beseech your ladyship to go on your course begun. . . . I venture my life and reputation it ends to your satisfaction at last. . . .[19]

Rather than someone subject to his orders, Cheyne's aristocratic patient was acknowledged to be an active partner in the therapeutic process: "You must ever follow the directions of nature and your own observation, for nobody can inform you so well as your own feelings what and when such evacuation is to be made, for nature and your feeling will point it out. . . ." And in venturing a suggestion that "cold bathing would relieve much, and a flesh brushing morning and night," Cheyne displayed all due diffidence and deference: "Begin on receipt of this the trial, I earnestly beg your ladyship. . . . and I shall expect by God's help, some considerable amendment soon."[20]

Cheyne's correspondence emphasizes the way in which contemporary physicians found it necessary to adopt a variety of often sharply conflicting approaches to their patients, on the one hand hectoring, cajoling, and even imperious, and, on the other, persuasive, negotiating, obsequious, and imploring. There is certainly evidence in his case book that Monro employed both tactical gambits, although it is the latter rather than the former that tends to predominate. Of course, comparing a physician's correspondence, which is bound to be more personal and negotiated, with his private case book jottings, which are recorded for his benefit alone, is not comparing like with like. One can safely presume that Monro also corresponded at length with many of his patients, and a variety of evidence suggests that, just like Cheyne and other eighteenth-century physicians, he often diagnosed and counseled patients by this means from a distance. If his correspondence of this sort had survived, we might well have discovered Monro in a rather different guise than the one we observe in the case book.

One should also be careful not to overstate the difference between the patients Monro and Cheyne saw in their private practices. Monro's case book demonstrates that, rather than the out-and-out maniacal, the majority of his customers were precisely the nervous, troubled, and worried individuals that Cheyne, too, mostly treated. Nonetheless, there seems little doubt that Monro was more emphatically recognized and called upon as a specialist "mad-doctor" than was Cheyne. Imploring or "begging" his patients was hardly Monro's style, and in any event, the patients with whom he dealt—or so he would have thought—regularly required sterner measures and a firmer approach. If most contemporaries probably would have conceded that severer methods were in order for the more seriously mentally troubled, there may have been less agreement with the mad-doctor when it came to distinguishing the milder cases from the truly mad.

Given that he specialized in the putatively irrational, one suspects that the mad-doctor was more inclined than any other contemporary physician to take his patients' words and inclinations (if not those of their families) with a heavy dose of salt. Monro's case book provides ample evidence of the Bethlem doctor disagreeing with and criticizing his patients and denying the reality of their symptoms. For example, Monro was highly mistrustful of Mr. Whitehead's own account of his case, dismissing his complaints as irrational, delusional, and self-inflicted:

> I found him full of complaints but could by no means trust to his own account of himself, with a countenance of good health he was dying, nothing would stay upon his stomach; he had no appetite, could not sleep, & was so weak he could scarce stand, these complaints the first excepted were without foundation; the sickness at his stomach was occasion'd likewise by his own management of himself, & sometimes I believe by his endeavours.[21]

The case book is notable for the detailed descriptions it presents of how Monro reported his patients' many and varied complaints. It also provides suggestive and valuable information about how such symptoms were interpreted by the physician, as well as by the patients, their families, and their friends. Thus, quite apart from its account of how medical evaluations proceeded, the case book allows us considerable access to individual, familial, and wider societal judgments about mental illness. In so doing, it facilitates the development of certain comparisons between lay and medical attitudes toward insanity.

ASSIGNING THE CAUSES OF MADNESS:
PATIENTS' ETIOLOGIES AND SYMPTOMS

In terms of the etiology of lunacy ascribed by Monro and other sources, a whole host of factors were mentioned. These range from essentially physiological causes such as bodily diseases and illness through things such as drink to emotional and environmental problems. Much of the discussion about these matters seems typical of the period, corresponding closely with the portrait others have already drawn from contemporary printed sources. Planetary or astrological explanations for mental disorder, common enough in the seventeenth century (if Michael MacDonald's findings may be generalized),[22] clearly survived with some vigor into the Augustan age. The "moon" is often mentioned in Monro's case book as a significant causative factor that needs to be given due weight in understanding patients' mental states, reflecting the traditional association of lunacy with lunar cycles. Accounts couched in these terms were readily accommodated in both lay and medical worldviews of the time and may have been especially appealing given the recurrent, cyclical nature of certain forms of mental disturbance.[23] The prominent society physician Richard Mead (1673–1754), a family friend of the Monros, had published an entire treatise on the effect of the sun and moon on the human mind and body and had been told by the former Bethlem physician Edward Tyson (d. 1708) that epilepsy was generally an accompaniment in "the *raving fits* of [those] mad people, which keep the *lunar* periods."[24] Yet although madness and epilepsy were often seen as especially likely to coincide with lunar cycles, some practitioners seem to have grown more skeptical of such beliefs during the course of the Enlightenment. The provincial mad-doctor William Pargeter, for example, remarked that he had "never observed in any maniacal case, that the disorder assumed any particular appearances at any particular phases of the moon, so as to make it of consequence in the cure." Indeed, he reported one case he had seen with Monro himself, and then "repeatedly, and at various times, in his fits," on whom "the lunar periods had no influence whatever, either in inducing or controuling the *epileptic* symptoms."[25]

Also commonly referred to in the case book as causative factors in the loss of one's wits were such calamitous and stressful moral events as impoverishment, upset, bereavement, love, fright, shock, rejection, physical and verbal abuse, and economic reversals. The resort to causal explanations of this sort is perhaps indicative of a more psychological and compassionate view of insanity than some historical accounts of eighteenth-century treatment of the mad lead us to expect. Such tragic events also regularly populate contemporary literary accounts of mental derangement. The writings of Smollett, in particular, temper the opportunity for comedy and ridicule that mental extravagance afforded with views of mental malaise and collapse as sad reactions to life's reversals and force of circumstances. Breakdowns and the loss of mental equilibrium were ineluctable social, emotional, and physical calamities, and "want of memory or judgement" was represented as a "natural defect" worthy more of "compassion than [of] reproach."[26] Monro occasionally gave more explicit testimony about his sympathy for some of his patients, referring to them as "poor" not merely because of their economic straits but also because of their perilous health and sociomoral circumstances. Thus, we learn of the case of the "poor man" Mr. Aspridge, who "told us he was pox'd [and] was so [and] died the next morning," and the "poor lady" Mrs. Pigot, who "has been in a bad state of health for some time past."[27] Occasionally, Monro was even able to acknowledge when circumstances were particularly difficult for his patients: Mr. Fitzgerald, for instance, who "seemed to me disorder'd," had nonetheless "said very few things out of the way and positively denied every thing laid to his charge" and could, in Monro's view, have been successfully managed at home; but the "fine Irishman" still found himself confined, at his family's insistence, in Miles's madhouse.[28] Yet such expressions of sympathy were exceptional. Monro's case book is more remarkable for the relative paucity of remarks of this sort, or indeed of any very explicit statements of compassion or sympathy by Monro for the patients he was called upon to attend.

The exception may have been in the occasional female case that Monro details. The breaking off of courtships and marital contracts was cited especially often among the women he treated. Doubtless this constituted a reflection of the extreme value women were conceived, and (to some extent) forced, to place on marriage, which for many was their major means of securing a propitious social situation and some degree of financial security in eighteenth-century society. Monro set down particularly long histories of such unsuccessful engagements and love affairs, implying that he, along with their families, may have shared a special empathy for these unfortunate women. He related in extensive detail over six pages of the case book, for example, the "whole story" of Miss Gilchrist—significantly, a woman of "small fortune"—who had suffered one disappointment after another in her relations with the opposite sex. In her first proposed match, the collapse of her hopes came about because her friends opposed it as improper; in her second engagement, her fiancé had fathered a bastard child with his maid and then broken off the betrothal; and in a third engagement, neither she nor her friends thought the man's financial circumstances sufficient, and she herself felt compelled to end the relationship. Monro also reported hearing of a recent renewal of correspondence from Miss Gilchrist's first love, written in ignorance of her last engagement, which he felt was sufficient on its own to have deranged her mind.[29]

That the afflictions of women were often attributed to challenges to the prospects or security of their marriages and to the hazardous consequences (or even the mere specter) of infidelity, and that marriage was not infrequently espoused as a cure for the nervous afflictions of single women, is highly revealing of the ways in which, and the extent to which, the marital contract was loaded with gendered physical, metaphysical, and moral significance. Consider, for example, Monro's record of the circumstances surrounding the mental troubles of Mrs. Hampson:

> Some 6 or 7 months ago a gentleman who was an acquaintance of her husband's, & visited in the family upon that footing an agreeable man, took in his head to make speeches to her, & address her in a particular manner. he was at last so troublesome to her, that she was obliged to inform her husband of it: but the surprise of the thing & the anxiety it caus'd brought her in to such a state of mind as made her very uneasy. . . .[30]

The space Monro reserved for such reports seems to imply a significant attention accorded to moral explanations of mental afflictions and a special gendered sympathy on his part, as well as on that of the families he attended, for affecting and tragic love stories involving women. Popular contemporary novels depicting women confined against their wills in brothels and madhouses, such as *Clarissa* and *The Distress'd Orphan, or Love in a Madhouse,*[31] clearly reflect this paradigm. Others among Monro's contemporary acquaintances certainly confessed to such biased understanding, Walpole declaring:

> I am very tender-hearted on love-cases, especially to women, whose happiness does really depend, for some time at least, on the accomplishment of their wishes: they cannot conceive that another swain might be just as charming. I am not so indulgent to men, who do know that one romance is as good as any other.[32]

Yet contemporaries, male and female alike, were far from universally sympathetic to the love affairs of "the fairer sex." Those considered to be displaying flighty or over-amorous dispositions received short shrift from a society deeply worried about artificial affectation and romantic abandon, one that tended to see madness, lust, and strumpetry as too often lurking behind the guise of *amour.* Whereas Lady Mary Wortley Montagu (1689–1762), for example, deplored the fictional excesses of Fielding's *Clarissa,* which she felt threatened to make foolish and mad passions moving and fashionable,[33] Mrs. Elizabeth Robinson Montagu (1720–1800) was for similar reasons thoroughly approving of the (factual) rumor in 1786 that the "pretty Miss" (or, rather, Mrs.) Barwell had been put into Monro's care by her husband, Richard (or "Nabob") Barwell (1741–1804). The latter had been a prominent East India officer in Calcutta (notorious for his bribery and intrigues) and one of Warren Hasting's (1732–1818) lieutenants on the Supreme Bengal Council. Mrs. Barwell (née Sanderson) had been renowned as the "reigning beauty of Calcutta" but became ill after passionately eloping with Richard. The disapproving Mrs. Montagu believed her to have been duped by a scoundrel and fortune hunter.

> . . . the amorous pair were found in a dirty Inn at or near Dartford, where they had passd 3 days, and I presume nights together: his apologies rather aggravate than extenuate his guilt, for it is easier for a man to resist the solicitations of another's passions than his own. . . . he married . . . a Woman with a fortune superior to his own. . . . The Gallant most basely charges the fair one with having from the first made the advances, and urged the elopement. . . . I find poor Miss Barwell was suspected to have an amorous disposition, and the men now say, they are not surprized at what has happen'd. . . . Some say Mr Barwell . . . put her under the care of Dr Monro, in which I think he did very wisely, for bleeding and a low diet wd do her good and a strait waistcoat cd do her no harm.[34]

Such accounts suggest how medical treatment, in taking on the bias of sociomoral disapproval, might itself be an effective tool of subjugation in these cases. An unrelated contemporary, Thomas Monro (1764–1815) of Magdalen College, Oxford, was certainly convinced that "the temper of the female mind may be warped by the violence of passion," even if "it cannot entirely divest itself of that tenderness which is its peculiar characteristic."[35] However, if John Monro likewise believed that love and madness were different for women, he was not always so accepting of accounts of illness pitched in these terms. Although gendered and other sociomoral ascriptions of mental derangement figure prominently in the lay and familial accounts detailed in the case book, Monro himself was sometimes disposed to deny the validity of etiological assessments such as these. Indeed, he tended to dismiss them as simplistic and superficial, if not ignorant and unappreciative of the physical symptoms the learned mad-doctor was better equipped to divine in the afflicted. The predominance of more mechanistic, physiologized accounts of mental ailments from early on in the century had undermined the credibility formerly accorded to explanations rooted in the passions and emotions. The

Newtonian physician and Bethlem governor Nicholas Robinson (1697[?]–1775), for example, repudiated the emphasis of some on the necessity of removing the disturbing original passion in mental and nervous patients, citing the following case to prove his point about the futility of trying to counsel the mad out of their corporeal illnesses:

> . . . a Gentleman who had one only Daughter, that was melancholy mad for Love of a young Gentleman: Her Father, by Advice from Friends, was prevail'd on to admit him to marry her, in hopes of her Recovery. . . . But Marriage did not abate the Lunacy. . . . So that at last they were oblig'd to confine her in a Mad-House . . . as strong an Argument, as can be given to prove, that these Disorders are more dependant on the perverted Motion of the Fibres of the Brain, than any absolute Stubborness of the Mind. . . .[36]

Although Monro may not have been as extreme a mechanist as Robinson, he nevertheless frequently disregarded moral in favor of physical etiologies, as when he dismissed as totally unfounded the family's understanding of what lay behind the mental condition of one eighteen-year-old young woman: ". . . it is imagined that she liked a young gentleman who . . . made his addresses to her elder sister about 2 years ago but I beleive [sic] all this is without any other foundation than that they have heard her mention him lately tho the affair broke off two years ago."[37]

Sedentary habits and solitariness, two particular bug-bears of eighteenth-century mad-doctors,[38] were also mentioned in Monro's case book as associated with the etiology of mental disturbance. Mr. Tonkin's "melancholy" was ascribed to "this poor man . . . having run out his substance, & possibly from his sedentary manner of life," and Mrs. Kinder, as described by her husband, "hates company, chooses solitude."[39] Other afflictions, however, were attributed to more overtly physical, or physiomoral, states, a number of which were clearly seen as more blameworthy, such as onanism (masturbation), dietary abuse, and inebriety. Sometimes, Monro may be found recording emotional and moral causes only to downplay them, preferring more physiologized accounts. Although, for example, the "flurried" and "hurried" state, "agitations," and insomnia of Mr. Molyneux were initially attributed to the death of his master and the shock of accidentally and temporarily losing one of his children, Monro subsequently learned that Molyneux had a mad son and concluded that it was "a family complaint" related to him being "in the decline of life" and having "drank hard"—a judgment that may have been confirmed by the patient's subsequent death.[40]

In recording some ascriptions of this sort, Monro appears to have been making independent judgments of his own or to have been informed by the views of professional colleagues before recording information in his case book. In the majority of cases, however, he seems to have relied heavily upon information about the history, origins, and progress of the disturbance that had been supplied by the family and other lay persons. Rather than reflecting any radical imposition of medical models of mental illness, the case book suggests the existence of relatively broadly shared and nonconflictual cultural assumptions that served as the basis for negotiating agreements about the nature and causality of patients' afflictions and the meaning of their speech and behavior. Yet, for all that, we may often discern Monro giving the family's account his own special spin.

CHAPTER 5

Diagnosing the Mad

GHOSTS IN THE MACHINE:
PATIENTS' METAPHYSICAL SIGNS AND SYMPTOMS

The Speech of the Mad

Monro's case book allows us, as one might hope, to obtain a relatively good idea of what both the mad-doctor and contemporary families considered to be the signs and symptoms of madness. The text reveals Monro to be someone who displayed considerable deliberation and a willingness to suspend judgment when diagnosing cases until more information had clarified matters. Generally, however, Monro's diagnostic concern is directed to the mental processes that appear to be suggested by patients' language and behavior, and it is notable that he attends very much to the form of their symptoms while not worrying very much about their content.[1]

Speech was predictably regarded as an especially firm indicator of mental state, verbal communications being often the first and most important point of experiential contact between doctor and patient and lying at the very crux of the consultative encounter. It was often and fundamentally on the basis of patients' spoken (or reported) language that the physician arrived at and evolved his diagnosis and his very means of proceeding. Patients who talked excessively "loudly," "incessantly," or too much, such as Mrs. Edge and Mrs. Holford; who were "full of talk" or prone to "ramble," such as Mrs. Elder; who "talk'd very insensibly," incoherently, inconsistently, nonsensically, or "without rhime or reason," such as Mrs. Holford, Mrs. Stone, Miss Hume, Mrs. Duncan, Mrs. Edge, and Mrs. Moreati; or who talked too vehemently or passionately, such as Mr. Sergison, presented vivid signs of mental disorder.[2] Patients who spoke too little or hardly at all were similarly marked out as disordered, their lack of words tending to distinguish them as idiotic, dull, melancholic, low spirited, and depressed, in contradistinction to the furious and the lunatic. Some patients were so resistant to the mad-doctor's probings that they can have given him little clue to their conditions, as when Monro complained of Mrs. Hobbes that "I could get very little more from her than that she wanted to get up & take a walk."[3]

For those, on the other hand, such as Miss Anther, who talked "pretty sensibly," or Miss Lovell and Mr. Whitby, who talked "very sensibly" or "very well" and were "able to give a good account of" themselves, speech might be a contraindicator.[4] In the case of others, such as Miss Campden, Miss Compton, and Miss Cutter, who not only talked to Monro "very rationally, & coolly" but "seem'd sensible" or "conscious" to some extent that they were "not well" and of the nature of their complaints, there were the clear suggestions of a better prognosis.[5] Such cases contrast with some of the "worst" patients Monro saw, including the attempted regicide Margaret Nicholson, "who did not seem sensible of having committed any crime."[6] The definitive association in this era between madness and various degrees of insensibility naturally led the mad-doctor to attend constantly to positive and negative evidence of sensibility in patients' words, deeds, and looks. The larger the remnants of sensibility that the mad-doctor could discern, the better the prognosis: just as Captain MacDonald was "in some manner sensible that he is not well," so Miss Compton was "at times conscious that she is not well & seems sensible what her complaint is."[7]

The alert reader may already have observed something else about this attention to patients' conversation: it is noticeable, as the balance of examples given above indicate, that disorders of speech seem to be much more commonly recorded for female than for male patients, perhaps implying a bias on Monro's part, or on the part of contemporary families, against women talking out of turn. It would be easy to suggest that other signs of a gendered evaluation of patients' behavior can possibly be discerned in the description of patients as "flighty," "full of gayety," "flurried," in a "high state/way," or "too full of spirits."[8] Such language is, after all, highly suggestive of prevailing expectations that women should conduct themselves quietly, demurely, and decorously. Yet matters are not so simple, for on closer inspection, it turns out that language of this sort is employed in the case book no more often to describe women than to describe men. If evidence of the mad-doctor's gendering of speech seems ambivalent, Monro's often dismissive attitude to such speech is certainly not. Disdainful terms such as "nonsense" crop up again and again to describe what patients said.

Some speech disorders were evidently connected to organic problems that in later centuries came to be understood as neurological and related to "General Paralysis of the Insane" (i.e., tertiary syphilis), to dementia, or to aphasia and stroke. Yet in the eighteenth century, phenomena of this sort tended to be more commonly linked (or confused) with more broadly conceived, life-threatening paralytic disorders, such as apoplexy and palsy, or with epilepsy and hysteria. Mrs. Lambert, for example, described as exhibiting "at times a faltring in her speech," was to die suddenly "Apoplectic" after being "seiz'd with a strong convulsive fit"; and Mrs. Duncan, who "had had 2 or 3 convulsion fits" and talked "incessantly without consistence & coherence," was correctly declared by Monro to be in danger of her life, and she died within weeks of his visit.[9] Yet contemporary mad-doctors also strove to some extent to distinguish madness from paralysis, as when Monro designated Mrs. Walker "mad enough, but at the same time seem'd to me to have many symptoms attending her complaint that were paralytic."[10]

The Delusions of the Deranged

Delusions and hallucinations are also frequently mentioned in the case book, and these were themselves normally revealed to the physician and patients' relations in verbal form. Monro was sufficiently objective toward and interested enough in speech of this sort to record it, and at times it appears in approximately verbatim form. Some historians and literary critics have interpreted most eighteenth-century writing about madness as signifying an emphatic disengagement with patients' speech and thought-worlds,[11] and Monro's case book furnishes much evidence to support these claims. On the one hand, the amount of verbatim testimony he produces reveals a significant space being accorded to patients' language and opinions within the case history narrative. On the other hand, rarely was such mad testimony seen as worth taking seriously, or as the grounds for any sort of "talking cure." For example, Mr. Moore was observed by Monro as "continually raving & talking to such fantastical beings as his imagination represents to him. 'Come forth ye ministers of death,' 'come from behind your intrenchments.' This he sd [sic] he spoke to the little insects, that were there crawling about in great numbers."[12] And perhaps, in this instance at least, Monro was right to treat these Lilliputian hallucinations as purely epiphenomenal, since the description he provides here clearly conjures up the spectacle of a patient in the throes of delirium tremens—a conclusion strengthened by the fact that Mr. Moore, like many habitual drunks, subsequently ended up drowning himself.[13]

In partial agreement with Foucault, Michael MacDonald[14] has argued for the enhanced significance of delusions as evidence of mental derangement in this period, as madness was secularized and as mechanistic, medical, and philosophical conceptualizations of insanity—whether as diseased judgment, distorted sensation, false imagination, or misassociated ideas—became more prominent. Delusions and hallucinations were accepted by Monro and the families he visited as one of the most distinctive signs of a more serious mental affliction. Thus, patients such as Mr. Moore, who spoke to imaginary, inanimate, or speechless beings, were often designated as profoundly deranged and were dispatched to confinement.[15] Those who were removed from their domiciles and sent to Bethlem appear not only, or necessarily, to have been poorer or violent cases, but to have been those who exhibited a more florid delusionary symptomology. Evidence of delusions or hallucinations was often enough on its own to convince Monro of the madness of the patients he saw. When called to attend on Mr. Pottinger, for example, after briefly detailing his station in life, Monro simply observed (not without a hint of amusement, and possibly remembering the earlier case of Cruden and countless others like him), "when I saw him he was rather feverish, but very mad: he talk'd & rattled very idly about being Sheriff of London, that he had laid great wagers upon it, & should win 300000£ I think, that there was near 3 millions laid on this event."[16] Likewise, nothing was reported of Miss Mombray, beyond the following thought and auditory impressions:

> . . . complained more than 3 months of designs against her, from what persons or for what reasons she knows not. sees often a flash like a flash of lightning. hears a noise like the ringing of bells under her windows. & imagines the people as she passes along look at her & laugh at her & take particular notice of her.[17]

The case book reports auditory hallucinations rather less frequently (in just five or six of Monro's cases)[18] than delusions of thought and visual hallucinations, but paranoid, persecutory delusions were relatively common. Delusions of grandeur (sometimes joined to such morbid suspicions) were also featured among thought disturbances, perhaps reflecting the significance placed by eighteenth-century medical and satirical writers on the follies of pride and vanity, which many felt so characteristic of the age (see below, pages 75–76).

More commonly, hallucinatory and delusionary symptoms were combined with other behavioral and physical problems, as in the following
anonymous case of a woman whose apparent paranoia seems to have
inflated her anxieties about a medical consultation with a renowned
mad-doctor:[19]

> Mrs— with Mrs Blinkhorn. she was appointed to have come the day before,
> but was so frighten'd at the thoughts of it that she ran away. she imagines she
> hears voices, that her friends have designs against her, & abstains from eat-
> ing is very indolent, & sleeps badly.[20]

The definition of madness as delirium without fever, so widely
accepted by mad-doctors in this period and further reinforced at the end
of the century by Pinel and Esquirol,[21] seems to have very much
informed Monro in his attempts to distinguish the truly mad from the
merely feverish. Significantly, Monro's library included many of the
most modern medical authors on fevers.[22] In most cases, including that
of the slave girl Flora, he cautiously suspended his final verdict on
patients' mental states until any suspicion or complication of fever had
passed.[23] For similar reasons, Monro also discriminated between the
"frenzied" and the lunatic, with the former tending to be associated with
raving, delirium, feverishness, bodily heat, and sweating—although the
commonality of the symptoms ascribed to both conditions made a clear
differentiation rather problematic. Mr. Moore, for example, was
described as having delusions, but "his distemper has more the appearance of frenzy than lunacy, he sweats much . . . in great agony sleeps little or none, is continually raving."[24] Monro also made distinctions
between hysterical cases and other nervous disorders, and full-blown
cases of lunacy. Monro made the diagnosis of hysteria in only two cases,
both females, just as he made the diagnosis of hypochondria (the virtual
male equivalent of hysteria) in only a single male case.[25] It is not precisely
clear what Monro saw as the main features of the condition, but among
the "many" "hysterical symptoms" he described in the case of one
anonymous woman (whose distemper was seen to originate with a previous childbirth) were somewhat imaginary (or psychosomatic) bodily
pains and sensations, such as headache, cold or chills, and turbid urine
apt to milky discoloration (implying a specific urinary or other dysfunc-
tion linked with childbirth), alongside other, more universal features
such as fear of becoming mad, sleeplessness, and anxiety or "hurry."[26]
Others with symptoms or delusions characterized by unwarranted
suspicions are regularly encountered in Monro's case book (recalling the

mad-doctor's earlier identification, in the Ferrers case, of suspicion and jealousy as idiopathic signs of madness).[27] In the 1766 case of Mr. Newport, for example, Monro placed special emphasis on Newport's unaccountable distrust of his nearest and dearest and the odd behavior that this provoked. Monro pointedly exposed the ridiculousness of the drama his patient had involved him in on his visit:

> He took me out of the room & I imagined he was going to trust me with some great secret, but after having shut the door with great precaution he told me little pitchers had great ears, he therefore open'd the door that led into the dining room again & desir'd his wife & Mr Williams to walk down stairs, he had nothing to communicate any further than that he had no notion of country Apothecaries.[28]

Although keen to discern the physical causes behind emotional and intellectual disturbances, Monro was far from being a materialist and was quite willing to accept that madness might have strong intellectual or ideational origins. He was plainly convinced that the imagination might be dulled or "hurried" and the spirits demoralized or raised by mere upsets, shocks, exhaustion, accidents, and other metaphysical events. For example, Monro recorded without overt question the etiological model offered for Miss Campden's mental indisposition, namely that she "was frighted some time ago by her brother."[29] His notes on the case of Mrs. Plow also imply a nondualist approach to mental disorder, although with a somewhat hesitant and unresolved tendency toward the divination of a primary physical seat. Soon after her marriage at the grand old age of sixty-eight, this patient had "imagin'd herself with child" and somewhat remarkably was able to persuade the self-satirically named physician Dr. Handasyde (probably a man-midwife) to examine her. Monro saw her two years later:

> She went two months beyond the time she had fix'd when a violent purging which came upon her, & continued near 8 months reliev'd her of her great belly. Whether this evacuation which in some measure still continues has weakened her faculties I know not but she now fancies her neighbours blow poisonous powders upon her, & that she is to be burnt & punish'd [in] various ways.[30]

Mrs. Plow may well have experienced a phantom pregnancy. Alternatively, or additionally, she may have experienced disorienting physical symptoms that could have been associated with a stomach ulcer, ectopic pregnancy, or cancer of the womb, and on one level her case seems indicative of the limited nature of eighteenth-century obstetric knowledge. Yet, speculation aside, such cases emphasize not only

Monro's preoccupation with delusions and hallucinations as symptoms
of bodily derangement, but also his willingness to suspend judgment
about the cases he was called to attend and about the precise factors
behind the weakening of his patients' mental faculties. In the case of one
patient (Mr. Rowley), by whose "present appearance" Monro was
"afraid of his becoming an Idiot," a certain compassion appears to have
stayed his diagnosis: "I think it is rather too soon to pass so heavy a
judgement on him."[31]

He was nevertheless at pains to bring to light the delusionary inau-
thenticity of some of the physiological symptoms his patients alleged.
Thus, the "various illnesses" Mrs. van Hock had reported over the previous two years (in particular, gout, headache, and loss of sight in one
eye) were recorded by Monro to have ultimately "vanish'd." Meanwhile
her mental affliction was shown to consist almost entirely in "fancy,"
with an underlying heredity:

> About 5 months ago she began to be wrong in her head & to fancy she shd
> come to poverty & to absolute want, that she shd not have a bed to lie on, that
> she had been wicked to a strange degree & such like. I attended her mother
> about 4 years ago in Glocester street in the same complaint, she told me this
> morning July 25 that she had not another gown or any Linnen or other nec-
> essaries to send for & was afraid she shd tear the flesh from her bones.[32]

Apt to be dubious about his patients' (and their families') opinions
with respect to the origins of their mental complaints, Monro often dismissed these judgments as exaggerated or merely imaginary, sometimes
exhaustively chronicling their attributions only to discredit them. The
long account of her complaints provided by one patient, Miss Lovell, was
quoted almost verbatim by Monro, but he clearly regarded most of
what she had to say as delusional. Simultaneously, the patient was criticized by the mad-doctor and her family for concealing her (supposedly
imaginary) symptoms. She

> says that being in the country last October she first eat [sic] some grapes
> which chill'd her blood, & afterwards some mushrooms which poison'd her,
> that she broke out in blotches, & has ever since been ill with various com-
> plaints, her inside is decay'd, she is in danger of a dropsy, of losing her nose
> & this morning she told me the upper part of the palate of her mouth was
> prodigiously swell'd but was now gone down again. & all these complaints
> are now upon her, & make her & her family uneasy. because . . . at first she
> did not relate all the symptoms of her complaint as she ought to have done.[33]

Monro likewise recounted at length the narrative of Captain Robinson, master of a Jamaica trading vessel, who, "fancying" he had con-

tracted venereal disease during his last voyage and claiming to have "been familiar with some infected person," believed he had communicated it to his wife. Moreover, "so far was he infatuated," as Monro put it, that he claimed—preposterously—to have "likewise infected" his ninety-year-old mother-in-law and "pretended to shew the marks of it in eruptions upon her face." Monro cast further doubt on this patient's narrative by recording that Robinson had been in "a low way for some time before I saw him" and that, on the day the doctor attended, the captain had just been cut down by the maid from a noose of his own devising.[34] Not only Monro but a number of contemporary authorities on venereal diseases, including Charles Hales (flourished 1760s), onetime physician to the Savoy Hospital, pointed to the frequency with which their patients falsely imagined they had been afflicted, maintaining that some were quite evidently distracted, and that, occasionally, both afflictions were combined in one sufferer. In fact, most of his patients, Hales averred, simply had "a poxed mind." Rather than any medicinal preparation, they required more of a talking cure—namely the "refuting of their groundless apprehensions" and persuasion that they "charge their eventual sufferings to their own account."[35]

At times, one can appreciate the canniness (and the difficulty) of the mad-doctor's efforts to sort out verifiable facts from fancy and pathology. For example, Monro presented a long account of the story of Mrs. Gordon, detailing how she had summoned him herself, having been bitten by her pet cat, "which she suppos'd to be mad." After the bite, she felt "a pain in the arm where she was bit, & a pain in her side, dreams of cats, and other such like things which she thinks the consequence of this bite." As her version of events makes clear, the combination of trauma, vivid dreams, high anxiety, and an accident provoking fears of death had produced a very frightened woman, someone seemingly in need of constant reassurance from her physician. Demurring from her account, Monro concluded instead that Mrs. Gordon's complaints "proceed from her imagination hurried with this disagreeable accident," noting by way of confirmation that another lady friend of hers, who was bitten at the same time, "has not the least complaint."[36]

The cat was characterized by her distressed mistress as "a great favorite for 2 years," although "at times wild & flying about, & sometimes surly." It had been put into an especial "fury" by the re-arrival of a dog in the household, who had formerly been "turn'd out" in order to keep "puss . . . quiet," but on whose return "the cat rais'd her back & erected her tail, at which she & the lady who was with her being fright-

en'd would have turn'd her out of the room but she flew at them both &
bit them in sevral places."[37] The anthropomorphism and high levels of
anxiety displayed in such accounts should not surprise us (indeed may
even strike a chord with the animal lovers among us). Eighteenth-century
literature was full of analogies between the emotions of animals and
humankind, and the wilder forms of madness had long been conceptual-
ized as a kind of animalistic atavism. It should also be pointed out that the
newspapers, magazines, and medical literature of the time were replete
with somewhat scare-mongering stories about mad or rabid dogs, cats,
and other animals (though not mad cows!), and the passage of diseases
from animals to humans—anxieties that went beyond whatever genuine
problems existed with the control of rabies and dangerous animals and
with the quarantining of pets and wildlife.[38] It might be expected, therefore, that some of the more nervously inclined in society would prove susceptible to excessive anxieties about the matter. Monro himself appears to
have been well read in the enormous literature relating to the madness
contracted via the bite of a mad dog.[39] Yet, however astute Monro's diagnosis may have been, he was evidently disregarding any wider contextual
meaning for his patient's anxieties, content with the judgment that what
he was witnessing was merely a delusion or an inflamed imagination.

Although extensively reported, delusions were far from invariably present, recorded, or emphasized in the cases Monro was called to. They
were often only a single, relatively minor, factor in a variegated combination of signs that the mad-doctor took into account in making an evaluation. Although Mrs. Hampson, for example, was assailed by "strange
& extravagant ideas crowding in upon her," she also (inter alia) "did not
sleep well was violently flurried at times, subject to a palpitation of the
heart, waked in hurries."[40] Monro had criticized in print Battie's attempt
to localize madness as fundamentally in the imagination and the connection of ideas, and had expressed his impatience with overly metaphysical
definitions of insanity.[41] Given his own view of madness as essentially
judgment vitiated by bodily imbalances (for evidence of which he was
constantly on the lookout), it comes as no surprise to learn that he was
wary of placing too much weight on delusions in the diagnostic process.

Crazy Conduct

Behavior of various kinds was plainly one of Monro's major criteria for
defining mental oddness. Quite a number of Monro's patients, as one
might expect, had committed acts of violence against themselves or oth-

ers, and in some cases such acts had clearly precipitated the summoning of the mad-doctor and/or recourse to a private madhouse or public institution. For example, Mr. Whitehead had cut off three of his own fingers; Mrs. Harris "had made to [sic] attempts to hang herself before she was brought to Mr Miles's"; Mrs. Holman had threatened that "she would either hang or drown herself" unless her future husband married her; and Captain Robinson was saved from death by self-hanging only by the timely arrival of his maid. A number of others (e.g., Mrs. Wilson and Mr. Hamilton) combined both suicidal and murderous inclinations. A few more added destructiveness to their behavioral abnormalities, Mr. Rowley pushing his head through the sash window so violently "that he drove out the glass entirely," as well as having "bit his own lip thro'." Others still were registered as being inclined to (often unspecified) "mischief" or "outragious" conduct of various sorts.[42]

John Monro's opinions on the larger sociopolitical and legal questions surrounding the confinement of such cases are difficult to chart from these and other sources. Other contemporaries and near contemporaries were certainly advocates of tougher action in terms of legislation and medical police[43] when it came to the dangerously insane. Writing in 1790, just months before John's death, the unrelated Thomas Monro of Magdalen College, Oxford, referred to such lunatics contemptuously as "monsters" and appealed for the law to take a wider

> cognizance of these mischievous and evil-minded madmen, of whom the number is by no means small, who are from day to day actively employed making attempts upon the property and the lives of their neighbours and themselves. Every man must in his life-time have been attacked by these monsters; and happy is he who has escaped without being wounded in his fortune, his health, or his reputation.[44]

Yet Thomas Monro's satirical target here was mainly the moral problem of "Libertinism" and the associated vices of "intemperance," "dissipation," and "debauchery," which had been long and widely condemned in eighteenth-century society as leading to violence, depravity, and madness. Furthermore, he clearly disagreed with certain "Moralists" who had confused the passionate, the foolish, and even the vicious with the insane, and was thus concerned to not apply "the spirit of confinement" too vigorously. For, if the mild and harmless insane, or those "who displayed the smallest symptoms of insanity," were "deprived of . . . liberty," there might be no one left in the world "to be indulged . . . without a keeper."

On the one hand, this kind of madman was deprecated as a "raving," "mean and squalid-looking . . . wretch," who, despite amusing the world, was a source of "distress" to "his friends by his absurdities." If the law was rendered "more rigorous," such a madman was apt to find himself in Bedlam, "reduced in his scene of action to a theatre of five feet square, and the catalogue of his property confined to little more than a bundle of straw and a wooden bowl." On the other hand, confinement was unnecessary, for whether a "moon-striken poet" or a "lord of thousands," "no danger need be apprehended" from such "harmless madmen": however "numerous" a "tribe," they could be tolerated, or even "disarmed" by being "humoured" in their "particular failing[s]." Rather, it was with violent and "mischievous insanity" that the legislature should concern itself.[45]

Whatever the extent to which John Monro shared these viewpoints, his case book confirms that the daily experience of the mad-doctor was more extensively preoccupied with the less florid and more harmless manifestations of mental disorder. Violence is, in fact, a rather rarer feature of John Monro's case book than one might perhaps expect, the illnesses of most of the cases he saw manifesting themselves in milder behavioral, emotional, and psychological difficulties. The most violent case that Monro mentions was actually someone the mad-doctor had not seen (or, possibly, had seen in an earlier consultation), the father of a patient he attended (Mr. Newport). This was the only case he specifies of someone who had actually been guilty of murder, or even of bodily harm.[46] Most of the violence we hear about in the case book consists of "violent flurries" and anxieties. Patients were much more often prone to worrying about external (or internal, as in mental or physiological) threats to themselves and their loved ones than they were inclined to commit violence or murder themselves.

Sometimes behavior was described too vaguely for us to know what was meant, as when little more was said of Miss Theobald than that she "behaved in a strange & unusual manner."[47] Often, however, the record is more transparent. Sudden, extravagant, or violent motions by patients were commonly noted by Monro and the families he attended, as were patients' attempts to run away from their domiciles or relations. Behavior of this sort was seen as especially irrational where relations displayed "the most tender concerns," even though some patients were clearly fleeing from their own confinement or restraint, however well meant. (Miss Campden, for example, was observed to "some times take a sudden jump, & run from them [her relations] as fast as she could.")[48]

Similarly, failure to observe the social etiquette and common decencies of appearance, personal hygiene, and dress strongly suggested a loss of rational control. Denudation and destruction of dress in particular were seen as signaling the mental degradation and degeneration toward a more brutish, uncivilized, antediluvian state, with which madness was commonly associated in this period. (Miss Campden, again, was observed "running into the yard with no cloaths upon her but her shift," and Mrs. Dibsdale was found "very much disorder'd, slavering & spitting upon her cloaths.")[49] Worse cases manifested themselves in more extravagant and offensive behavior. Mr. Mitchell was adjudged "exceeding mad" when Monro saw him because he was not only silent and "refusing to eat" but was "spitting, sulky . . . tumbling & tossing about," so that he was "obliged to be tied down in his bed"; Mr. Rowley's abnormalities included being "extremely nasty" (i.e., dirty).[50]

Passions and Emotions

Emotional disturbances that seemed excessive, disproportionate, and unjustified by any "reasonable" cause were also regularly reported in Monro's case book. Exaggerated agitation, fears, restlessness, and incongruous anxieties were taken as eloquent signs of mental disturbance, as when Captain Macdonald was described as "in constant agitation," or Mrs. Harris was observed to be "at present in violent hurries," or Miss Theobald was described as "restless, passionate."[51] Occasionally, however, such symptoms suggested deeper physical problems, as when Mrs. Duncan was found on a second visit from Monro "in a most violent agitation, & as they told me had had 2 or 3 convulsion fits."[52] Patients who could not account for their emotions or actions, whose emotions appeared incongruous or contradictory, who laughed, cried, or sang without cause, or were sad and melancholy without discernible grounds, were generally recognized as mentally deranged. For example, Monro recalled that on a first visit to Mr. Newport, the patient had "said very little but laught at times," and Miss Compton, he remarked, "falls into violent passions, & then dissolves into tears."[53] Mr. Bevan was observed to merely laugh in the face of those who asked him questions, "tho at the same time he is extremely melancholy," with "thoughts of destroying himself," and yet he says he knows no reason for his "melancholy" and "feels as if he was a fool."[54] Captain Macdonald was found "sitting in his bed sometimes singing, & sometimes imitating dancing, & making a strange kind of noise."[55]

Religiously articulated or associated melancholy and more secularly framed despair, low spirits, and depression were also regularly reported by Monro's patients. Indeed, rather than manic, outwardly violent, paranoid, or delusional disorders, it was the despondent and the depressed, the self-blaming and self-hating, the self-harming and suicidal, the unhappy and the uneasy, who predominated among the cases Monro was called to attend. However prominent the raving, animalistic maniac in contemporary literary and artistic portrayals of madness, in the private practice of this leading member of the mad-doctoring fraternity such cases are conspicuous by their relative absence.

Mental distress that involved domestic disputes, or husbands and wives inexplicably or unreasonably abnegating their responsibilities as breadwinners and heads of households or as wives, mothers, and housekeepers, also figured relatively prominently in the case book. Such models of disturbed and disturbing conduct included the occasional reference to extravagant spending. Indeed, the proverbial lunatic wasting his estate and the spendthrift wife wrecking the household economy found more poignant echoes in patients such as Mrs. Kinder. According to her husband's account, she displayed irrationally antisocial and irresponsible conduct, behavior that today might be seen as symptomatic of a manic depressive psychiatric condition. She continued

> for 3 weeks in a high state during which time she is very talkative; expensive buying many things she does not want & full of acquaintance, after that moderate & as she should be, & then she falls into a low state of despondency, hates company, chooses solitude, & is angry with her husband for suffering her to run into expence when he knows, she says, very well that she is not right.[56]

Women were clearly expected to behave with a certain degree of modesty and moderation, and those who contravened such behavioral norms were often reported as deranged. Those who became immoderately disaffected toward themselves or relatives they had formerly loved, or who contravened those emotional ties, conduct, and duties conventionally seen as natural to familial and social relations, were also apt to appear as irrational. Mrs. Hampson was observed to have lacked "that Regard for her husband, her children or her family that she used to experience."[57] In an age before medical men had begun to articulate concepts of puerperal insanity, let alone postpartum depression, mad-doctors and families were still appreciative of the pathological nature of problems of affect. Monro recorded of Mrs. Wilson, for example, that she "thinks herself very wicked, & is afraid she shall murder her husband, or herself or her child, for whom she says she does not feel the affection she formerly did tho she loves her beyond any thing."[58]

Women seem to have been recorded in Monro's case book with a range and proportion of depressive symptoms considerably in excess of those detailed for men. The large number of Monro's female patients who were reported to be sad, melancholy, and suicidal, to have felt morbidly guilty, sinful, or low in self-esteem, prompts us to ask whether women—or, more particularly, women from families with private means—may have been more prone to depression in this period. Alternatively, were eighteenth-century women more likely to acknowledge and (classically constructed as "the weaker sex") to be diagnosed with forms of mental disease characterized by over-emotionalism, sadness, self-loathing, tearfulness, and despair? For example, although Mrs. Harris was observed "talking much of having done wrong," Mrs. Brooke was said to have been "in a low spirited way these six months past, her thoughts are desponding to the last degree at some times in the day, & she is so much afraid of doing mischief."[59]

Such cases might be said to accord with current psychiatric experience of the higher proportion of women than men presenting with depressive illnesses. However, we cannot determine here to what degree this gender disparity represents something of a transhistorical, or an illness-specific, phenomenon. Women were regularly portrayed in both contemporary literary and artistic representations (figures 6–8) as distressed, melancholic, and suicidal, romanticization of feminine emotions and frailty tending to vie with more censorious accounts of women perverted and destroyed by their passions and weak intellects. However, precisely where the social construction of illness begins and genuine illness behavior ends in the representations of this period is difficult to say. Antique representations of melancholy, which were revived and widely disseminated in eighteenth-century culture, had long associated the affliction with women. Although melancholy as a disease was originally and frequently personified as an old rather than a young woman, it was younger women, as the afflicted, who predominated in such depictions. Of course, women were far from being the exclusive carriers of melancholy, and there was a strong class and modish dimension to such characterizations.[60]

On the other hand, early-eighteenth-century writers such as Pope had caustically parodied the dullnesses, "splenetick" cheerlessness, and hypochondriacal affectations of the aspiring elite and fashionable crowd, male and female alike. Furthermore, problems of nerves, sensi-

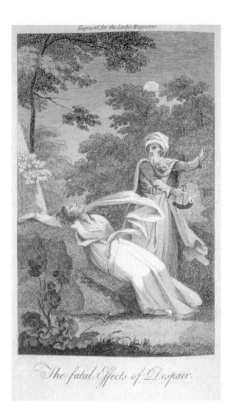

FIGURE 6. "The Fatal Effects of Despair."
Engraving from the *Lady's Magazine* (20
[1789]) accompanying the fictional story (on
pp. 171–73) of Louisa de Baumelle, driven to
despair and drawing a "poinard" from her
pocket to stab herself, after her lover, the
Chevalier de Molu, was confined in a Turkish
dungeon. Molu is shown here disguised as a
Turk. Reproduced with kind permission of the
Bodleian Library, University of Oxford, Per.
2705 e. 1279 (1789), page 171.

bilities, and mood, or rather temperament and spirits, could also be
fashionable in this period. The rather more contemporary examples of
Samuel Johnson's well-publicized "gloom" and Boswell's somewhat
melancholy *Hypochondriak* suggest that similar avenues for the sick
role were far from closed to men in late Augustan times.[61] Moreover,
times were gradually changing for those whose nerves and sensibilities
appeared vulnerable or who displayed susceptibilities to mental disorders. Monro's case book dates more or less from the period when the
(rather disingenuous, and oft-parodied) cult of sensibility had begun to

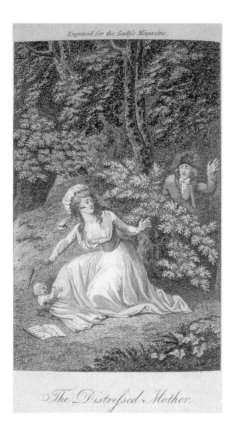

FIGURE 7. "The Distressed Mother"—"a picture of conjugal and maternal distress." Engraving from the *Lady's Magazine* (19 [1788]) accompanying the fictional narrative (on pp. 361–63) of Mrs. D—, who had "worked herself into a state bordering upon insanity" after reading a letter falsely announcing the death of her husband, Captain Charles D—. She was said to retire regularly with her baby, avoiding compassionate friends, "to enjoy the miserable luxury of solitary affliction." Saved at the last from a desperate act of self-murder, she is depicted dropping both her baby and the knife she had drawn on being hailed by her husband, who has arrived in the nick of time. Reproduced with kind permission of the Bodleian Library, University of Oxford, Per. 2705 e. 1279 (1788), page 360.

allow more scope for men of feeling to display emotional frailties, to be sad, mortified, and wan, and to faint and weep in public. Previous Augustan enthusiasm for the virtues of stoicism was steadily tempered during the second half of the century, as part of a wider Enlightenment critique of classical philosophies and a reassertion and rearticulation of the benefits of feelings and passions. Notably, by the 1790s, men such as

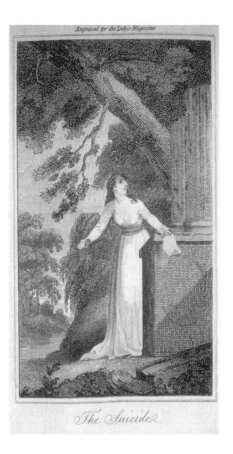

Engraved for the Lady's Magazine

The Suicide.

FIGURE 8. "The Suicide." Engraving from the *Lady's Magazine* (19 [1788]) accompanying another unsophisticated moral tale (on pp. 585–86). This was the story of Mrs. Amelia Hantley, who, by contrast with Mrs. D— (see figure 7), carried through her suicidal intent, after being "driven to desperation" by receiving a false letter from a woman, Arabella Dalton, accusing her husband, Harry, of inconstancy. Reproduced with kind permission of the Bodleian Library, University of Oxford, Per. 2705 e. 1279 (1788), page 585.

Thomas Monro of Magdalen College were expressing trenchant criticisms of stoical responses to distress, attacking such reactions as a form of "hardened insensibility." Indeed, echoing a broadly shared anti-Enlightenment discourse, Monro argued for a legitimate place for grief, tears, joy, and the other passions (at least when "restrained within due bounds"), defending them as innate capacities that were vital to the cementing and preservation of societal bonds and of humanity itself.[62]

Writing thirty years or so before this, John Monro had rather less to say in defense of sensibilities and feelings, although one should not, perhaps, expect to find much philosophical disquisition either in a chronicle of his private attendance on patients or even in his *Remarks* (1758), his published response to rival mad-doctor William Battie's *Treatise* (1758).[63] Like many other contemporaries, medical and lay, however, he regularly employed the language of the "spirits" in his case book. Phrases such as "low spirited," "dispirited," and "depression/ dejection of spirits" are especially conspicuous, and (though less commonly) inverse terms such as being "in high/full of spirits" can also be found.[64] Here, nonetheless, Monro was probably echoing again what his clients reported, rather than relying himself on the notion of "animal spirits," although he had emphasized in his *Remarks* how in some species of madness, high or low spirits were "the first symptom" of the disorder.[65]

By this period, most doctors, under the influence of new "iatromechanical"[66] ideas, had lost faith in earlier theories that stressed the significant role of these notional entities as so-called messengers to the senses and memory. A 1735 publication, *Epidemical Madness,* addressed to the College of Physicians, was one of a number that had satirized this doctrine of "the moderns," whose belief in "these invisible Agents," it alleged, merely "satisfies their curiosity by confounding all ideas, and increases opinion of faculty members in proportion to their ignorance of our inability to account for the inexorable mysteries of nature."[67] Although John Monro was content to use the language of "the spirits" to describe his patients' emotional states, it is perhaps not surprising that he avoided using the term "animal spirits" itself and that he refused to assign precise physiological meaning to such language.

At the opposite extreme from the downward-spiraling emotional disturbances we have been discussing, also featured in Monro's case book were those who thought themselves well above their actual station in life. People of this sort were pictured as being out of touch with reality and as having diseased imaginations. A vigorous tradition of Augustan satire attacked the folly and madness of the vain and bombastic, those who paraded their delusions of grandeur, and this genre may well have encouraged the closer identification of pride and self-delusion with insanity. Thomas Monro of Magdalen College was certainly apt to joke about the madness of pride when a young man at Oxford: the *Olla Podrida* (1787) he edited with others included, for example, a derivatively Swiftian account of Mr. Afflatus, a "scribbler . . . that was once a man" who, having imbibed the "furor poeticus" from a reading of Sir Richard Blackmore's poetry, "instantly mistook himself for a genius, and communicated his mistake to the public."[68] Monro's account of such deluded hubris was, at times, positively scornful, as when, in another collection of essays in 1790, he discussed pride as "the cause of deranged intellects": "When this is the case, the readiest mode to protect yourself from disagreeable altercations with a madman, is to give the poor object the wall, and salute him with the profoundest respect, which he returns with a shocking grin of satisfaction."[69]

What then of John Monro? Strongly influenced by classical theories about the origins of mental disorders in the passions, contemporary mad-doctors in general viewed excessive pride as one of the classic forms of madness. They were apt to dismiss claims of being (or of being associated with) eminent persons, and other impressions and expressions of a vainglorious sort, as pure "nonsense" and often saw them as signaling mental unbalance. Specific examples of such views are assuredly, to some extent, available in Monro's case book. There was Dr. Macham, for example, who when visited by Monro "enquired if his Sovereign was well"; and Mr. Ryan, whom Monro found poring over the Bible for things he "wanted to communicate to the King." Alternatively, there was Captain Macdonald, whom Monro described as hearing "a voice telling him he is anointed D[uke] of Gordon & nonsense of such like"—and Monro went on to note in marginalia that he "thinks the people in the street all look . . . at him & know his thoughts by a glance of his eye."[70] There was also the doomsday-prophesying distiller whose delusions included the belief that he had "kill'd a hare which he did not think to be a common hare but was something he knew not what of infinite power."[71] Yet on the whole, despite their prominence in literary and artistic representations of the mad, examples of delusions of pride and grandeur that were explicitly taken as such by the mad-doctor are actually rather few among the one hundred cases Monro details, and he accorded pride little emphasis in his assessments.

THE MACHINE WORKING THE GHOST:
MADNESS MANIFESTED IN THE BODY

Physical signs, by contrast, were given considerable emphasis by Monro, and it is here that one sees the mad-doctor most transparently revealing his particular standpoint and rewriting the narratives with which he was provided. He noted general abnormalities in body temperature or pulse, and determining these must, of course, have demanded a certain degree of hands-on intervention. He recorded, for example, that Mrs. Duncan's "hands & arms were remarkably cool, rather cold" and her pulse was "much agitated," and Mrs. Harris was "in great sweats."[72] However, rather than attending to the obscurities of the body's internal workings, Monro's diagnostic techniques were almost exclusively directed toward exterior physical signs that were observable by the naked eye at some remove: such things as demeanor, weight, and pallor of skin.[73] In this, of course, he was entirely typical of the physicians of his age.[74]

Facial and motor oddities and abnormalities of gait and posture, from winking and grimacing to tottering, were remarked upon in some patients. Of Mr. Griffin, Monro noted that he "winks all the time he is talking," and of Mr. Whitehead he observed that "when I desir'd him to walk into the room, tho seemingly as well able to do it as I was myself; yet he made as if he could scarce support himself, & totter'd every step he took."[75] Captain Macdonald was described in terms that verged upon the disdainful; he was "in constant agitation bowing his head towards his feet, & had every absurd ridiculous appearance of a mad man."[76]

The eyes of patients were regarded as especially telling windows to the diseased mind, with staring, expressionless eyes betraying the Lockean, "insensible" madman with his attention fixed on one object. Indeed, Monro's description of some cases implies a conviction that "true" or emblematic madness, although more rarely encountered than more minor nervous afflictions, consisted essentially in a combined debility, if not a total lack, of affect and of intellectual power, and in insensibility and absence of capacity for rational thought. Mr. Tonkin was observed to have "had the true mad stare with his eyes, that is they seem'd fix'd as if regarding the <u>object they were directed towards</u>, & yet at the same time without sensibility & shewing a vacancy of thought."[77] Most contemporary mad-doctors appear to have shared this belief in the eloquence of the eyes as a diagnostic sign. Indeed, Monro details how in the case of Mrs. Mackenzie, William Battie had also regarded "a particular look in her eyes" as having "express'd distemper in a very strong manner to him."[78] With the increasing sophistication of physiognomy as the century progressed, fueled in particular by the researches of Johann Caspar Lavater (1741–1801), the expression of the eyes and other facial features came to be distinguished by mad-doctors such as Pargeter as particularly telling signs of both madness itself and the approach, or "*pathos animi,*" of the disease. In his *Observations on Maniacal Disorders* (1792), Pargeter claimed never "to have been deceived in my diagnosis" on these grounds.[79] Yet, even in the 1790s, physiognomy remained an uncertain tool of rather limited application in terms of any strict diagnostic science.

Much of the time, Monro's musings on his patients' outward manifestations of disease appear hesitant and vague, perhaps reflective of the elasticity of eighteenth-century medical theories. He was careful to record what he considered to be remarkable in each case, but quite evidently the minds and bodies of his patients were often something of a mystery to him. Monro was obviously influenced by mechanistic approaches that encouraged contemporary physicians to attempt to pinpoint disease more specifically in various bodily sites and in disordered mechanical bodily processes and functions. Yet the vigorous survival of ancient humoral medical models still frequently allowed him to situate derangement in non-localized physiological media and processes, such as the blood, the spirits, and the humors. For example, Captain Prowsett's mental affliction was linked to "his blood [being] totally broke with liquor," and Miss Lovell ascribed her own complaint in part to having eaten some grapes "which chill'd her blood."[80]

Monro's report of his suspicions in Mrs. Cookson's case typifies this diagnostic pliancy and preoccupation with external bodily signs:

> She had some time ago a humour in her nose which was thought to be cancerous, on which account she came to town, but that was not the case it seems however I cannot but suspect her blood to be contaminated for her pulse is rather too quick, her tongue is dry, her flesh too warm, tho neither of these in any great degree. but her hands of a most remarkably pale colour when she squeezes them close wch she is apt to do & by no means such as I have ever before observ'd: a deadly pale with a bluish livid cast in no ways inclining to red, & seems confined to her hands & wrists.[81]

Examination of bodily excretions and secretions was also a vital part of contemporary diagnosis, and Monro paid plenty of attention to these matters in the case book. Incontinence was seen as an especially telling sign of insensibility in the mentally deranged, and constipation or "costiveness" was also assessed negatively, tending to be viewed in quasi-humoral terms as deriving from blockages and loading of fluid and solid parts with heavy, corrupt, and viscous matter. Recovery of control over such functions was closely associated with remission and recovery of mental faculties and rational powers of self-control.

Changes in the smell, color, and consistency of bodily excretions were likewise closely attended to. Sometimes these signs were accorded a more definite diagnostic meaning, as when Monro counted the fact that one woman's "water" was "often turbid & after standing turning milky" as one among "many other hysterical symptoms."[82] As the royal physicians were to do when attending George III at the end of the century,[83] Monro pored repeatedly over the frequency and (more rarely) the quality of his patients' stools. For example, Mrs. Duncan was observed encouragingly to be "not insensible of her stools"; but Bella Tuten was said to "evacuate both way[s] in the room standing," Mrs. Stone was said to have "made water, & parted with her stools in general in the bed without notice," and Mrs. Cookson was said not to "go to stool" at all.[84]

For similar reasons, what patients took into their bodies was also considered of profound import. Dietary abuses and abnormalities figured again and again as symptoms and causes of disease, and recovery of normal appetite was seen as vital to regaining normal physical functions and mental health. It was noted positively of Mrs. Duncan that "she took . . . her nourishmt," and Mrs. Cookson's appetite was deemed "tolerable."[85] Refusing to eat is an especially prominent symptom recorded in the case book. Behavior of this sort is often ascribed to delusions, such as that the food was "poisoned," that a patient was "dying," or that eating would increase a patient's "fever." Alternatively, attitudes toward eating were seen as so unusual and unwarranted in themselves as to be plainly irrational. Mr. Rowley, for instance, was said to be not only "afraid to eat lest he should be poison'd" but "so absent that he would drink hot water if not prevented."[86]

Monro said little in his *Remarks* about diet, which—by contrast with contemporary physicians such as Cheyne—he clearly regarded as a relatively straightforward matter of moderation in all things. On the other hand, Monro was highly skeptical of Battie's belief that gluttony (and idleness) could give rise to madness, and seems considerably less concerned to stress dietary privations. He advised that patients' "meals should be moderate, but they should never be suffered to live too low, especially while they are under a course of physick." The presence of medical dietary guides in his library and comments he made in the case book itself suggest that he gave regular advice on this subject to his patients.[87] Mental conditions were generally associated in contemporary medical texts with depraved appetites: the maniacal tended to be perceived as eating too much (their voracity being one emblem of their loss of humanity, their atavistic link with animality) or as having morbid cravings for peculiar foods or drinks, whereas the melancholic were seen as eating too little. The entries in Monro's case book very much mirror this basic distinction. Mrs. Lambert was observed to have had at times "a most voracious appetite"; contrariwise, Mrs. Manley's "low despairing way" was connected with her "not caring to eat." As for "the dull" Miss Graham, she was found "emaciated to a great degree from having eat very little & that very unwillingly."[88]

This conception of mental problems as deriving quite considerably from willful, or avoidable, self-starvation or, at the opposite extreme, intemperance and irregularity, was apt to render patients all the more blameworthy for their afflictions. The occasionally harsh tone adopted by Monro in his case book toward some patients is again broadly reflected in medical treatises of the time. Speaking of Miss Graham, for example, Monro declared that "she had no other complaint than being costive, whch [sic] proceeded probably from her having starved herself, & being negligent in the performance of all that nature requir'd."[89]

Then, too, alongside disturbances of appetite, disruptions of sleep patterns were also regularly reported. The centrality of abnormal sleep patterns to the mad-doctor's evaluations of mental disturbance, and their actual importance as disruptive influences on the family, is emphasized by the fact that they are mentioned in about 20 percent of the cases in the case book. For example, Mrs. Holford was recorded as having "slept very little" and Mr. Moore and Mr. Sergison "little or none"; Mr. Whitby "cannot sleep"; likewise, Mr. Molyneux suffered from "want of sleep," Mrs. Cookson "does not sleep well," Mrs. Winter "sleeps but indifferently," Miss Compton "sleeps but little till towards morning," and others, such as Mr. Fitzgerald, actively refused to sleep despite attempts by their friends (and the mad-doctor) to persuade them to do so.[90] Often, Monro recorded more explicitly what was keeping his patients up at night: in the cases of a servant girl and Mrs. Harris, it was "wicked" or "bad & blasphemous thoughts"; Miss Greaves was sleepless as a result of being "plagued" by similarly "bad" and sinful thoughts, alongside fearful visions of "knives, bits of string. &c."[91] Other cases were detailed whose depressive illnesses took the form of loss of energy and motivation for life's duties, often manifested in wanting to sleep too much, as with Mrs. Holman, who was "very happy while she is sleeping has no dreams to disturb her, but as soon as she wakes she is thoroughly unhappy. she does not care to rise, & when she is persuaded, she does not know how to employ herself."[92]

Sleep, speech, and eating disorders were, for some patients, actually (or virtually) the only symptoms of derangement reported in the case book, as in the case of one eighteen-year-old woman of whom Monro noted merely that she "sleeps uneasy some times not at all is much flurried & at times will talk inconsistently."[93] Likewise, Mrs. Hobbes, apart from being "in a low despairing way," was simply said to take "very little nourishment" and to be difficult to get any words out of beyond the expression of a desire "to get up and take a walk."[94] Here, as elsewhere, Monro is far more concerned to describe the form of the symptoms and to delineate the kinds of disturbances experienced by his patients than to attend in detail to their content.[95]

It would be wrong to treat the case book as if it were intended to be a comprehensive record of patients' every symptom or a complete documentation of the variegated nature of Monro's consultations. Often Monro was merely jotting down and summarizing his observations and conclusions about cases, rather than precisely mapping the processes by which he had reached them. Yet, despite and because of their somewhat elliptical nature, his notations are highly suggestive of the particular preoccupations of this mad-doctor, of what he felt was significant or insignificant about a case, and of the often very circumscribed nature of his inquiries into his patients' circumstances.

The style of Monro's consultations lends very limited support to arguments by historians such as Nicolson that tactile examination was more crucial to eighteenth-century doctors than previous historiography has held.[96] Although it might be argued that mad-doctoring was somewhat inevitably disposed to look to external signs, being primarily concerned with patients' behavior and mental states, most physicians were still preoccupied with the corporeal basis of the distemper. It seems significant, therefore, that Monro makes no mention at all of percussion, palpation, or any other methods of diagnosis that required manual examination. Signs played an important part in the diagnostic process, but for the most part Monro employed only those that were discoverable without close or continuous contact with the body—the pulse and the temperature of the skin, but not much more. Notably, when testifying in the Ferrers case in 1760, Monro had dismissed the pulse as an unreliable sign when diagnosing lunacy, putting the onus instead on "the irregularity of" behavior: "the pulse discovers nothing in general."[97]

CHAPTER 6

Religion, Madness, and the Case Book

ENTHUSIASM, FANATICISM, AND FRENZY: DIVIDING INSANITY FROM INSPIRATION

A Tory in his political sympathies and an Anglican in his religious observances, a man who in his youth had flirted with Jacobitism and who came from a family tainted by Jacobitism, John Monro was unlikely to have had much sympathy with "enthusiastic" forms of Protestant belief. And in his suspicion of the religiously transported and obsessed, he was at one with much of polite society in this period. As we shall suggest below, the Hanoverian elite was deeply mistrustful of unorthodox religious belief, whose potential for making mischief and subverting the social order marked it as a dangerous form of heterodoxy. To be sure, Methodists and other evangelicals secured a few prominent supporters among the aristocracy, but for many more of the "better sort," these preachers were in the business of propagating superstition, misery, and despair. The satires of Swift, Pope, and Hogarth, and of hack dramatists such as Samuel Foote, lampooned the movement's leaders—George Whitefield and John Wesley—as pious frauds and hypocrites and portrayed their followers as the credulous and naïve, whose misplaced enthusiasms smacked of irrationality if not outright madness. The notion that certain forms of religious belief and observance might provoke insanity or even constitute marks of it was, moreover, more than a conceit of the satirist: "methodical madness" was considered by a variety of medical authorities to be a real and not rare phenomenon, and many claimed that mentally frail folk were being driven out of their wits by melodramatic representations of hellfire and damnation. An obvious question, therefore, is to what extent such concerns surfaced in John Monro's practice and in his case book.

The most famous religious "enthusiast" with whom Monro came

into contact was Alexander "the Corrector" Cruden, whose obsessive indexing of every crevice and cranny of the Bible to create a *Concordance* that remains in print to this day was matched by an equally obsessive pursuit of a succession of inappropriate potential marital partners (which on at least two occasions led to confinement in madhouses) and by an irrepressible conviction that he was divinely appointed to reform the morals of his licentious fellow Londoners. John, like James Monro before him (and to the discomfiture of both of them), found himself drawn into Cruden's circle and charged with supervising his confinement and treatment. What Cruden regarded as a divine calling Monro plainly viewed as signs of madness. Yet one must confess uncertainty about the extent to which it was Cruden's religious convictions (peculiar and even pathological as Monro may have found them), rather than other aspects of his behavior, that dictated the decision to lock the strange Scotsman away.

If the conclusions that can be drawn even from Monro's extensive involvement with Alexander Cruden's religious extremism and obsessions remain somewhat ambiguous,[1] one might hope that his case book would shed a little further light on the doctor's views on religion and madness. There is, however, no mention here of Methodism and little reference to other sectarian beliefs. If Monro shared orthodox Anglicans' prejudices toward Methodism and other forms of so-called religious enthusiasm, few indications are given in the course of his case records that he had similar qualms about the only sectarian denomination he does remark on, Quakerism.

Monro is very matter-of-fact in the comments he makes about the two Quaker patients he attended in 1766, and one assumes that his aid would not have been summoned if their families had considered him unsympathetic to their religion. Monro does not explicitly associate the problems of either patient with their particular sectarian beliefs. Only physiological details were recorded in connection with Miss Lovell's complaints, although Monro seems to have regarded some of these as rather fantastic. Nothing was mentioned of Miss Cutter beyond self-harm and a rapid recovery.[2] One is not sure quite what to make of his response in these cases, however, for it may simply reflect the reality that the comparison between Quakers and Methodists is unhelpful in this context. After all, although "methodical madness" was a volatile new ingredient in the denominational melting pot, Quakerism, removed in time from its turbulent beginnings, had entered a somewhat quietist phase by the mid-eighteenth century and had lost much of its earlier

overtones of disruption and social threat. Still, it has to be said that elsewhere in the case book are scant signs of any particular antipathy
toward religious nonconformity influencing or clouding Monro's clinical
judgment.

The evidence, to be sure, is susceptible to more than one interpretation. Monro remarks, for example, that one of his patients, a Captain
Knackstone, was "when well of an enthusiastic turn in religion."[3] He
makes no explicit connection between the man's "enthusiasm" and his
mental affliction, so one might take this as negative evidence. Alternatively, however, one might argue that Monro would not have
thought the fact worthy of comment if he did not consider it of possible significance in explaining the patient's symptomatology and the etiology of his disease. Similar conclusions may be drawn from Monro's
record of the weaver Mr. Ryan, whom the doctor attended at Miles's
madhouse and described as "fond of reading the bible, where he told
me he found some things which he wanted to communicate to the
King." Such an entry may well suggest that the mad-doctor was prone
to seeing those who took the application of biblical messages too far as
likely to be insane, although Ryan was also "very talkative &
flighty."[4]

Historians such as Michael MacDonald, who rather sensationally
depict the eighteenth century as something of a "disaster" for the insane,
nevertheless have argued convincingly that the benefits of spiritual
physic and individual claims to spiritual inspiration were not only held
in a more dubious light after the Restoration, but were more commonly
dismissed as signs of irrationality, if not full-blown madness.[5] Religious
zeal had decidedly negative associations for the English ruling classes,
who had witnessed, not so long before, the consequences of letting
enthusiastic religion loose upon the land—the Ranters and the
Levellers, the Muggletonians and the Diggers, the Fifth Monarchy Men
and all those other sectarians who threatened to turn the world upside
down—and they exhibited a positive aversion to the pious emotionalism
of the radical Protestant sects.[6] Preferring "rational" forms of religion
and fearing the subversive potential of claims to possess divine inspiration, the Anglican-sympathizing elite had come to equate evangelical
fanaticism with "delusion, obsession, madness."[7] To be sure, some came
out in defense of revelation against the putative sufficiency of reason and
Anglican doctrinal and social conformity.[8] Others, however, inveighed
against the folly, if not madness, of such views. From their perspective,
enthusiasm itself was "nothing but the effect of mere madness, and

arose from the stronger impulses of a warm brain,"[9] and Methodism was one of the prime producers of candidates for the madhouse.[10] At the seemingly opposite end of the religious spectrum from these Protestant sects, Anglican and nationalistic disdain for the "foreign" doctrines and practices of Catholicism and popery strongly identified veneration of the saints, exorcism, and transubstantiation with idolatry, diabolism, possession, superstition, and irrationality.

Monro and the families of many of his patients certainly seem to have regarded those who talked loudly of religion and manifested eschatological delusions (particularly if they also had diabolic visions) as deranged. A Mrs. Edge, for instance, was recorded to have been "calling out & making a noise in a seeming religious way" and to have "talk'd of seeing the Devil," and Mr. Tonkin was observed to be "much afraid of the Devil."[11] The mental afflictions of other patients were routinely associated with their preoccupations with the religious realm, especially for those who spoke about such matters disconnectedly, repetitiously, or with excessive passion, and for those who implied or identified the existence of supernatural powers in the doctor himself and in others around them. Mrs. Duncan, for example, was said to have "wander'd very much in her discourse, calling me her Saviour, & repeating, I know my redeemer liveth."[12]

Monro was far from alone among contemporary specialists in adopting a suspicious attitude toward the religious visions and agonizing of his patients. Writing in the 1780s, William Perfect, for example, opined that if insanity was on the increase, this

> owes much . . . to the absurd tenets and ill-founded notions of an epidemic enthusiasm, whose type is absurd and gloomy notions of God and religion derived from vulgar prejudices, which excites the attention of the weak understandings to points of religion, which they contemplate without comprehending, to the entire subversion of their rational faculties.[13]

Perfect went so far as to prescribe total isolation from spiritual media and conversation of any kind for some of his melancholy patients. In the case of one woman who "talked of religion in a confused, timorous, and mistaken manner," Perfect described how

> all books of religious tendency, I caused to be removed from her sight; forbade her the use of the testament, which she had been suffered to have continually in her possession, and ordered the servant not to answer any interrogations she might propose upon pious matters, or even to speak to her thereon.[14]

The "dangerous state of fanaticism" of another such woman meant that:

religious objects had so far gained the ascendant of her mind, as to impel her to words and actions of the most maniacal kind, and she had imbibed a fixed belief in the manifestation and interference of the deity in her behalf, although her conduct was ever so reproachable or criminal. . . .

Perfect's treatment amounted to an utter disregard for and negation of her religious experience: he banned "her religious sectaries" from visiting her and permitted no one "to pay the least attention to her extatic [sic] reveries."[15]

THE RATIONAL BOUNDS OF RELIGIOUS SENSIBILITIES: BLASPHEMY AND FEAR, DESPERATION AND INSPIRATION

A number of prominent contemporary physicians and Anglican divines had devoted considerable time to providing natural and mechanical explanations for putatively diabolical phenomena, publishing reinterpretations suggesting that the witches and the demoniacs of the Old and New Testaments were in reality suffering from hysteria and other nervous illnesses.[16] Monro himself was plainly an avid consumer of this sort of literature, his library including many of its leading examples.[17] Elite opinion in general in the eighteenth century stigmatized folklore, superstitions, and beliefs in the unseen and diabolic as irrational, if not mad. Superstition became something of an Enlightenment shibboleth, typified by Smollett's description of the theater manager Mr. Vandall as having a head "not naturally clear, disordered with superstition" and laboring under "the terrors of hell fire."[18] The seventeenth-century philosophy of Rosicrucianism, which posited the reality of a vibrant spirit world of fairies and ghosts and other unseen forces, although popular in some quarters during the century that followed, was held up to ridicule by many leading Enlightenment thinkers and Augustan satirists.[19]

Monro himself was not reluctant to offer (or substantiate) secularized, physiological accounts of his patients' supernatural experiences. Mrs. Hooper's opinion that she was "bewitch'd by her mother in law" was passed over as one of a number of false beliefs or fancies, Monro according greater significance to the fact that her own mother was "disorder'd" at the time.[20] Monro was equally convinced that the sensations of one young lad, who had "fancied the Devil had been talking to him," were explicable in naturalistic terms: in the first place by reference to the "epileptic fit" that his patient had suffered, according to "the account I received of him"; and secondarily by lack of sleep and other unspecified "irregularity" in his habits.[21] Similarly, Monro's explanation for the condition of Mr. Darby, whom he found "in frights attended with violent tremors & convulsive twitchings, & much afraid of the Devil," was that his trouble "is generally brought on by drinking" and "soon gives way to evacuation."[22]

Not merely excessive religiosity but opposite behaviors such as profanity, impiety, and blasphemous words and thoughts were often reported by contemporaries and regarded by eighteenth-century maddoctors as signs and symptoms of mental disturbance, betraying a loss of rational control and restraint. To have "roared like a mad bull, danced, cursed, blasphemed," or to have behaved in some similar fashion, was repeatedly represented and understood in a wide range of contemporary literature as the quintessence of "a frantick bedlamite."[23] At other times, blasphemous tendencies were associated less with mania than with a quasi-Burtonian[24] religious melancholy, with unhappiness, loss of religion and faith in God, atheism, religious despair, despondency, depression, and suicidal inclinations. For example, Mrs. Harris was recorded in Monro's case book to be "in a low melancholy way, troubled with bad & blasphemous thoughts which kept her from sleeping & made her very uneasy & unhappy."[25]

In this and other cases, Monro provides a register of symptoms of depression that might be recognized by psychiatrists today and that shows concern for both the physical and emotional consequences of such symptoms. It would be inappropriate, of course, to assess his medical acumen in accordance with modern clinical standards. Yet, in his own contemporary terms, Monro seems to have been prone to interpret such melancholy spiritual thoughts as not merely unhealthy but unjustified imaginings. He indicates on occasion, and generally seems disposed to consider, that his patients had not really been wicked, or so wicked as they believed. As always, Monro seems to have been less concerned with the nature or content of such thoughts and feelings than with the physiological disturbances and hereditary predisposition that he commonly suspected, found, or attempted to demonstrate were the primary underlying and causative factors.

Miss Jefferies, for example, was noted to be "very low, imagines herself to have been very wicked, & her distemper to have been brought on by her own imprudence & has attempted, & talks very deliberately of putting an end to her life." Monro's response was to point to evidence that her illness was a matter of heredity: "her brother was either an Idiot or a lunatic & died under confinement."[26]

Even more evidently, in recording that Mrs. Cookson was "troubled with blasphemous thoughts, & imagines herself . . . to have been very wicked," Monro was most interested in the observable and verifiable physical facts that she was sleepless and constipated ("does not sleep well, nor does she go to stool"), despite a "tolerable" appetite, and that she had been suffering from "a humour in her nose." Moreover, he emphasized her rapid pulse, dry tongue, higher than normal temperature, and "remarkably" or "deadly pale" hands, "with a bluish livid cast no ways inclining to red, & seems confined to her hands & wrists," such as he had never before observed, all of which led him to "suspect" that her blood was "contaminated."[27] (Descriptive terms such as "blasphemous," although often applied to notions of personal wickedness and potentially sinful impulses toward self-harm, might also be rather nonspecific in meaning or provide the moral loading for putatively unbecoming or indecent sexual propensities.)

In making such observations, Monro was plainly centering and displaying the craft of the physician in the way that made him and most other conventional mad-doctors most comfortable: in the identification of bodily imbalances, more than in the evaluation or diagnosis of problems of a metaphysical order. Physicians such as Monro tended to subsume problems of moral or religious worth, self-loathing, self-abuse and self-destruction, and other peculiarities of feeling, fancy, and ideas beneath those of the body. In doing so, they were simultaneously medicalizing, rationalizing, and subordinating the metaphysical, and secularizing the sensibilities of sinfulness. Studies by MacDonald and Murphy have shown that, although still theoretically conceived of as a mortal sin and a statutory crime, suicide was itself being secularized and medicalized in this period, and gradually being emptied of its eschatological associations.[28] Monro's case book provides further evidence that self-destructive impulses, attempts, and acts tended to be seen as quintessentially irrational and as signs of underlying mental disease.

Still, one should be careful not to exaggerate the mad-doctor's inclination to secularize and physiologize his patients' complaints. The wickedness and mental deviations of many patients were reported without any (or much) reference to physical pathology. Monro's observations in Miss Compton's case were (apart from her sleeplessness) exclusively confined to the emotional and metaphysical plane. Miss Compton

> has fancied for some time past that she has been more than ordinarily wicked, & that she is malicious & tells lies & thinks ill of others, she hears voices, & will some times return answers, falls into violent passions, & then

dissolves into tears, sleeps but little 'till towards morning, & is at times conscious that she is not well & seems sensible what her complaint is.[29]

Likewise, Mrs. Bromfield "is very bad. thinks herself too wicked to live & many such desponding notions," and Miss Greaves, attended by Monro on "the 3rd or 4th relapse . . . imagines nothing she does is right, & that she is thus plagued for the sins she has been [i.e., done?]. has bad thoughts Sleeps but little & is afraid of seeing knives, bits of string. &c."[30]

Religious manifestations and sacred subjects in general figure prominently in Monro's reporting of patients' delusions. However, this was perhaps more a reflection of the intensely religious way in which many ordinary lay folk understood and articulated distress, guilt, and discomfort than it was a matter of any construction, medical or otherwise, of the nature of mental disease. Irrespective of Monro's evaluation of such cases, the frequency with which his patients referred their psychosomatic experiences to the supernatural confirms what historians from MacDonald to Harrison have said about the tenacious survival of beliefs in hellfire and damnation, diabolic power, and the spirit world among the laity well into the late eighteenth century and beyond.[31]

It may be significant that Monro's case book has very little to say on the matter of divine inspiration, though such issues do surface on rare occasions. Mrs. Trecothick, for example, was quite evidently viewed as deranged because she "has been for some time fancying that her husband intercepts blessings design'd [for] her by Providence, & fancies that she sees God & Jesus Christ in visions. . . ." Monro (and presumably her husband) seems to have dismissed such notions as "fancy." Nevertheless, we can see that the patient herself was far from confident about this interpretation, alternating between perceiving these visions "sometimes as the effect of a deluded imagination, at other times beleives [sic] all real." (It is tempting to wonder whether Mrs. Trecothick may have been jealous or resentful of the busy and successful city career of her alderman husband, but such psychological conjectures must remain purely speculative given the limitations of the surviving evidence.)[32]

The case of the Huntingdon clergyman Mr. Stanfield, meanwhile, may have reminded Monro somewhat of Alexander Cruden. Here, too, the patient sought to involve the mad-doctor in his religious agonizing, mistaking Monro for a divine messenger and falling down on his knees. However, Stanfield's state of mind took more of a depressive than an elated turn: "he told me he knew very well I was a superior being, & come to inflict eternal punishment upon him, went down on his knees, to beg I would respite him for a short space, tho he knew it must come at last. . . ."[33]

More broadly, it seems likely that contemporary stigmatizing and secularizing of the visionary as "deluded" encouraged tension between those still inclined to see such folk as engaged in spiritual strivings and those disposed, on the contrary, to assign them to the sick role and dismiss their religious transports as a conclusive sign that they were mentally troubled. To be sure, claims to be subject to visions and supernatural inspiration had long been liable to the accusation of folly and madness. Now, however, such interpretations were becoming routine in some quarters.

Monro does not seem as single-minded as some of his contemporaries in this respect. Rather than seeing religious torments and troubles as necessarily irrational, he appears at times to strive to distinguish between justified feelings of sinfulness and exaggerated, unspecific, or unfounded feelings of a superficially similar sort. Mr. Jones, for example, came to Monro "very much confus'd & frighted he said he had seen a print he beleiv'd of the devil as he came along. he talk'd in a strange manner of not having done his duty to God tho' he could not accuse himself of any actual sin."[34]

The matter-of-factness with which Monro frequently reports such beliefs implies a degree of nonjudgmental professional detachment. Nonetheless, he was thoroughly primed as to the potential irrationality in his patients' convictions of personal wickedness. As with their claims to peculiar sanctity, worth, or wealth, he was far from slow to expose their religious foibles. His agile summation of the case of a servant maid who came to see him provided him with an occasion to generalize on this matter and offers us an eloquent illustration:

> . . . her case a low melancholy, fancying she had not been righteous enough tho' like most others in the same way, she could lay nothing positive to her charge, but wicked thoughts which hinder'd her from sleeping, & kept in hurries & at some times put her quite into agonies.

Yet, to establish how irrational the depressed feelings he encountered were, he found himself forced to assess not only their extremity and vehemence, but also how far they exceeded their apparent immediate causes. For example, Monro observed Mr. Aspridge to be "low from circumstances wch [sic] tho' not so bad as to make him reasonably despair had yet confused his understanding."[35] Defining the reasonableness of despair was thus not simply a matter for independent assessment by the mad-doctor, but required attention to the entire history of the case as supplied by the patient's family and friends, and to how well the patient could account for his or her feelings and actions. Thus, to an extent, Monro and his medical colleagues could not ignore lay narratives of mental distress and were obliged to engage in detailed discourse with patients and to embark on close inquiry into patients' histories and symptoms.

Patients who could not explain or adequately articulate the causes of their depression to the mad-doctor were especially likely to be declared mentally unsound, and inconsistencies, contradictions, and confusions in their narratives served only to confirm the diagnosis. Thus, Mr. Hamilton's affliction was designated by the patient himself as "an excessive depression of spirits without reason, thus far he himself allow'd & told very freely." Nevertheless, the fact that he "denied any thought of hurting himself, which however I find he has more than once attempted, & has likewise at times been very outragious," persuaded Monro that the patient was more ill than he was wont to recognize.[36]

Monro was not unsympathetic to the mental torments and agonies his patients put themselves through, but once he had revealed them as unreasonable to his own satisfaction, there is scant indication that he ever felt it worthwhile actually to engage with, contest, or further plumb the meaning and the content of patients' thought-worlds. This stance would seem to provide further support for Allan Ingram's assertion that rational disengagement was at the heart of most medical and educated writing about madness in eighteenth-century England.[37] Patients who bothered Monro with long narratives of their circumstances, however faithfully reported, were often heard with rather deaf ears. Mr. Ramsay, for instance, an Edmonton butcher whom Monro saw at Miles's madhouse, was described somewhat derisively as "a long story teller," having recounted to Monro "how he beat & abused several people, particularly one woman, his barber who had shav'd him for 30 years & several others of his old acquaintance us'd him ill & had a spite against him for no reason."[38]

In recording patients' statements and the conversations he had with them in an apparently almost verbatim way, Monro appears to have felt that their accounts more or less spoke for themselves and were manifestly irrational. In this respect, he resembled subsequent Bethlem practitioners, such as the apothecary John Haslam, who were prepared to address the language of their patients as scarcely more than illustrations of madness, self-evidently the mere symptoms of disordered brains.[39] Other than their role in the diagnostic process, the patients' words were of scant interest, amounting to little more than the epiphenomenal manifestations of their madness.

CHAPTER 7

Treating Patients and Getting Paid

PREFERRING MANAGEMENT TO MEDICINE

Monro devotes considerably more space in the case book to discussing patients' symptoms and histories than he does to recording treatments. This adds further weight to the view generally taken of all the Monros: namely, that they had very little interest in therapeutics or experimentation and remained steadfastly conservative in their espousal of the standard evacuative and antiphlogistic remedies—bleeding, purging, and vomiting—that were the current orthodoxy.[1] When purging and vomiting are referred to in the case book, these are more frequently spontaneous, or disease-prompted, motions in the patient's own body. Monro notes their existence for their diagnostic significance—to imply, for example, some vitiation of the blood or of other parts of the patient's physiological system. If one may judge by what is recorded in the case book, it appears that Monro gave his patients very little medicinal treatment at all.

It is quite possible, of course, that Monro may not have considered that the case book was an appropriate place to go into much detail about treatments. By contrast, we know that he was prepared to discuss treatment in some detail in his *Remarks*. Those medical treatments that are mentioned in the case book are mostly orthodox contemporary therapies for mental and nervous disorders, confirming the general impression that Monro would rarely be caught recommending adventurous or "quackish" alternatives. In other respects, too, what the case book teaches us of his practice seems to correspond quite closely with the approach he had recommended in his *Remarks*. Monro mentions bleeding just once, in the case of Mrs. Edge, noting its good, if temporary, effects ("continued very peaceable till towards evening when she began to be again very furious").[2] Unspecified evacuation is also referred to once (Monro elsewhere used the term to encompass both vomits and purges), when Mr. Darby's delusions are said to soon give way to this form of treatment.[3] Monro does note down a number of instances of patients taking medicines, some of which he had clearly prescribed, but precisely what drugs he had ordered, and in what dosages, is not recorded. Likewise, evidence (as introduced earlier in this volume) showing that Monro advised patients on their diets is often only tantalizing, as the case book provides us with few details about the substance of such advice. As a general rule for Monro, as for many other contemporary practitioners, the maintenance and restoration of health, mental or physical, had more to do with dietetics, and with preserving or restoring normal bodily functions and routines, than with anything else. As he observed with respect to Alderman Richard Peers, what was most important was having a "good appetite," taking "proper exercise," and being "regular and temperate."[4] In his *Remarks,* Monro had made similar recommendations about "moderate diet," "using exercise," "breaking all ill habits," and obliging patients "to observe regularity in their hours."[5]

The frequency of sleep deprivation and disorder among his patients meant that Monro's ministrations were often directed at simply procuring sleep for them—although this desirable objective might be achievable through practical advice as much as via opiates or other medicinal preparations (the use of which is never actually recorded in the case book). For example, Monro advised Mr. Bevan, whose "complaints had always attacked him" at midnight, when the moon was full and "when he was asleep," to try sleeping "in an easy chair & in an erect posture" instead of in bed, which "he did for two nights & had no return."[6] Sleeplessness was often attributed to nothing more than irregularity in habits, such as staying out late and carousing, so that the mad-doctor often simply advised getting back to more regular patterns of living. In the case of one young lad with delusions about the devil, for example, Monro recorded how "a hearty sleep made a great alteration in a night or two."[7]

In his public *Remarks,* of course, Monro had insisted that medical treatment was far less important than management in dealing with cases of insanity,[8] and the slight attention given to medical prescriptions and interventions in the case book should be read with this point of view firmly in mind. Specialists such as Monro seem to have adopted a strikingly noninterventionist, hands-off consultative approach to their richer patients. However, this pattern of clinical practice cannot easily be interpreted as revealing an empathizing and sympathetic approach to the moneyed mentally troubled. On the contrary, the cursory, elliptical, and sometimes dismissive way in which Monro often wrote up these cases strongly suggests that a certain aloofness, if not negligence and complacency, was constitutive of the very ethos and praxis of mad-doctoring at this time.

Despite this whiff of arrogance, Monro was far from being generally or uniformly either highly critical or blatantly disregarding of the opinions of his patients and their families about the nature of their afflictions. He was frequently reliant on his clients, after all, for the histories of each case, as well as for the implementation of his prescriptions, to say nothing of getting paid! What does emerge at times in the case book is the way in which the mad-doctor's interventions had to be, on occasion, negotiated with the individual patient or the patient's family. Although some patients who declined to be treated, to eat, or to be restrained were forced to comply, others were persuaded to do so. Mrs. Edge, for example, is said to have "submitted to be blooded," while Sir Francis Chester "very readily submitted" to his physician's advice (but not to that of his family), and a few of Monro's patients even summoned him themselves.[9] Many other patients, however, refused to speak to Monro, while some declined to let him examine parts of their body, from their tongues to their faces.[10] All too often, such responses and tactics served only to confirm a patient's irrationality and provided further justification for confining them and ignoring their wishes.

More generally, it has to be said that overt evidence of patients effectually negotiating their treatment is rarely evident in the case book. It is distinctly less common than one might expect if Monro had considered it a priority to gain his patients' confidence or to involve the family very centrally in effecting a cure. In his *Remarks* of 1758, Monro had emphasized talking to his clients "with authority," making them "accustomed to obey," fostering "a kind of reverence" in them for the mad-doctor's knowledge of their complaints, and gaining "an ascendant [i.e., ascendancy] over them," rather than gaining their confidence. It was the family, rather more than the patient, who were required to "put . . . much confidence in the physician."[11] This suggests that (apart from the physician himself) it was the family, and not the patient, who were (and were regarded as) the prime arbiters in determining treatment—a reflection, presumably, of the fact that it was they who had most frequently summoned the mad-doctor in the first place, and it was they who continued to pay for his services. On the other hand, the importance of the distinctive craft of the mad-doctor and the object of winning the patient over through persuasive means were also highlighted in Monro's brand of practice. This is implied by his concurrent concern that patients, as well as being dealt with authoritatively, "should be used with the greatest tenderness and affection" and that "great art should be made use of" to correct their bad habits. Even more explicitly, he was able, on occasion, to recognize the need to "endeavour in every instance to gain their good opinion" and even to see the role of the honorable and humane mad-doctor as one requiring him to "act as much like a friend as a physician."[12]

As a first principle in his *Remarks,* Monro had observed the importance, in effecting a cure, of confining the nervous patient, and his preference was to do so away from the influence of family and friends and at some remove from the familiar, but morbid, associations of home. As might be expected, confinement does indeed figure prominently as a strategy in Monro's case book. Yet, even so, it is employed in only a minority of cases. Most patients received no more than a consultative visit and the odd piece of advice or prescription. Monro's case book thus adds further ballast to the arguments of historians critical of the Foucauldian concept of a "Great Confinement" in the eighteenth century.[13]

Although provision for the mentally afflicted in public hospitals, private madhouses, and workhouses certainly expanded in this period, it remained very limited. More often than not, whatever the preference of the mad-doctor, patients were treated and cared for in their own domiciles. Occasionally, as the case book confirms, a home confinement might be recommended as the first recourse, but such a tactic depended heavily on gaining the cooperation of the family. Family members might be keen to avoid the stigma of extra-domestic confinement, given its considerable costs and risks; but, conversely, they might reasonably object to having to cope with a deranged member under their own roof.

Monro's case book reveals a mad-doctor who—perhaps because he was so established and secure in his clientele—was not as thoroughly at the service of his patrons as some accounts of eighteenth-century doctoring would have it.[14] Monro was prepared to contradict the viewpoint of the family and actually to withdraw from the case if a family persisted in a course of action at odds with his advice and assessment of the patient's best interests. For example, the case book records Monro washing his hands of one patient, a linen draper, Mr. Fitzgerald, after he had failed to persuade the family to try confinement at home.[15] The family insisted instead on sending Fitzgerald to Miles's madhouse, where "he behaved himself so well for 3 days" that Monro "would have nothing further to do with his confinement," and then the patient returned home. In the aftermath of the 1763 Madhouses Enquiry, where Monro had heard and given evidence substantiating the frequent occurrence of false confinement, here is a case where the doctor may well have been exerting rather more caution than had been customary before the inquiry.

In addition, the limited space available in contemporary madhouses and public hospitals, and many families' prejudices against such confinements, probably made Monro more reliant on domiciliary-based treatment than he would have preferred to be. As Mr. Fitzgerald's case indicates, he was by no means opposed to home confinements, especially in milder cases of mental distress. Yet, although mild courses of physic and small changes in regimen might be recommended for merely nervous cases, in more serious or acute cases of madness, particularly where poorer patients were concerned, Monro (like other mad-doctors) was more than willing to resort to strong-arm and highly interventionist tactics. In this sense, strictness in confinement was often matched by equal vigor in dosing. Although in his *Remarks* Monro had cautioned practitioners "not to be too hasty in . . . evacuations, nor to carry them beyond the strength and constitution of the patient," there were unquestionably some doctors who displayed rather more serious scruples and hesitation on this front.[16] There were others, furthermore, such as the physician and Bethlem governor Nicholas Robinson, a dedicated Newtonian mechanist, who prescribed particularly strong doses of evacuative medicines. These practitioners accused their medical brethren of cruelly letting down their patients and allowing their diseases to become grave through excessive caution in treatment.[17] The term "heroic medicine"[18] seems particularly apt when applied to certain kinds of mad-doctoring.

Traditional early modern therapeutics for the insane, as espoused by a range of specialists from Willis to Mead, had conceived of the patient as perverse, atavistic, and insensible, or dulled in sensibilities, and had long stressed the need for harsh measures to tame the will, correct the depraved appetites, and restore the corrupted physiology of the maniac. The case book partially reflects this perspective on the mentally disordered. Monro, for example, referred to some self-starving and otherwise uncooperative patients in loaded or censorious terms such as "obstinate" or "sulky."[19] Casual references to the force-feeding and force-dosing of patients indicate a relatively common recourse to coercive and bullying tactics to overcome the resistance of patients who refused to eat or take their medicines. Mr. Aspridge was said to have "grown much worse not caring to eat, & refusing both that and physic unless forced to take them," and Mrs. Alcock was observed to "willingly not eat any thing if we would permit it."[20]

There is limited evidence, however, of Monro recommending such forcible methods independently or against the wishes of patients' families. Both Monro and the families themselves appear to have been prepared to allow self-starvation to persist for considerable lengths of time before countenancing sterner methods. His comment, for example, that Mrs. Alcock "has by this means [i.e., unwillingness to eat] lived extremely low for some time past" is indicative of a degree of tolerance for behavior of this sort before compulsion was resorted to. Here, Monro's recorded practice agrees with the position he puts forward in his *Remarks*, where he endorses compulsion where eating and taking medicine were concerned, but only in cases where he deemed the life or health of the patient to be seriously at risk. Although, as mentioned above, Monro spoke of the importance of gaining ascendancy over patients and commanding them in some cases, he also underlined the need for them to be "soothed into compliance" and to never to "deceive them in any thing" nor to persuade them "by frightening them," but to talk to them "kindly."[21]

Similarly, whereas earlier historiography depicted mechanical restraint and beatings or lashing as relatively staple fare for the insane in this period, Monro's case book suggests that such methods were more the exception than the rule, at least for the moneyed classes and their dependents whose treatment is recorded here. No mention is made of any patient being beaten, except as an instance of ill-usage, and Monro had expressly outlawed such means in his *Remarks*.[22] On the other hand, Monro is never found in the case book actively appealing for kindness on the part of relatives or keepers in the treatment of mental cases, and rarely appears to have intervened to prevent or mitigate any harsh usage of his patients. Furthermore, for a few of the more extremely maniacal patients, Monro certainly seems to have thought some measure of restraint necessary, and in individual cases the form in which this was administered appears to have been quite severe.

When Monro "first saw" Mrs. Dibsdale, for example, she was "raving & held down in her bed by 4 or 5 people, talking nonsense [i.e., the patient, not her attendants!]."[23] Monro was concerned about this woman not because he perceived the methods being used to restrain her as excessively violent or severe, but because he "thought [her] in danger from the violence of her distemper." Similarly, Mrs. Manley's "hands

were obliged to be confin'd" because she was "picking & scratching herself to such a degree," and the "exceeding mad" Mr. Mitchell was
"obliged to be tied down in his bed."[24] There is, it should be pointed out,
only one apparent instance of Monro actually prescribing any form of
restraint in this case book. In this case, that of the aforementioned Mr.
Fitzgerald, Monro had "desired" the family "to send for proper persons
to secure him." It was not until the following day, however, that the family took steps to ensure that Fitzgerald was "secured" (and, even here,
"secured" might possibly have connoted something milder than
mechanical restraint). Despite acknowledging Fitzgerald as "disorder'd"
and "very much flurried," Monro nevertheless regarded him as "one of
those people who are seemingly cured by a very little restraint which they
bear with the utmost reluctance," and recommended a less extreme
form than the family ultimately decided on. Monro plainly considered
the family to have overreacted. He had been "sent for in a violent hurry,
to come & see this man . . . who was described as a very dangerous &
desperate man & one who would in all probability murder some of his
family if care was not taken to hinder him."[25]

Mechanical restraint was probably considered less advisable or necessary in Monro's private practice than in the public arena of Bethlem. In
the latter context, low staff-to-patient ratios made it seem less dispens-
able, and the putatively degraded social origins and circumstances of
patients made it seem more appropriate. Just as mechanical restraint is
seldom overtly prescribed in his case book, Monro's *Remarks* makes
even fewer references to the subject. On the other hand, this seems less
to reflect any serious reservations about its use than it does an acceptance
of its uncontroversial and common or garden nature. One passing
observation Monro makes in the latter work certainly seems to imply a
pretty realistic acceptance of the necessity for forcible methods such as
restraint for more serious cases of madness and of the futility of providing such patients with the normal creature comforts. Here he commented on certain patients he had seen

> where . . . every other quality, which distinguishes a man from a brute, seems
> totally obliterated . . . for months (I may say years) together, lying in straw;
> not suffering even a rag of cloaths on [them] . . . and without showing any
> signs of discontent . . . maintain an inviolable silence against all the applica-
> tions of persuasion and force. . . .[26]

Comments such as these underline how much coercive methods and the
poor conditions in contemporary institutions for the insane were justi-

fied and sustained by the association of madness with insensibility and animality.

If Monro rarely recommended mechanical restraint in his private practice, he equally rarely appears to have objected to its usage when others deemed it necessary. Of course restraint was written in more broadly to the very nature of confinement, and it was often more general constraints on patients' liberties and movements, as well as the fact that they were deprived of the normal things available to the free person, that aroused most objection from patients. The ready availability of such techniques in the madhouse, coupled with the rough-hewn, often ill-motivated and poorly educated nature of madhouse-keepers, may have rendered Monro's explicit order or sanction simply redundant. Mechanical restraint was almost certainly a more regular recourse in these establishments than the physician himself would have either realized or liked.

There were, besides, other means of restraint, deprivation, and coercion beyond strait waistcoats and chains. These included secluding patients and locking them in rooms, providing them with vigilant guards, isolating them from families and friends, or depriving them of pen and ink—tactics that feature prominently in the protest literature on confinement and that also appear occasionally in the case book. While in Duffield's madhouse, for example, the suicidal Mrs. Brooke was attended by, "besides her own maid," "a maid of Mr Duffield's [who] constantly lies in the room." In addition, "the doors of the bedchamber are lock'd & the keys taken out of them."[27]

There was obviously a genuine demand for such treatment from contemporary families and (if less so) even from patients themselves; and there was a growing consensus in contemporary society, and not just among mad-doctors and madhouse proprietors, that such methods were sometimes necessary to control and cure the mentally affected. Far from every confinement was a source of intense conflict, or met with resistance from patients. The nature and quality of medical treatment of the deranged (including the extent of restraint it involved) were negotiable and variable factors. Class, social connections, and other considerations of status, occupation, and the domiciliary environment played a vital role in such negotiations. In general, for example, Monro thought it "doubtless unreasonable to appoint a servant to be his master's governor," thinking it much more preferable and easier for the insane to be "managed by strangers over whom they have no authority."[28] Despite such preferences, nevertheless, many of his better-heeled patients, including Mrs. Brooke herself, were permitted to be attended by their own personal servants while under confinement. As a result, they were capable of enjoying considerable freedoms, if not, at times, of directing operations. To be sure, these servants could also be extra organs of confinement, employed by families to maintain a firmer control of their wayward members. Yet they might additionally ease the pains of that confinement, granting those they waited upon some of the attention they were accustomed to receive at home, while helping the family to secure greater discretion over patients and to ensure better means of access to patients while they were in the madhouse.

The case book offers some hints and impressions of other types of treatments patients sought, beyond and before the specialized attendance offered by a mad-doctor. Many of these interventions, as one might suspect, appear to have received little sanction from Monro, who often recorded the failure of alternative treatment options. Although bathing was one of the most popular and fashionable recourses for the sick, the nervous, and the hypochondriacal in this period, it is conspicuous by its relative absence from the cases Monro details. Only Mrs. Holman was recorded to have been at the baths (at Ramsgate), and one other patient went to a mechanical bath in Chelsea (see below). Furthermore, neither embarked on bathing at Monro's explicit recommendation, and both failed to procure "any relief" from this operation.[29]

One must seriously question how far treatments such as bathing should be seen as the province of irregular medicine. They were prescribed, after all, by Monro himself at Bethlem and by a host of other elite physicians. However, a number of distinctly less orthodox treatments were available to patients, and only a few of these are mentioned in Monro's case book. Some of these less orthodox treatments were evidently embarked upon by patients more or less independently. They can be seen as examples of the frequency of self-dosing and the manifold opportunities for enterprise that historians have traced as part and parcel of an expanding and relatively non-policed medical marketplace in this period. However determined certain members and aspiring members of the medical elite were to identify and outlaw quackery and to persuade patients to seek only regular medical advice, the boundaries between regular and irregular medicine were far from clear at this time. Irregular practitioners plied their trade, if not with impunity, then with considerable freedom from prosecution, signaling, perhaps, the limited faith many evidently possessed in the orthodox doctor's armamentarium.[30]

As Porter has shown,[31] eclecticism abounded in the way patients shopped around for health, and Monro's patients appear to have constituted no exception to this general pattern. One of those who consulted Monro had tried the bathing machine of the Italian doctor Bartholomew di Dominiceti (flourished 1735–82). Another relied on Robert James's famous Fever Powders, a powerful mixture of antimony and mercury. Both treatments were extremely popular in this period and were used by thousands of contemporaries for all kinds of bodily as well as nervous disorders. A myriad of sufferers flocked to Dominiceti's hydropathic establishments in Bristol, in Westminster, and finally in Cheyne Walk, Chelsea, seeking relief from a variety of real and imaginary ailments in the opulent and soothing surroundings the entrepreneurial Venetian exile strove to provide. For those more inclined to trust in the pharmacopoeia, James's Powders were especially likely to be prescribed in mental cases because of the frequency with which feverish symptoms were involved, or confused, with mental derangement—and this despite contemporary efforts to distinguish the delirium of madness from that produced by a fever.[32]

Treatments of this sort, nonetheless, had strong overtones of quackery. Both Dominiceti and James had patented their "inventions" and had stirred up considerable tensions with, and criticism from, rival practitioners in the course of purveying them. Some of the orthodox spoke of severe doubts about the efficacy of either treatment, even as others showed themselves keen to copy or pirate them.[33] Elite physicians were especially critical of the dubious, if not dishonest, way James and those who represented him had patented, and become the monopolistic vendors of, the medicine. They were equally censorious of the inconsistencies and mystery surrounding the preparation and ingredients of the powder. William Battie was particularly hostile toward James and his powders on these grounds, resolving, according to the JP George Hardinge, "never to meet him at a consultation" and "never" to prescribe the drug—even going so far as to have "declined attendance in fevers upon this account."[34] On the other hand, although Battie confessed to detesting James, whom he regarded as "a good for nothing dog," he nevertheless felt duty bound to support James's candidature when (as acting president) he examined him at the College of Physicians, quarreling "with half the College" in the process.[35]

Monro was somewhat less extreme in his attitude toward James and toward such "empirick" remedies. He records rather matter-of-factly that in neither of his cases were such treatments successful: in the one case, Dominiceti's "operation" had been essayed "without effect"; in the other patient's complaint, James's Powders were likewise "tried in vain."[36] Yet, whereas Dominiceti's treatment had been embarked upon by the patient before Monro had been called in, the doctor himself evidently had agreed to prescribe James's powders, perhaps because the compound had already been credited with curing the patient in a previous trial.

A number of contemporary physicians who expressed severe reservations in print about James's Powders simultaneously complained that they had been obliged, against their better judgment, to consent to the prescription. Their patients, asserting their own authority over the treatment of their maladies, simply insisted on it, and the professionals lacked the wherewithal to resist. The most notorious and controversial instance of this sort of thing was the case of Dr. Goldsmith, who—as some orthodox practitioners delighted to point out—died after insisting that his apothecary give him the drug.[37]

Apart from the nature of the methods of management and treatment Monro employed, the mad-doctor, at least for a time, regularly recorded the outcomes of each case. Unfortunately, however, his resolve (or else his knowledge of the outcomes in each case) seems to have deserted him as 1766 progressed, and after about June, Monro seldom recorded any outcome whatsoever. This fact alone obviously limits the extent to which the case book can be used by medical historians or historically minded clinicians for any sort of survey of the epidemiology of madness or of Monro's clinical effectiveness. Nevertheless, a number of other conclusions may still be ventured.

What seems immediately apparent from a simple arithmetic of those forty-three outcomes Monro does record is the large numbers of his patients who died, but also the quite significant number who recovered. Monro records the death of fourteen patients in total (seven men and seven women), the recovery of about twenty (a ratio of ten to ten), and the unaltered state of about six (a ratio of two to four). A fair number of Monro's patients appear to have died "suddenly," and rather unexpectedly. Notably, in his *Remarks* Monro had contradicted the opinion, not infrequently encountered in other medical works, "that the generality of madmen are long lived," dismissing it as just another "vulgar error."[38] One should also emphasize how rarely in the case book Monro employed terms such as "cured" or "uncured/incurable," preferring to designate patients "well," "better," "recovered," and (occasionally) "perfectly/very well," or alternatively "not well," "no better," "rather better, but not well," and even "as bad as she came." These findings suggest a number of things. First, they indicate how candid Monro's private record was about outcomes. Second, they suggest that Monro was often called in at a late stage in cases with somewhat advanced physiological pathology, which itself may have been at the root of many of the mental problems he confronted. Rarely was cause of death recorded, though a number of patients evidently died in the midst of convulsive fits, and occasionally causes of death such as diarrhea and pox (or venereal disease) are mentioned. Finally, an examination of the outcomes of Monro's cases appears to underline how limited the efficacy of his ministrations was.

On the other hand, even when patients are recorded as cured or dead, how much this had to do with Monro's interventions is almost invariably impossible to say. Rarely is enough information provided to be sure of cause or effect in these cases, and many may have entered remission or decline almost irrespective of what Monro did or advised. Although the relapse of cases was sometimes mentioned, and one patient (Mr. Moore) sadly committed suicide six months after being declared well by Monro,[39] this seems more revealing of the mad-doctor's fastidiousness in keeping tabs on his patients than it tells us about either how actively harmful or how beneficial Monro's attentions were. If, then, Monro's case book might not permit a clinician to systematically or reliably hazard some sort of assessment of the clinical effectiveness of the mad-doctor's ministrations, it might at least, one hopes, provide the historian with some clues as to what tended to be recognized as full or partial recovery from a mental affliction in this period. The return of patients such as Mr. Bevan to Monro three or four times after relapses, and the occasional tantalizing references to patients as "well [but] drinks," suggests the rather circumscribed nature of these recoveries and implies that some were plainly more recovered than others. This was a circumstance that Monro was fully prepared to acknowledge in his *Remarks:* "It [madness] is a complaint the most liable to a relapse even where the cause is known."[40] Yet here, too, on the whole, the case book record is often disappointingly brief and elliptical. Monro generally seems to have recorded the outcome in his cases as something of an afterthought in the marginalia or at the end of a case entry, rarely detailing how that outcome came about, or (in the case of a recovery) was assessed.

PROFESSIONAL TIES, REFERRAL NETWORKS, AND REMUNERATION

The references to colleagues in the case book tell us a little about the medical circles Monro moved in, the general practitioners he consulted with, and the physicians from whom he received referrals. We have dis-

cussed elsewhere his sometimes fraught relations with his chief metropolitan rival, William Battie.[41] Other sources tell us that, during the
1780s, he fraternized with the physicians William (1711–91) and David
Pitcairn (1749–1809) and Bethlem's surgeon, Richard Crowther (d.
1815), at the Paul's Head dining club, which met every Tuesday.[42] We
learn from the case book, not surprisingly, that his circle also included
old Oxford classmates such as Swithin Adee (1705–86) and other
Leiden-trained London hospital physicians such as Thomas Reeve
(1700–80), M.D. 1732, who had been president of the Royal College of
Physicians (1754–63) and physician to St. Thomas's (1740–60), and
who had employed madness as a metaphor in his work of 1744 attacking tar water as a quack remedy.[43] Reeve had thrice selected Monro as
one of the censors at the college, so it seems safe to assume that the two
physicians were on relatively good terms.[44] Encountering a patient recommended to Monro by a Dr. Southwell, we can conclude that this was
most probably Thomas Southwell, who had practiced for a time in Paris
and had just written a book on its medical faculty. Yet references of this
sort are on the whole tantalizingly brief and reveal little about the precise
nature of Monro's professional connections and associations.

Turning to the question of remuneration, it is not clear what Monro
charged for a consultation, although his standard fee was probably comparable with the guinea per visit charged by his colleague and friend
Richard Mead.[45] According to Alexander Cruden, who was perhaps
Monro's best-known and certainly his most clamorous patient, Monro's
fee was only half this amount for visits to patients at Inskip's Chelsea
madhouse, but Cruden also alleged that he additionally "makes near 20
guineas a week from the 2 academies of Mr Duffield [Inskip's uncle]."[46]
More than likely, Monro was prepared to occasionally reduce or even
forgo his fees for poorer clients, a relatively common practice among
eighteenth-century medical men. Yet even for routine functions, such as
regularly certifying the insanity of patients at madhouses such as
Bethnal Green, Monro, like his father before him, must have been making considerable profits. Cruden alleged that in the case of a French sol-
dier confined for years at Bethnal Green's White (or pauper) House in the
1730s, James Monro "signed an Attestation of his being a Lunatick
twice a year, that his friends might receive his pay" and received "a
Guinea for each Subscription."[47] We know that James often charged the
wealthy astronomical sums in return for his attentions, and one may be
sure that John was not slow to follow his example in this as in other matters. Joseph Girdler, for example, the Sergeant-at-law of the Inner

Temple,[48] had complained bitterly to Lord Fermanagh in 1733 of "Dr [James] Monroe alone demanding for himself and assistants about £130 though we think not a Quarter could be due or deserved." Girdler protested that, at this rate, his father's entire estate was "ready to be Devour'd by the mad Doctors."[49]

Cruden was certainly convinced that John was every bit as avaricious and grasping as his father, suggesting that both were more preoccupied with their pockets than with their patients.[50] Having been treated by both father and son, he might seem to have been peculiarly qualified to know about their fees and motives. However, a word of caution is in order: Cruden was also peculiarly liable to exaggerate all the various injustices he conceived himself to be enduring at the hands of the Monros and was perhaps not as knowledgeable as he claimed to be about what his family was paying the Monros. There is, moreover, a generic quality to these allegations of mad-doctors' avariciousness (an image often and widely applied to elite medical practitioners more broadly). In the late seventeenth century, James Carkesse—whose narrative, composed while confined in Finsbury madhouse and in Bethlem, was told in poetic form in the book *Lucid Intervalla* (1679)—had accused the former Bethlem physician Thomas Allen of haunting both houses "like a louse."[51] Even more vividly, perhaps, the stereotype was captured a few decades later in William Belcher's portrait of the mad-doctor as "a smiling hyena":

> This animal is a non-descript of a mixed species. Form obtuse—body black—head gray—teeth and prowess on the decline—visage smiling, especially at the sight of shining metal of which its paws are extremely retentive—heart supposed to be of a tough kind of leather. N.B. He doth ravish the rich when he getteth him into his den.[52]

Perhaps such images convey the weight of cumulative evidence. However, one must question whether another accounting is also possible: that all mad-doctors were bound to be somehow culturally constructed in this fashion by their disaffected patients; that all or most were tarred with the same brush, and all or most were inevitably pictured as profiteering from human misery.

Some may have found the Monros' fees exorbitant, but they were far from exceptional compared with those of other elite metropolitan physicians. Battie, for example, demanded outstanding fees of almost £750 from the estate of one of his private patients—an extraordinary sum.[53] We may confidently assume that John's wealthiest patients, such as Lord

Orford, Lady Dorothy Child, and Sir Charles Hanbury (or their families), paid him handsomely for his attentions.

One measure of the profits John made from all this business is his wealth at his death. Besides valuable leasehold property in Clerkenwell and Clapton (including his own madhouse, Brooke House, which had opened in 1759, and the Clerkenwell madhouse previously operated by William Battie), he left family legacies totaling £12,500, and his will instructed his sons to pay his widow an annuity of £500 from part of the proceeds of what was clearly an extremely lucrative business. The lucre presumably went a long way toward compensating for the stain on one's status that mad-doctoring inevitably brought in its train.

CHAPTER 8

Being Mad in Eighteenth-Century England

Patients' Views of Their Own Illnesses

When patients consulted physicians about all forms of illness in Monro's time, the clinical encounter bore little relationship to its modern counterpart. Conversation was as a matter of routine quite central to the diagnostic process, for patients' own accounts of the history of their disorders were considered of far more moment than anything that might be learned from the doctor's direct examination of the body before him. Those bringing their complaints to the physician expected and were expected to not just talk at length of their pains and their suffering, but to offer up vital information concerning their habits and regimen and any unusual events or behaviors that might have helped to precipitate their disorder. Within the broadly shared universe of discourse about disease that existed in the Augustan age, they often went further and even offered their self-diagnosis of what was wrong. Physicians had learned to expect these features of the encounter with their patients; more than that, they were deeply dependent upon them for the performance of their most central tasks. Part of what distinguished the skillful physician was, in fact, his ability to draw out his patient and, by subtle and sophisticated inquiry and inspired reading between the lines of what he was told, to elicit and interpret the evidence considered crucial to rendering an informed judgment about the nature of the malady in front of him. By contrast, physical scrutiny of the body was, as Porter has noted, "extremely perfunctory [and] conducted primarily by the eye—not by touch . . . [indeed,] the reliance upon 'taking the history' was a positive mark of the confidence felt by the expert clinician in his personal ability to assess a case solely from the patient's story and gross visible signs."[1] Seen in this broader context, it is unsurprising that Monro's case book records that more than a handful of those who consulted him ventured their own opinions about the nature and sources of their troubles.

To be sure, the mad-doctor was not disposed to place much credence

in the stories he heard from what were, for him, evidently suspect
sources. Yet even when Monro discounted his patients' etiological
ascriptions and prognostic musings, the fact that he recorded them presents us with some idea of the wide range of moral, supernatural, and
mental processes (beyond or alongside the bodily realm) that contemporary lay people saw at work in reproducing and determining their
afflictions. Unintentionally and inadvertently, therefore, the case book
provides us with not inconsiderable insight into the actual experience of
being mentally afflicted in eighteenth-century England and into the ways
in which sufferers themselves articulated and understood their mental
problems. Many nineteenth-century asylum case records tell us more
about the judgments of medical men than they do about the behavior,
views, and inner worlds of patients. By contrast, Monro's occasionally
detailed and often imperceptibly edited reporting (despite and because of
its aptness to conceal the precise nature of the doctor's own opinion of
the various cases and mental manifestations he was witnessing) allows
the historian considerable purchase on the speech patterns and thinking
processes of those deemed to be deranged.

Monro's notes provide us with telling portraits not only of patients
who were existentially suffering, but of those who were causing anxiety
and misery to their close relations and of the reasons they were doing so.
Occasionally, as we have seen already, we are afforded insights into how
patients negotiated their sick roles and the various strategies they used in
an attempt to get their way with relatives and the mad-doctor. Although
many were severely incapacitated and disabled by their illnesses, some
seem to have used (or derived some solace from) their mental afflictions—as a means of gaining attention in the family, for example, or of
achieving exemption from ordinary social and economic demands and
obligations.

Not all owned their troubles and conditions as illnesses or as medical
problems, of course, some positing alternative explanations and believ-
ing that they were ill used. Although a few, as detailed earlier, harbored
high hopes for Monro's interventions, seeing him as an agent of God or
of their restoration and liberation, others refused to cooperate with the
mad-doctor and occasionally even accused their caretakers of being
their persecutors, of being agents of diabolic forces, or of simply being
mad themselves.

Quite apart from these issues, Monro's case book also allows us, in
the many glimpses it provides of the language of patients and their families, to appreciate the significant extent to which madness (like illness

more generally)[2] was a shared discourse in this period. Far from being an entirely medical matter, the etiology, diagnosis, and appropriate management of the insane appears to have been, in many ways, something for both the mad-doctor and his patrons and clients to discuss. Thus, what Monro records is substantially and repeatedly derived from the accounts of each history he has received, often directly from the family and from the individual patient.

Of course, whatever glimpses Monro offers us of the lives of his patients and their families, the version he gives us of his patients' own thought-worlds is inevitably selective, biased, and distorted, and using the evidence he provides us, we can only partially and cautiously reconstruct their genuine viewpoints and experiences. Yet Monro's detached recording style often succeeds in providing a surprisingly vivid portrait of particular cases. Take, for example, the case of Mr. Walker, which Monro summarized as follows:

> ... told me the Devil left him this morning about 4' o'clock that he had been with him 7 years, was brown & of a size between a mouse & a rat. He inform'd me that there were but 2 starrs left, the rest having fallen that he had seen them, that the world was near it's end, that the mist we had some days since was not a common mist, but the smoke of the fewell which was to destroy the world taking fire, but that it was put out, & it might now last some 2 or 3 years longer. that about 27 years ago he saw the fall of mankind, in company with a very good man, who keeps the Sun Tavern in Westminster, that many years ago he kill'd a hare which he did not think to be a common hare but was something he knew not what of infinite power.[3]

The case book allows us to see how patients themselves explained their own ailments. Several patients proffered supernatural explanations of their state, evidently concluding that their melancholy, low spirits, and the like were punishments for their sins.[4] Still others spoke of being bewitched by a mother-in-law[5] or being possessed by the devil.[6] Psychological and emotional traumas, such as "a sudden fright"[7] or "a sudden fit of Passion"[8] or even the stress of "being upon the Jury at the old Bailey the last Sessions,"[9] were invoked alongside a variety of environmental, circumstantial, and somatic events that were more or less directly connected to the loss of mental equilibrium, and it is quite apparent that it was accepted in this period that some predisposing psychological event could be crucial in the generation of nervous disorders and outright madness.

Additionally, the case book often presents us with a moving and poignant account of the physical pain and unease, torments and suffering,

mental confusion, and disorientation that were very much the experiential core of many mental afflictions. In this sense, many of Monro's
patients' symptoms might be relatively easily recognized, not only by the
psychiatrists of today, but also by any ordinary lay person with some personal experience of mental illness. Mrs. Hampson's anxieties about an
unwanted but persistent suitor "brought her in to such a state of mind as
made her very uneasy, she did not sleep well was violently flurried at
times, subject to a palpitation of the heart, waked in hurries, had strange
& extravagant ideas crowding in upon her. . . ."[10] The delusions some
patients suffered under were plainly terrifying to them, and to their nearest and dearest. Physical and mental discomforts often combined,
patients expressing all kinds of worries about bodily ills and bizarre bodily processes that caused them pain or distress. Some reported fears about
their bodies being transformed into material objects, which may well
have been closely related to intense unease about their own immortal
souls, or more generally to an existential crisis that eroded the boundaries
between mind, body, and the external world (cases that resonate with the
findings of modern scholars such as Gill Speak on the "glass delusion" in
early modern Europe).[11] Others, such as Mr. Whitehead, Miss Gilchrist,
Mrs. Alcock, and Mrs. Fludger, were convinced that they or their friends
were in various states of bodily and mortal peril, were physically sick, in
prison, in danger of being murdered, "dying," or actually dead—those
more drawn to religious conceptions of their conditions in life being
more prone to express such impressions in terms of various states of
grace.[12] Although, for example, the clergyman Mr. Stanfield was "sure he
had not died," he nonetheless "look'd upon himself as in a state of separation among the dead, & waiting for the reward of his evil doings."[13]

   The worries of most patients were rather more prosaically bound to
the earthly sphere of household and family or to socioeconomic concerns, but were not necessarily any less acute for that. Women's terrors
often gravitated toward threats to their families and to their domestic
security and welfare, as when Mrs. Wilson was frightened she would
murder her spouse or child, or when Mrs. Winter was recorded as saying "she knows her children were then actually tied to a stake to be worried by the beasts in Smithfield."[14] In quite a number of these cases, the
social context seems more amenable to historical interpretation, but in
others there may be more for modern clinicians in terms of the post-diag-
nosis or epidemiology of historical patient populations. For example,
paranoia might be surmised to be the dominant affective condition
behind many such patients' impressions, as with the lawyer Dr.

Macham, who, the night before Monro saw him, "got up & threw up the sash calling out murder" and who latterly "hoped he should be punish'd; & was full of ideas of treason & such like & people having designs against his life, that the doors of the room, & the wainscoat flapp'd about, that his sister was murder'd."[15] Quite a number of patients are recorded as ascribing their mental states to the problems of poverty and impoverishment, or as having extreme (and often, evidently, unfounded) fears and anxieties about loss of material goods and well-being—as in the previously mentioned case of Mrs. van Hock, who was beside herself with thoughts that "she shd come to poverty & to absolute want, that she shd not have a bed to lie on . . . [and] that she had not another gown or any Linnen or other necessaries to send for. . . ."[16] Although some received disapprobation and blame from their families or from Monro for their disorders, a few (especially those suffering from depression and low spirits) blamed themselves, as when Miss Jefferies declared "her distemper to have been brought on by her own imprudence."[17] Not infrequently, one encounters fears of material loss combined with kindred fears of a more metaphysical nature: fears of loss of status or becoming a social outcast; or, more threatening still, fears of loss of one's identity or very soul and of being plunged into eternal damnation. Such anxieties often accompanied self-punishing and self-destructive impulses, self-harm, suicidal thoughts and acts, and other symptoms of depression, as in the case of Mrs. Manley, whose talking "of being ruin'd" seems to have been but one constituent of a profound depressive illness that threatened to entirely consume her sense of self.[18]

Men often worried similarly about their business affairs, though they were perhaps more prone to blame others and outside circumstances than themselves, as when Mr. Fitzgerald complained that "his wife & the servants neglected his business. That he loved to see every one in his house diligent as the bee & hungry to work."[19] Others, such as Mr. Rosat, a Swiss-born merchant who was trading in Turkey (from whence he had recently returned when Monro saw him), looked to more stereotypical prejudices to explain their misfortunes: Rosat declared that he had become especially "low spirited" after "he met with great losses, by putting too much confidence in a Jew who deceiv'd him."[20]

The eighteenth century witnessed a major growth in overseas trade and the paraphernalia of a capitalist currency-led economy—the full-fledged emergence of credit exchange, banking, and investment in fluctuating stocks and shares.[21] Partly as a result, it was characterized by considerable collective and individual bouts of boom and bust, typified by the "bursting" of the South Sea Bubble during the 1720s amid the inevitably shifting vagaries of international (especially Atlantic) trade. Such developments may well have increased levels of anxiety about material welfare in this period, but what seems certain is that some of the genuine and ascribed victims of this flux of credit and commerce found their way into Monro's case books.

In some cases, the insanity of another family member is also adverted to in order to explain patients' own mental states. On several occasions, however, when Monro was aware that there was a family history of insanity, patients failed to mention it. Perhaps this hints at a reluctance to acknowledge a hereditary component to their disorder on the family's part, both despite and because this was a connection that Monro was convinced existed. Wherever such evidence surfaced, he was quick "to conclude that it was a family complaint."[22]

SELF-REFERRAL AND
PATIENT/DOCTOR RELATIONS

In an age when contemporaries were generally (and with good reason) skeptical of doctors and available medicines, and few would have believed in a right to health or treatment, it should not surprise us that occasionally patients also appear to have seen the affliction they were under as iatrogenic; that is, medicine itself was to blame for making them nervous and mad. Captain Macdonald, for example, opined that his complaint "has been occasion'd by some medicinal preparations given him 6 months ago"; and an anonymous female patient blamed her emotional upset in substantial part on being "improperly treated by her nurse giving her some spirituous liquor, during her lying in about a year ago."[23] Monro never openly disputed such views and was apparently quite prepared to attribute his patients' afflictions to bad medicine and nursing, although at times he clearly suspected that other somatic causes were to blame.[24] He might also register the failures of rival practitioners, as when Dr. Battie was observed to have treated Miss Jefferies "to little purpose."[25] Yet, notably, he was never overtly critical of any of his professional colleagues in the case book—perhaps indicative of some degree of instinctive restraint when it came to crediting his patients' aspersions against other practitioners. Problems were more likely to be attributed to patients having taken bad advice from quack or unqualified practitioners, or to their own self-dosing, than to be blamed on bad doctoring by any properly educated, orthodox physician.

It was not just his professional rivals, however, who occasionally mistreated their patients, for families also do not always emerge with much credit from the records of the case book. The way in which some patients were brought into confinement, for example, suggests the abusive responses that must have characterized some domestic settings, as when Mrs. Winter was said to have arrived at Miles's madhouse "with a black eye," saying that she "was never mad but is extremely ill us'd & sure her friends do not know of her confinement."[26] In other cases, as we have seen, families fearful of the stigma associated with insanity seem to have procrastinated and fought against consulting a mad-doctor, even when their afflicted relations sought such counsel.[27]

This reminds us, as we have already highlighted, that not all patients had to be compelled to seek medical assistance for their troubled minds. The case book, on the contrary, is replete with examples of those who came to Monro's consulting rooms of their own accord, convinced that their mental turmoil might benefit from his expert assistance. Mr. Bevan, for example, who reported that his symptoms of melancholy and "dejection of spirits" had first come on when he lost his father, and had recurred after he "was afflicted with the dry-belly-ach" in Jamaica two years previously, repeatedly sought Monro's advice about his condition. Bevan, like many of the seventeenth-century folk whose moping and melancholy are recorded in Michael MacDonald's *Mystical Bedlam*, was equally as willing to invoke astrological as psychological or somatic sources of his troubles and had observed a close correlation between his emotional state and the waxing and waning of the moon. (Monro, in fact, was to term his case "the most particular case of Lunacy, in the true sense of the word, I ever remember.") Bevan's final recorded visit to his mad-doctor was prompted by his worry that the approach of the full moon would bring about a recurrence of his symptoms, something he evidently had no qualms in consulting a physician about.[28]

Mrs. Godwin, who previously had been treated with some success by Monro's father, James, for her hysteria, showed up once more, hoping her wide array of physical complaints and psychological troubles would yield to the younger Monro's ministrations.[29] Still another female patient, whose name Monro did not record, came in on her own to discuss the sleep disturbances that often "put [her] in a flutter" and acknowledged she was "very much afraid of losing her senses."[30] AB, a "servant maid came to consult me upon her case a low melancholy," her "wicked thoughts" disturbing her sleep and causing her intense anxiety.[31] These women also had their male counterparts, such as Mr. Alderman

Peers, who "called upon me often with complaints strongly hypochon-driacal," spoke feelingly of waking constantly at four in the morning "in violent hurries and in great horror," and was "much afraid he shall lose his senses."[32] Alternatively, there was Mr. Jones, a grocer, who came in voluntarily to see Monro "very much confus'd and frighted" at having seen "a print he beleiv'd of the devil";[33] or still another anonymous patient, who "came to me to relate his case which was of the low spirited [type,] proceeding, as he said, from having been guilty of Onanism to a great degree when young."[34]

These, of course, were (generally) patients suffering from some of the milder varieties of nervous disorder, rather than those suffering from full-fledged madness. Among the latter, many were so disturbed, so violent, or so withdrawn that their families were the ones who sought outside intervention. Mrs. Stone, for example, "talk'd very insensibly" and never appeared cognizant of her condition, and Mrs. Moreati "has lain about a fortnight, & is extremely mad, incessantly talking nonsensical incoherent stuff."[35] We mentioned earlier another occasion, when Monro arrived to see Mrs. Dibsdale in Horsley, finding her "raving" and "talking nonsense" and being restrained by as many as five people, "& I thought, in danger from the violence of her distemper."[36] Mr. Mitchell was a somewhat similar case, "exceeding mad when I saw him, spitting, sulky, saying nothing tumbling and tossing about, grinning, and obsti-nate refusing to eat, & obliged to be tied down in his bed."[37] As for Mr. Rowley, the eldest son of Sir William Rowley, he had always been "weak & rather wanting in understanding." Having convinced himself that he was "not well cur'd of a clap he contracted 18 months ago," he at length "broke out in so violent a manner that the family were obliged to send him up from Bath immediately." With delusions that those about him were trying to poison him, he had been "very sulky and mischie-vous," mutilating himself and showing signs "of his becoming an Idiot."[38] Patients such as these, or the almost insensible Bella Tuten,[39] scarcely acknowledged the doctor's ministrations, let alone requested his presence. Others, however, including patients who were suicidal, highly disturbed, or delusional, were "very sensible" of being disordered in their wits and appear to have welcomed his interventions.[40]

Not always, though, for a handful of those Monro was called upon to treat vigorously denied that they were insane. Mrs. Fludger, for instance, conceded that "her friends had thought her mad but [insisted they] were mistaken [and] that she had indeed been a little so, but was now very well." (Monro noted dryly that, in his view, Mrs. Fludger remained "violently Mad.")[41] Mrs. Winter, who appeared to him to be equally clearly disturbed, likewise "tells me she is not mad."[42] Mrs. Elder, meanwhile, although disposed to concede that she herself "was not always right," countered that it was her family, friends, servants, and Monro himself who were the truly mad ones, an opinion she persisted in even after being taken into confinement outside of her domicile.

> When I saw her first, she was full of talk & told me all the house her husband the servants & the ladies were all wrong in the head at times, & that she was not always right. Mrs Elder upon being removed into lodgings on Lisson green has still the same fancy that her maid, myself, & the people of the house are all wrong in the head at times.[43]

Her complaints, however, like those of the Restoration poet Nathaniel Lee—who protested, "They said I was mad; and I said they were mad, damn them, they outvoted me"[44]—remained the minority view. One suspects, though, that these patients would probably also have seemed mad to any culturally competent eighteenth-century observer who took the trouble to become acquainted with their peculiar beliefs and behaviors.

With few exceptions, then, Monro's patients either were so disturbed that they were scarcely capable of coherently challenging the legitimacy of his ministrations, or else they actively sought and welcomed his advice and nostrums. Gothic novellas and noisy Alexander Crudens notwithstanding, remarkably few of the customers of this particular corner of the mad-trade spent their time protesting their sanity and the iniquity of their captors. Therapeutically unadventurous Monro may have been, but his were interventions that, more often than not, were eagerly embraced by either the patients' families or the patients themselves, and often by both parties at once. His experience gave him the authority to provide vitally important reassurance to his clientele, for he had seen so very many cases of disturbance, knew what was delusion and imaginary, and could recognize patterns of behavior that were strange, upsetting, and unfamiliar to those who consulted him. The burgeoning fortunes of the mad-trade were, when all was said and done, securely rooted in the demands and desires of its patrons and customers. The mad-doctor might be the butt of satirical commentary, his social standing diminished by the stigma surrounding his speculative trade and its sorry subjects, and his motives and clinical competence routinely questioned and lampooned in pamphlets and the popular press—but when mania and melancholia manifested themselves, increasingly it was his services that were sought, his institutions that were patronized, and his expertise that was implicitly or explicitly acknowledged. Here, after all, resided the essential foundations of the cultural authority of medical practitioners like Monro, the social roots of their economic success, and their intellectual authority over the identification and treatment of the mad.

PART TWO

John Monro's
1766 Case Book

1766.∼

January.∼

8.   Flora an Indian girl, slave

_I   to Mrs Denne, sent to Mr Miles's[1] from

Mr Dudley's Bloomsbury Square;[2] her

well   mistress alledged she had been frighten'd

by the ill usage of some servants in

the house where she had been; however,

as she had been guilty of several

peices of extravagance, & had re:

:fused both Physic[3] & nourishmt, for

fear of being poison'd; they not know:

:ing how to manage her sent her

to Mr Miles's, but as the girl had also:

lately some remains of fever upon

her I think it better to await the

event of that before I sh^d pronounce

her mad. She afterwards proved mad
enough, but got well.
——Mr Aspridge a Taylor in Wild Street

2   low spirited from circumstances w^{ch}

tho' not so bad as to make him rea:

died suddenly
:sonably despair had yet confused

his understanding.—sent to Mr Miles

he is since his coming grown much

worse not caring to eat, & refus:

ing both that & physic unless

forced to take them. on Tuesday Jan:

         man   seeming reluctance
21. this poor ∧ with great ~~unwillingness~~ told us he was pox'd
                                        ∧

he was so, but died the next morning.——

3.   Case from Scotland by Mr Douglas

3   answer'd the 17.th ——

6.   Mr Molyneux[4] in White's yard in

        White:cross Street? tells me, that he

4   was very much flurried at first

died
suddenly   death of
        by the ₍ₐ₎Mrs Whitbread[5] (he was cooper

        to Mr W.) & that going out afterwards

        with one of his children he had

        the misfortune to lose her in the

        streets, that this affair hurried

        him so much that altho' he

        found the child again, he still

        continued to feel the effects

        of this accident, by frequent

        & violent agitations of his

C-3

want of sleep, & a prodigious de:

:pression so far as to meditate mis:

:chief to himself. But I have since

learn'd that he had a son con:

fined at Mr Devic's^6 at Hoxton

& have therefore reason to con:

:clude it a family complaint

& may have seiz'd this poor man

who is in the decline of life & has

as I am inform'd drank hard.

he died suddenly.

6.   Miss Jefferies Welbeck Street a

5   maiden Lady aged 46. has

been afflicted once before in

this way[?]; when she ^{was} attended

by D[r] Battie[7] to little purpose, she
was afterwards cured as her
mother thought by the use of
D[r] James's powder.[8] This has been
tried in vain since the return
of her complaint; she is now
very low, imagines herself to
have been very wicked, & her
distemper to have been brought
on by her own imprudence
& has attempted, & talks very
deliberately of putting an
end to her life. her brother

was either an Idiot or a lunatic

& died under confinement.

7.   Mr Hamilton. a Scotch gentle:

6

better

:man some miles north of

Edinburgh turn'd of 60. sent

to Mr Clarke's by his friend

Mr Dempster, very sensible

of his complaint, viz an ex:

cessive depression of spirits

without reason, thus far he

himself allow'd & told very

freely, but denied any thought

of hurting himself, which

however I find he has more than

once attempted, & has likewise

at times been very outragious.

this gentleman was continued un:

:der my care, one fortnight only, &

then set out for Scotland with

a man to take care of him.—

8.   Mrs Walker a servant of Mr Goupy

7.

brought
to the
hospital   the painter, whom I call'd upon

(by desire of Dr Southwell)[9] at

Mr Inskip's in little Chelsea,[10] she

was mad enough, but at the

same time seem'd to me to

have many symptoms atten:

ding her complaint that were

paralytic.—

18   Mr [blank] came to me to relate

8   his case which was of the low:

:spirited proceeding, as he said,

from having been guilty of Ona:

:nism[11] to a great degree when

young. he was once before in

this way.—

22.   Sr Francis Chester. I was de:

9.   sir'd to call on him by

died
of a   Sr Geo: Robinson[12] who was
Diarrhoea

one of his relations that

had the care of him, he had

been long disorder'd, was very

weak & grown unruly in some

measure not caring to do any

thing without the advice of

a Physician to which he

very readily submitted.—

24.   Miss Compton Argyle street.

10   I visited this young lady
better
with Dr Adee.[13] she has fancied

for some time past that

she has been more than

ordinarily wicked, & that

she is malicious & tells lies

& thinks ill of others, she

hears voices, & will some times

return answers, falls into vio:

:lent passions, & then dissolves

into tears, sleeps but little 'till

towards morning, & is at times

conscious that she is not well

& seems sensible what her

complaint is.

26. Mrs Stone was some years

11   ago disorder'd in her sen:

died   :ses, from which she recover'd,

one of her daughters,[14] ha:

:ving been in the same way

I think it may fairly be look'd

upon as a family complaint.

She had been deliver'd about

ten days before I saw her,

& every [word missing] had happen'd regu:

:larly & fortunately, nor had
                       about two days
she wander'd at all till,
before
,I saw her. She was ~~by~~ hot

but not to a degree of fever.

talk'd very insensibly &

very much, slept little or

none, made water, & parted

with her stools in general

in the bed without notice.

She continued in this state

till thursday morning, at

which _{time} I found her more cool

than before, but still talking

incessantly & almost insen:

:sibly. at one time in the

following remarkable man:

:ner.—I—can—not—

turn—my—head—on

—that—side.—She sit

up two hours this day but

about nine in the evening

was taken with a fainting &

frequent convulsive twitchings

& continued incessantly tal:

:king & growing weaker till

Saturday morning that

she died.

28.   Miss Hume a young lady

12.   born in the Island of Antigua [last four words

partially deleted]

well.   aged 24. was taken about

a fortnight before I saw

her, nor could the family

give any reasonable acc[t]

of the cause, unless it was

a sudden fright from one

of the servants getting a fall

on the stairs, without any bad

consequence, but if this was

really the case it was not

perceived at the time. She

talk'd extremely incoherent,

so much, that she seldom fi:

:nish'd any sentence she

began, but run into some

idea quite different from

that she sit [i.e., set] out with, laugh'd

& cried at times, but both

without reason. She got well & I
took my leave of her June 6.—

February. ⁓

2.   Mr Bevan Clerk to Messrs

13.   Drake & Long[15] says that
better.

some years ago, he being

at Madrid with his father

had the misfortune to lose

him, that this & some other

accidents ruffled him so

much that he became melan:

:choly, but recover'd from

it; that afterwards he was

in Jamaica, where about 2

years since, he was afflicted

with the dry-belly-ach. that

ever since his recovery from

that complaint he is gene:

:rally afflicted either at the

new moon or the full with

a kind of stupidity & dejection

of spirits which makes [him] quite

unfit for business; that he nei

:ther knows what is said to him

nor how to give proper answers.

he has no bodily complaint,

unless an uneasiness or pain

in his head at the time he

is first seiz'd.—

3.   Mr Walker[16] a distiller in Shoreditch[17]

14.

well   whom I call'd upon this mor:

:ning told me the Devil left

him this morning about 4'

o'clock that he had been with

him 7 years, was brown & of ~~th~~ a

size between a mouse & a rat.

He inform'd me that there were but

2 starrs left, the rest having fallen

that he had seen them; that the

world was near it's end, that the

mist we had some days since was

not a common mist, but the smoke

of the fewell which was to destroy

the world taking fire, but that it

was put out, & it might now

last some 2 or 3 years longer.

that about 27 years ago he saw

the fall of mankind, in compa:

:ny with a very good man, who

keeps the Sun Tavern in West:

:minster, that many years ago

he kill'd a hare which he did

not think to be a common hare

but was something he knew not

what of infinite power

8. Miss Greaves[18] the 3^d or 4th relapse

15

well

a family misfortune, imagines

nothing she does is right, & that

she is thus plagued for the sins

she has been[?]. has bad thoughts

Sleeps but little & is afraid

of seeing knives, bits of string.

&c.

10. Miss Mombray of Stanhope

16. Street Clare Market. has com:

plained more than 3 months

of designs against her, from

what persons or for what reasons

she knows not. sees often a flash

like a flash of lightning. hears

a noise like the ringing of

bells under her windows. &

imagines the people as she

passes along look at her

& laugh at her & take par:

:ticular notice of her.

4   Mr Buckley was brought to

17.   Mr Miles's where he had been

confined once before about

a month, whether his misfor:

:tune proceeded from irregu:

:larity I do not so well know

but I sh[d] imagine it did, as

it disappear'd so suddenly

that he went away very well

in less [than] ten days time.—
& was brought back again in a fortnight.
15. Miss Lovell. a Quaker in Red lion

18.
Street Clerkenwell.[19] talks very sen:
well.

sibly & is able to give a good acc[t].

of herself, but says that being

in the country last October

she first eat some grapes which

chill'd her blood, & afterwards

some mushrooms which poison'd

her, that she broke out in blot:

:ches, & has ever since been ill

with various complaints, her

inside is decay'd, she ~~his~~ in

danger of a dropsy, of losing

her nose & this morning she

told me the upper part of the

palate of her mouth was

prodigiously swell'd but

was now gone down again.

& all these complaints are now

upon her, & make her & her

family uneasy. because she

at first she did not relate all

the symptoms of her complaint

as she ought to have done.

16.   Mr Coltman.[20] a young gentleman

¹⁹   of 20 y^{rs} of age lodging in War:

well   :wick court Holborn; has been

for some time past in a low

depress'd state of mind: he

went this morning to the Grecian

coffee house,[21] where he said some:

:body had affronted him and

us'd him ill, on coming home

to dinner, he order'd the serv^t

to fetch him a bottle of white

Port, this (which usually lasted
him 2 or 3 days) he drank up
at, & soon after his dinner, out
of a large tumbler, & became
soon afterwards both drunk
& mad going out of the room
soon after dinner, & returning
again he imagined some of
the company had been talking
disrespectfully of him. he was
so outragious when I was with
him, that no less than three
chair:men were employ'd to

keep him in bed, whom he attem:

:pted to bite whenever they gave

him an opportunity.—His un:

:cle informed me he had ~~an~~

near relation under my father's

he got very well in 3 weeks.
care.

19.   Mrs Edge[22] at the king's wine cellar

20.   in St James's Park in a very violent

died. manner calling out & making a

noise rather in a seeming religious

way, incessantly talking, & furious

tho not attempting to do mischief

talk'd of seeing the Devil, entire:

:ly inconsistent, was prodigiously

furious ~~after~~ the whole night after

I left her, which continued till ten

o clock the next morning, at w^{ch}

time she grew calm got up, & walk'd

about the room after she had dress'd

herself, submitted to be blooded &

continued very peaceable till to:

wards evening when she began to

be again very furious, & continued

so the whole night, & the next day

doing every thing under her. slept

she died on the monday   very bad.
following.—

20. Bella Tuten. a girl of nine years

21   old & a fine girl of her age was

brought to me she had been from

her birth in the state I saw her

not able to give answer unless

by choice rather than design, upon

my asking her what the fire was

she said green trees, but she spoke

very plain most of her words, &

sometimes came out with a whole

sentence quite consistent as, I

have lost my glove—Molly you _{have} ^

got a new necklace.—but in

the general what she said was

incoherent & without notice,

& by the acc^t given of her she

would ~~do~~ evacuate both way in

the room standing slept well in

general sometimes not at all.

20.   Dr Macham[23] Drs Commons. He was

²²   ill about 4 years ago, & is rather

well.   apt to be delirious whenever

he is feverish. but I cannot [word missing]

his pulse was high, or the heat

extraordinary; the night before

I saw him he got up & threw

up the sash calling out murder

& went [*sic*] I came to him enquired

if his Sovereign was well, & hoped

he should be punish'd; & was

full of ideas of treason & such

like & people having designs

against his life, that the doors

of the room, & the wainscoat

flapp'd about, that his sister

was murder'd & such sort

of imaginations slept little.

26. Mrs Lambert in the old Bailey

23.
died

I attended this lady who is a

Dutch woman, about two years

suddenly

ago, she was then in a high

way, & full of gayety, but got

well in six weeks or thereabouts

She is now, in the opposite

extreme, sits moping all

day long by the fire side

& does not care to stirr or

She had at times a faltring in her
to speak. speech & a most voracious appetite
She was seiz'd with a strong convulsion fit on Tuesday
June 3 & died Apoplectic the next day.

March

2. Mr Bevan who first came to

me the 2d of last month call'd

upon me this morning, & told me ^he^ was

seiz'd with his complaint on wednes:

:day last, the 2^d^ day after the full of the

moon; that it seiz'd him as it gene:

:rally does in bed, that he is better

as soon as he can raise his head.

that he cannot answer, if a per:

:son asks him a question, but laughs

in their face; tho at the same time

he is extremely melancholy & had

even the last time thoughts of

destroying himself, & yet says he

knows of no reason for his me:

:lancholy; in short, he says he feels

as if he was a fool. he had call'd

upon me about a fortnight ago

C-30

& was then perfectly well. I think

his case is the most particular

case of Lunacy, in the true sense

of the word, I ever remember.

he call'd upon me this morning

Sunday. March. 9th. perfectly well.

6.   Mem: Miss Howard wrote to her

[24] brother to desire to speak with

him & to ask him if there

was no conspiracy against her.

9   Mrs Cookson[24] at Mr Duffield's[25]

25.   a Maiden lady about fifty

or turn'd of that age, is

troubled with blasphemous

thoughts, & imagines herself, to

have been very wicked, she does

not sleep well, ~~but in other re~~

nor does she go to stool: but

her appetite tolerable she

had some time ago a hu:

mour in her nose which

was thought to be cance:

:rous, on which account

she came to town, but that

was not the case it seems

however I cannot but sus=

=pect her blood to be contami=

=nated for her pulse is rather

too quick, her tongue is dry,

her flesh too warm, tho nei=

=ther of these in any great

degree. but her hands of a

most remarkably pale co:

:lour when she squeezes them

close wch she is apt to do &

by no means such as I have

ever before observ'd: a deadly

pale with a bluish livid cast

no ways inclining to red, &

seems confined to her hands

& wrists.——

15. Mrs Duncan in Laurence Plane

26.
died.   was pretty quiet when I first

visited her, but at times

wander'd very much in

her discourse, calling me

her Saviour, & repeating, I

know my redeemer liveth &

her hands & arms were re:

:markably cool, rather cold:

they were much the same

the next time I saw her, tho'

she was herself in a most vio:

:lent agitation, & as they told

me had had 2 or 3 convul:

:sion fits; she was at times very

furious, talking incessantly

without consistence & coherence

her pulse likewise much agi=

:tated: but at the same time

she took both her nourishmᵗ

& her medicines, & was not

insensible of her stools.—

her complaint has more

the appearance of frenzy

than madness, & I cannot but

think her life in danger.—
She died April. 3ᵈ.

18.   Mʳˢ Pigot. in North Street Red

27.
well.   Lion Square. this poor Lady

has been in a bad state of

health for some time past

having been much afflicted

with bilious complaints; whe

:ther her head is affected

from weakness, or from any

other cause I will not pre:

          to say
:tend₍ₐ₎, tho from the manner

I should suspect weakness.

while I was in the room she

was apprehensive of people

being in the room with her,

or in the next room with a

design to murder her, they

were blacks, & she was sure

meant to do mischief.

She got very well in 3 weeks.

— Mrs Holford an old woman

28.
went
away as
bad as
she
came

brought to Mr Miles's very

talkative, & at first rather

mischievous slept but

little, & talking without

rhime or reason.

— Miss Anther. at Mr Miles's.

29 talks pretty sensibly, but is

well

rather flighty & too full of

drinks

spirits.

19. Mrs Williams^26 in Carnaby

30.

Street was brought to bed

went to the
Hospital &

got well. about 3 months ago of twins,

& has not been in her senses

from that time, when I saw

her she was in bed between

2 & 3 in the afternoon & to

most of the questions I ask'd

she return'd for answer I

do not know.

14. Mʳˢ Shoreland brought back to
31. Mʳ Miles's where I was first
well.   attended her before she was

married. she has several times

relapsed, & is now very bad

talking & acting very insen

:sibly.—

21. Mʳˢ Mercer brought to Mʳ Miles's
32
well.   in a very low:spirited way,
drinks.
& as I was informed had

attempted to make away

with herself.

23. Mʳ Bevan call'd here very

well.

April.11. Mr Moore. I have attended

this gentleman once before, who

33.

has labour'd under the same

well but

relapsed complaint several times; I ap:

in the

:prehend it may be caused by

month of October

drink, but the times I have

& drown'd

himself. seen him he has been exces:

has

:sively bad, & his distemper

more the appearance of frenzy

than lunacy, he sweats much

is in great agony sleeps

little or none, is continually

raving & talking to such fan:

C-40

tastical beings as his imagina:

tion represents to him. "Come"

"forth ye ministers of death"

"come from behind your intrench

"ments. this he s.[d] he spoke to

the little insects, that were there

crawling about in great num:

bers.—

17.   M[rs] Moreati[27] the wife of an

34.
brought Italian employ'd in designing
to the Hospital
& got
well.   for the King by M[r] Dalton.[28]

She was M[r] D.s maid & mar:

:ried to this man some time

ago she was frighten'd by an

ox, has lain about a fort:

:night, & is extremely mad.

incessantly talking nonsensi:

:cal incoherent stuff.

She got well in the hospital.

27. Mr Bevan call'd upon me last

Sunday & communicated to me

his fears on the approaching

change of the moon wch was to

be at the full about midnight

his complaints

the 24th as ~~it~~ always had attackd

when

him at that time ~~& more~~ he

was asleep & more especially as

he imagin'd from the declining

posture of his head. I advised

to sleep in an easy chair & in

an erect posture. he did so for

two nights & had no return.—

22.   Miss Graham.[29] the sister of a

35.   Scotch merchant residing in
not better.

London. I saw her at M[r] Thutton's/Strutton's [?]

Bethnal green,[30] extremely dull

barely answering yes or no to

such questions as were ask'd

her skin extremely dingy,

emaciated to a great degree

from having eat very little

& that little very unwillingly

She slept tolerably, & had no other

complaint than being costive, w^{ch}

proceeded probably from her ha:

:ving starved herself, & being

negligent in the performance

of all that nature requir'd.

28.   Mr Tonkin[31] a watch engraver

36
brought in Kirby street Hatton garden.
to the Hospital

this poor man from having

run out his substance, & possi:

:bly from his sedentary manner

of life had fallen into a me:

:lancholy which had afflicted

him at times for 2 years. he

had the true mad stare with

his eyes, that is they seem'd

fix'd as if regarding the ob:

:ject <u>they were directed towards,</u>

& yet at the same time without

sensibility & shewing a vacancy

of thought. ^{much afraid of the Devil.}

M[rs] Worth.[32] vid: last year.

May   M[rs] Godwin. her case

37.
well.   rather hysterical than any

way tending to lunacy, but

having rec.[d] benefit from

my father's advice, many

years ago, & one of her sisters

having been unfortunate in that

manner she chose to tell me

her case.

Mrs Harris. from Hendon her

38.

not well

husband some years since a

baker in Turn:stile had re:

:tir'd there. in a low melan:

:choly way, troubled with

bad & blasphemous thoughts

which kept her from sleeping

& made her very uneasy & un

:happy. she had been afflicted

in the same manner about

twenty years ago.

3.   Mrs Theobald call'd on me about

39. her daughter who according

to her account was restless, pas:

:sionate & behaved in a strange

& unusual manner.

9.   Miss Cutter.[33] a quaker. when

40. I first saw her had cut her

well hands in several places, by

striking them thro a sash

window the day before in

a violent hurry, she was very

sensible of her complaint, &

by keeping quiet, got so well

as to return home in 3 weeks.

10.	Capt.ⁿ Robinson.[34] Master of

41.

better

a ship in the Jamaica trade

had been in a low way for

some time before I saw him

fancying himself infected

with the Venereal distemper.

which he imagin'd he had

contracted in his last voyage

to Jamaica where, according to

his own account, he had been

familiar with some infected

person; this, he said, he had

not only ~~gi~~ communicated to

his wife, but so far was he

infatuated, that he had

likewise infected his wife's

mother aged about 90, and

pretended to shew the marks

of it in eruptions upon

her face. the day before

I visited him, he had fairly

hanged himself but was

cut down by the maid.

12.   Mrs Mackenzie.[35] I was directed

42.

not better

by the court of king's bench to

visit this Lady in conjunction

with Dr Battie & report my opi:

:nion of her to the court.

Dr B.s acc.^t of her was as fol:

:lows. that about 7 years ago

he was sent for to visit a

lady in Poland street, who

was at the time he saw her

very mad, that he order'd w^t

he thought proper, & saw her

no more 'till last January

when upon being call'd in

again he found her very

mad, he then advised her

husband to confine her; but

not chusing to take her into

his own house, he recom:

:mended Mr Mackenzie to

Duffield; he went there &

made an agreement with

Mr D. but never sent his

wife there, nor was Dr B. call'd

in afterwards 'till April last,

when he again found her

very mad, with a particular

look in her eyes which ex:

:press'd distemper in a very

strong manner to him; he

advis'd M^r M^{c}kenzie again

to confine her; but having

reason to imagine she had

contracted some acquaintance

who might create difficulties,

he advised him not to send

her to any private Mad: house

but to keep her in his own house

& sent him a nurse accordingly:

& he paid her another visit

himself, & when Mr Mackenzie

complain'd that she made too

much noise for him to bear

her in the house, he advis'd

the sending her to a private

lodging, & recommended one

Day[36] who had just taken

a house at Paddington

for that purpose. Mrs M.—

was carried thither & confined

but in 4 or 5 days was set at

liberty by one Sherratt[37] accom:

:panied by Justice Miller.[38] Both

parties appeall'd to the court of

King's B.[39] & I was in consequence

directed to visit her as above;

but was not able to discover

from the examination she

underwent before us any marks

of Lunacy. 'tho I must own the

examination was such as I

was not thoroughly satisfied

with.

13.   Mr Frazer.⁴⁰ vid: last year's acc.^t

43   rather better, but not well.

14.
      A B. [blank] a servant maid came
44
      to me to consult upon her case

      a low melancholy, fancying

      she had not been righteous

      enough tho' like most others

      in the same way, she could

      lay nothing positive to her

      charge, but wicked thoughts

      which hinder'd her from

      sleeping, & kept in hurries

      & at some times put her

      quite into agonies.—

16.   Mr Whitehead.[41] this gentleman's

45   brother I had formerly attended

       about a month, he is still in

       the same way he then was, as

       I have been informed, as is

       likewise the sister. at that

       time, this gentleman was

       confined at Mr Duffield's,

       under the care of Dr Heberden.[42]

       he had cut off or render'd use:

       :less 3 fingers of his right

       hand. he continued at Mr D.'s

       about a twelvemonth & at

the time of my visit was atten

:ded by a man of Mr D.⁓s. I found

him full of complaints but could

by no means trust to his own

account of himself, with a

countenance of good health

he was dying, nothing would

stay upon his stomach; he

had no appetite, could not

sleep, & was so weak he could

scarce stand, these complaints

the first excepted were without

foundation; the sickness at his

stomach was occasion'd likewise

by his own management of himself,

& sometimes I believe by his endea:

vours; for almost the whole time

I was with him, he was constantly

sighing & moaning to himself;

& when I desir'd him to walk

cross the room, tho seemingly

as well able to do it as I was

myself; yet he made as if

he could scarce support

himself, & totter'd every step

he took.

17. Mr Rowley[43] eldest son to S^r

46. W. Rowley. I visited this gen:

:tleman with Dr Pringle[44]

I am inform'd he was always weak

& rather wanting in understanding

for some time past he has ima:

:gin'd himself not well cur'd of a

clap he contracted 18 months ago.

Mr Hawkins,[45] Dr Pringle[46] & Dr Relhan[47]

have been employ'd to satisfy him

in this point but without success.

About 3 weeks ago he broke out in

so violent a manner that the fa:

:mily were obliged to send him

up from Bath[48] immediately.

He is afraid to eat lest he should

be poison'd, is at times, & that

quite suddenly very sulky & mischie:

:vous, has bit his own lip thro' is ex:

:tremely nasty, & so absent that he

would drink hot water if not pre:

:vented, walk out of the door in:

:stead of the window, & the day

before yesterday the 27th, he suddenly

jump'd up from his seat, & with

the utmost violence thrust his

head thro the sash, very luckily

the violence with which he did

this was so great that he drove

out the glass entirely, & by that

means got no further hurt than a

few scratches on the face, ~~but~~ by

his present appearance I should

be afraid of his becoming an Idiot

but I think it is rather too soon

to pass so heavy a judgement

on him.—

19.   Mr Sergison.^49 a coach maker

47.   at Kensington had been disorder'd

well   about a fortnight before I saw

him. I believe it to be a family

disorder, but they told me it took

                his

its rise from ~~the following~~ acci:

:dentally being upon the Jury

at the old Bailey the last Sessions

he was very mad & furiously so
when I saw him talking very
incoherently & with great vehe:
:mence slept little or none &
sometimes refused both physic
& nourishment.

19.   M[r] Alderman Peers[50] has call'd

49   on me often with complaints
strongly hypochondriacal, but
is much afraid he shall lose
his senses, he constantly wakes
about 4 o'clock in the morning
is in violent hurries & in great

horror, which does not go off till

he gets up, he is then very well, He

has a good appetite & uses pro:

:per exercise, & is regular and

temperate.——he died suddenly

23.   Mr Inge near Tunbridge in

49.   Kent aged 70 & upwards, is

very full of lunatic imaginations

according to the account given

to me, his father was confined

in the Hospital near 40 years

ago.

June.

7.   Mr Whitby tells me that from a

50.   sudden fit of Passion some time

ago he is become very low spirited

cannot sleep & is subject to hurry &

confusion but talks very well & is

able to give an account of himself.

13.   Miss Sutton sister to a Baker

51.   in Wood street whom I attended

the last year in the same way

I doubt not of her lunacy at

times by the acc^{ts} I have rec^d

but when I have attended

her she has had a fever, which

this time made a very serious

part of her complaint but

she however got very well in

a fortnight or less.

74.   Mr Ryan a weaver at Mr

e

gs

iger

was more calm but still very

much disorder'd, slavering &

spitting upon her cloaths. she
died the 5th day after I last saw her.

24.   Mrs Manley.[51] had been for some
54

time in a low despairing way

not caring to eat, picking

& scratching herself to such

a degree that her hands were

obliged to be confin'd, she talk'd

of being ruin'd & having de:

:stroyed herself eternally.

—   Mr Cawthorne[52] was brought
55
up with an intention to be

put into the hospital, but

74.   Mr Ryan a weaver at M^r

52.   Miles, very talkative & flighty,

fond of reading the bible, where

he told me he found some things

which he wanted to communi:

cate to the King.

16.   Mrs Dibsdale in Horsley down

53.   was when I first saw her ra:

:ving & held down in her bed

by 4 or five people, talking

nonsense, & I thought, in danger

from the violence of her dis:

temper, in 4 or 5 days she

was more calm but still very

much disorder'd, slavering &

spitting upon her cloaths. she
died the 5th day after I last saw her.

24.   Mrs Manley.[51] had been for some

54

time in a low despairing way

not caring to eat, picking

& scratching herself to such

a degree that her hands were

obliged to be confin'd, she talk'd

of being ruin'd & having de:

:stroyed herself eternally.

—   Mr Cawthorne[52] was brought

55

up with an intention to be

put into the hospital, but

his friends chose to leave him
for some time at Mr Miles's
he appears quite harmless, &
good:natured is sensible that
he is not right; it is said
by his relations to have been
the consequence of inoculation[53]

— Mr Hudson.[54] at Mr Miles ex:

:tremely mad & raving at
:times, then tolerably quiet
but talking in a manner
that shew'd he was quite
lost, his complaint has the
appearance of frenzy.

24.   Mrs Winter.[55] incessantly talking

57.   something very p[?]
but with coherence was never

mad but is extremely ill:us'd

& sure her friends do not know

of her confinement sleeps

but indifferently. came with

a black eye to Mr Miles's.

Capt. Macdonald. has been

58.   for some months in a low

dispirited way, but when

I came to him, he would

not answer any question I

ask'd he was sitting in his

bed sometimes singing, & some-

times imitating dancing, & ma

:king a strange kind of noise

& in constant agitation bowing

his head towards his feet, &

had every absurd ridiculous

appearance of a mad man.

26.   M^{rs}— with Mrs Blinkhorn.[56]

59.   she was appointed to have

come the day before, but was

so frighten'd at the thoughts

of it that she ran away. she

imagines she hears voices, that

her friends have designs against

her, & abstains from eating is

very indolent, & sleeps badly.

— M^{rs}— came to me at

home to ask my advice.

She was improperly treated

by her nurse giving her some

spirituous liquor, during

her lying in about a year

ago, since which she has been

afflicted with a pain on the

top of her head, a coldness

which begins in her left leg

& at last spreads a chilliness

all over her body with many

other hysterical symptoms

her water often turbid & after

standing turning milky,

is very much afraid of

losing her senses. sleeps

badly & wakes hurried is

easily & often put in a

flutter.

* Mrs Winter has something very

particular in her voice talks

very loud & with great energy

tho' she is rattling about such

nonsense as does not require it.

at the same time that she tells

me she is not mad she says

she knows her children were

then actually tied to a stake

to be worried by the beasts

in Smithfield.

— Captn Macdonald in some man

:ner sensible that he is not

well says it has been occasi:

:on'd by some medicinal pre:

:parations given him 6 months

ago. [Word deleted but illegible] hears a voice telling

he is anointed D[uke]. of Gordon

& nonsense of such like.— thinks the
people in the street all ~~are all employ'd to~~ look at him & know
his thoughts by a glance of his eye.

C-72

July 1. Mr Kinder[57] consulted me about
his wife, who was frighted ten years
ago by a fire which consumed his
house since which time by several
accidents which have happen'd suc:
:cessively, she has never been quite
right, she was overturn'd once &
broke her arm, another time she
broke her collar bone & a rib by
a like accident. he thinks she
grows rather worse, & says she is
for 3 weeks in a high state du:

61.

ring which time she is very tal:

kative; expensive buying many

things she does not want &

full of acquaintance, after

that moderate & as she should

be, & then she falls into a low

state of despondency, hates

company, chooses solitude, &

is angry with her husband

for suffering her to run into

expence when he knows, she says,

very well that she is not right.

— Mr Jones a grocer in Fleet street

62 came to me very much confus'd

& frighted he said he had seen

a print he beleiv'd of the devil

as he came along. he talk'd ~~so~~ in

a strange manner of not ha:

:ving done his duty to God tho'

he could not accuse himself

of any actual sin. he slept

tolerably well till 2 o'clock

but not afterwards.

4. Captain Prowsett's at his brother's

63 the corner of Fleet Market a grocer

2.   Mrs Law[58] a baker's wife the cor:
64   ner of Peter's street Cow cross.[59] she

is undoubtedly incapable of ta

:king care of herself or her

family, but all her complaints

seem to be paralytic & if I

may judge from the acc^t. I

rec^d the effect of concussion

she got a fall about 18 months

since & visibly came off with

some few bruises but her me:

mory has fail'd since that time

& I think her right side weak.

4.   Captain Prowsett at his brother's

a grocer the corner of the Fleet

Market. This gentleman had

drank very hard tho' a young

man, had been afflicted with

the dropsy had at this time

a jaundice on him & his blood

totally broke with liquor. He

seem'd very apprehensive, of

the people round him. wan:

:ted to go out of the house with

me tho not able to walk, ask'd

me if I had brought instru:

:ments & dressings proper for

him for he had receiv'd a very

large cut in his belly a little

before I came. he w^{d} not eat &

had slept but little for 3 or 4

nights, he was apprehensive that

poison & improper things were

given him. & seem'd to have

more confidence in me than

his own brother & sister.

8.   Miss Printer the bottom of fleet

65   ditch. incessant talk & pretty

fast, but with some coherence

sleeps little; very outragious the

next time biting, & would not let

me see her face. she died the next day.

8. Mˢ Griffin who has been my patient

66. 3 or 4 times, in high spirits, talks

incoherent, & winks all the time

he is talking. at Mˢ Miles's.

9. A young lad brother to a Tallow:

67 :chandler the corner of Jewin

Street, had by the account I

recᵈ of him an Epileptic fit

after which he fancied the

Devil had been talking to

him, but this seem'd to have

been occasion'd by irregularity

& a hearty sleep made a great

alteration in a night or two.—

9.   Mrs Alcock[60] wife to Clergy man

68   in Sussex, has a notion that she

       must not eat least she should

       increase her fever, she has by

       this means lived extremely

       low for some time past, she

       thinks herself dying, & would

       willingly not eat any thing

       if we would permit it. at

       the same time she sleeps well

       & talks tolerable well. at M^r

       Clarke's

10.   Mrs Bromfield daughter to

69   Mrs Wilson[61] who was in Bethlem

about 4 or 5 years ago. she is
very bad, thinks herself too wic:
ked to live & many such de:
:sponding notions.

—   Sarah Peace at the Craven
70 head in Drury lane, was mad
enough but had a fever at
the time I saw her.

—   Mr Newport I saw twice at
71 Mr Williams's[62] an attorney in
Castle yard who told me the
following story of his father
He was a lunatic, but never
confin'd & look'd upon as

harmless, however one he run after ^{day}

a country girl who was going with

his children to take a walk, &

ask'd her [what] she meant by carrying

the children to the wood, saying

you B.—h I see you have a mind

to murther them, & I will be

even with you, upon which he

drew a knife from his pocket

& struck her on the forehead

but the poor girl's tears & en:

:treaties, satisfied him so far

that he put up his knife & s^d

he was sorry, he was so mistaken;

The girl was thus luckily saved
but her mother was not so for:
:tunate, she saw what pass'd at
a distance, & standing at the
door of her own house, cried
out to her daughter to come &
save herself under her roof;
Mr Newport hearing this runs
up to the mother immediately
& drawing his knife cries out
Oh! you old B—ch, then it is
you, says he, that are the
cause of all this, I will be
reveng'd on you, & plunged

his knife in her side & kill'd her.

he was tried for this at Hartford[63]

& tho brought in a lunatic, con:

:fined in Gaol till he died.

the first time I saw this gentle:

:man he said very little but

laught at times. the second time

he took me out of the room

& I imagined he was going

to trust me with some great

secret, but after having shut

the door with great precaution,

he told me little pitchers had

great ears, he therefore open'd

the door that led into the dining

room again & desir'd his wife

& Mr Williams to walk down

stairs, he had nothing to commu:

:nicate any further than that

he had no notion of country

Apothecaries.

11. Mrs Wilson[64] a gingerbread baker's

72 wife near 3 crown court in

the borough, has been complai:

:ning some time, was attended

at first by Dr Reeve[65] got pretty

well & was sent into the

country, but relaps'd within

the week, thinks herself very

wicked, & is afraid she shall

murder her husband, or herself

or her child, for whom she says

she does not feel the affection

she formerly did tho she loves

her beyond any thing.

— Mr Fitzgerald a linnen draper at

73   the 7 dials; I was sent for in

a violent hurry, to come & see

this man the evening before,

who was described as a very

dangerous & desperate man

& one who would in all probability mur:

:der some of his family if care was not

taken to hinder him: I desired them to send

for proper persons to secure him, which

they still neglected to do; however the next

day he was secured & I saw him. he

was very much flurried & tho' he seem'd

to me to be disorder'd, yet I thought

at first he was one of those people

who are seemingly cured by a very

little restraint which they bear with

the utmost reluctance, he said very

few things out of the way & posi:

:tively denied every thing laid to

his charge, tho' I believe true, that

bore hard upon him. he told me

that he would not sleep, nor take nou:

:rishment, that he had been in that

humour ever since the Saturday be:

:fore I saw him, that he was mad &

out of his senses at times, that it

was ill usage was the cause of it.

That his wife & the servants neglec:

:ted his business. That he loved

to see every one in his house dili:

:gent as the bee <u>& hungry</u> to work.

He was a fine Irishman in his

expressions, I did advise them to

keep him at home for 2 or 3 days

that I might see what effect a

confinement at home would have

upon him, his family not seeming

willing to consent to it, he was

carried to Mr Miles that evening

but behaved so well for the 3 days

after he came there, that I told

Mr M. tho' I did not think him

well I would have nothing far:

:ther to do with his confinement

he accordingly went home that

day.—

15.   Mrs Hampson of Hitchin in Hert:

74   fordshire. Some 6 or 7 months ago

a gentleman who was an acquain:

:tance of her husband's, & visited

in the family upon that footing

an agreeable man, took in his head

to make speeches to her, & address

her in a particular manner.

he was at last so troublesome to

her, that she was obliged to in:

form her husband of it: but the

surprise of the thing & the anxie:

ty ~~of~~ it caus'd brought her in

to such a state of mind as

made her very uneasy, she did

not sleep well was violently

flurried at times, subject to a

palpitation of the heart, waked

in hurries, had strange & extrava:

gant ideas crowding in upon her

had not that Regard for her hus:

:band, her children or her family

that she used to experience.——

—— Miss—— with Mr Taylor from

75 Rotherhithe about 18. sleeps uneasy

some times not at all is much flurried

& at times will talk inconsistently.

it is imagined that she liked

a young gentleman who þ made

his addresses to her elder sister

about 2 years ago but I beleive

all this is without any other

foundation than that they have

C-91C-91

heard her mention him lately tho'
the affair broke off two years ago.—

18. Mrs Gordon[66] a young lady by her

76   appearance about 20. sent for me

to consult me, she was of some

bad consequence from the bite

of a cat wch she suppos'd to be

mad but wch was immediately

kill'd. She says that a cat which

she had kept as a great favorite

for 2 years, but wch us'd to be at

times wild & flying about, & some:

:times surly, about 2 months ago

was put in a fury by the entrance

of a dog, who ~~being~~ ^{was} soon turnd out

& puss remain'd quiet, but not

long afterwards the door being

open'd, the cat rais'd her back

& erected her tail, at which she

& the lady who was with her being

frighten'd would have turn'd her

out of the room but she flew at

them both & bit them in sevral

places, the Lady has not the least

complaint, but Mrs Gordon ima:

:gines, she feels a pain in the

arm where she was bit, & a pain

in her side, dreams of cats, and

other such like things which she

thinks the consequence of this bite,

but, which I cannot but think,

proceed from her imagination

hurried with this disagreeable

accident.

22.   Mrs Van hock sister to Mrs Sheeles[67]

77.   in Queen's square Ormond street.

for 2 years past

has been ᶺ afflicted with various

<u>illnesses</u>, but particularly the

gout & a pain in her head

to such a degree as to lose the

sight of one eye, at last these

complaints vanish'd & about

5 months ago she began to be

wrong in her head & to fancy

she sh^d come to poverty & to abso:

:lute want, that she sh^d not have

a bed to lie on, that she had

been wicked to a strange de:

:gree & such like. I attended

her mother about 4 years ago

in Glocester street in the same

complaint; she told me this mor:

:ning July 25 that she had not

another gown or any Linnen or

other necessaries to send for

& was afraid we sh^d tear the flesh

from her bones.

28.   Mrs Elder a Scotch lady in the

78.   seventh month of her pregnan:

:cy. was in the beginning of June

seiz'd with a complaint of

an acidity at her stomach

vomited a deal of sower stuff,

sometimes had a purging

& at other times very costive.

about the middle of July

she was first perceiv'd to ram:

:ble, she complain'd of her head

& loss of memory. She then com:

plain'd of cruel usage she met

with from a companion of

her own in the house who

endeavour'd to sow dissenssion

between her & her husband.

when I saw her first, she was

full of talk & told me all

the house her husband the

servants & the ladies were

all wrong in the head at

times, & that she was not al:

:ways right. Mrs Elder upon

being removed into lodgings

on Lisson green[68] has still the same

fancy that her maid, myself, &

the people of the house are all

wrong in the head at times.

Aug: 16.

Miss Campden daughter of Mr C.

79   who keeps the 3 tuns on Snow=hill[69]

was frighted some time ago by

her brother, since which time

she has been much indispos'd

in her head at times, running

into the yard with no cloaths

upon her but her shift, she

talk'd to me very rationally, &

coolly, seem'd sensible that she

was not well; but Miss Preston

told me that she w^{d} some times

take a sudden jump, & run from

them as fast as she could.

19.   Mrs Hobbes the upper end of lea:

80   ther lane, in a low desponding

way, & took very little nourish:

:ment. I could get very little

more from her than that she

wanted to get up & take a

walk.—

20.   Miss Gilchrist at a hatter's

81.   in Cross lane near the Monument.

had bewilder'd herself very much

about a gentleman who had

made his addresses to her, &

was thought by her friends &

herself to be an improper

match, which had hurried

her extremely, she gave a

very good acc^t of herself but was

a little hurried, & fancied

herself dying. I had afterwards

an opportunity of learning her

whole story which was as follows.

She was very agreable both in per:

:son & understanding, & when very

young was for many months

together in the same house

with M^r St.— frequent oppor:

:tunities of seeing & conversing

with each other, made the young

people who were both agreable

conceive a liking for each other.

this was put an end to by his

friends from prudential motives

as the world calls them, her

fortune being small. They

were separated; & some years af:

:ter Mr Beecher[70] who was then re:

:turn'd from India with a con:

:siderable fortune paid his ad:

:dresses to her[71] & was receiv'd as

he c.^d wish; every ^thing was agreed on;

& when she thought herself on

the point of being married to

him; it broke out that he had

an intrigue with his maid

who was with child by him, &

he was so intangled with the

maid, that he broke off the

match with Miss G. offer'd her

a 1000£ which she disdained

to accept, & married his maid.

Some time after this 3 or 4 years

she took an inclination to

Captn D——n^{72} in the E.I.^{73} service

& things went such a length

that they were engaged & a

correspondence was on foot

between them after he sail'd

from England; after his depar:

:ture she began to imagine that

he was not a man proper to

make her happy, not being a

person of such understanding as

she w^d choose, & her friends not

thinking his circumstances such

as they lik'd seconded her incli:

:nations & she was resolvd to break

off the match accordingly; of

which she wrote him word

& this was first told me as the

cause of her discomposure.

but I sincere learn'd another

circumstance which if true,

seems to me to have been cause

sufficient for this misfortune

which is that M^r St.— ignorant

of her engagement with Captn D.

had wrote her a letter lately, on

the subject of their first mutual

inclination.—

September. 3.

82.   Mr Mitchell at Mr Allwright's[74]

near the Turnpike at Westminster

was exceeding mad when I saw

him, spitting, sulky, saying

nothing tumbling & tossing

about, grinning, & obstinate

refusing to eat, & obliged to

be tied down in his bed.—

3.   Captn Knackstone at Mr Duffields

83.   This gentleman's [*sic*] was a patient

of my father's once or twice, &

likewise of mine, for a short

time. He is when well of an

enthusiastic ^turn in^ religion but a

very odd compound when

ill. He talks very well & with

~~much~~ coherence, & seeming

composure upon the subjects

of his confinement, & the

ill usage he has met with

on that account, & might

in all probability succeed in

making people unacquainted with

him or his story, beleive that

he was confined without reason;

& they would conclude, if they

enquir'd no farther, that liber:

:ty was terribly [word missing[75]] by the usage

he rec[d]. but tho he can talk

with consistence & seeming

moderation, let him but alone

his talk is without end, even

to tire himself & bring him

into flurries: his actions if

carefully observ'd without letting

him know it, are all trifling &

childish : & by those who are ac:

:quainted with him he may be

brought into inconsistencies, he

fancies that he has been charg'd

with being register'd as a free:

:Mason at the Devil Tavern,[76] &

on this point, if press'd, he

cannot talk, so as to make

himself intelligible.

5.   Mr Pottinger.[77] at Mr Miles this

[84]   man was a bookseller & some

years since became a bankrupt.

when I saw him he was rather feve:

:rish, but very mad: he talk'd &

rattled very idly about being She:

:riff of London, that he had laid

great wagers upon it, & should

win 300000£ I think, that there

was near 3 millions laid on

this event.

9.   Mrs Hooper wife to Mr Hooper[78]

85   of Ramsgate captain of a

trading vessell in the

merchant's service, has

been disorder'd some months,

she fancies herself bewitch'd

by her mother in law, her

own mother is disorder'd now

by[?] in such a manner as

not to be confined.—

11.   Mrs Plow an old woman of 70

86   in king's gate street was mar:

:ried about 2 years ago & begin:

:ning to swell about 2 months

after imagin'd herself with

child, &, as they told me, was

search'd by Dr Handasyde;[79]

She went two months beyond the time

she had fix'd when a violent purging

which came upon her, & continued

near 8 months releiv'd her of her

great belly. Whether this evacuation

which in some measure still con:

:tinues has weakened her facul:

:ties I know not but she now fan:

:cies her neighbours blow poisonous

powders upon her, & that she is

to ^be^ burnt & punish'd various ways

24.   Mr Ramsay a butcher from Ed:

87   :monton brought to Mr Miles's, a

long story teller how he beat &

abused several people, particular

:ly one woman, his barber who had

shav'd him for 30 years & several

others of his old acquaintance

us'd him ill & had a spite

against him for no reason.

— Miss— from Chichester.

88

an acquaintance of Mr Richard:

:son's[80] of Mr Pleasant. was brought

to me rather to see her than

any thing else. she was herself

much more willing to call her

unhappy complaint by its true

name, than her friends seem'd

to be. She had been ill for 6 years

3 years of which time she had been

continually in bed. She felt no

joy, seem'd a burthensome crea:

:ture in the world, & if she attempted

to amuse herself, seem'd much

the worse for it afterwards com:

:plain'd of great tightness round

her head, & gave a very regular

good account of herself without

the least inconsistency.—She had

been at Chelsea, & undergone the

operation of D[r] Dominiceti's

father,[81] but without effect.

— Mr Walker[82] a distiller in Horton:

~~89~~ falgate a relapse vid: Feb: 3. N° 14

30. Mrs Harris. she has been my

89. patient twice before in the

time of her first husband

Mr Jackson. she is at present

in violent hurries, talking

much of having done wrong

is in great sweats, & had

made to [*sic*] attempts to hang

herself before she was

brought to Mr Miles's

— A Case from farnham

about a woman.—

October. 7.   Mrs Fludger at Mr Devy's[83]

90.   Hoxton, violently mad, talking

with vehemence & great incohe:

:rence saying that her friends

had thought her mad but were

mistaken that she had indeed

been a little so, but was now

very well, asking ^(after) some friend

of hers whom she fancied

dead or in bonds.—

8.   Mrs Trecothick[84] John street in

91.   the King's road. of a very thin

delicate habit, has been for

some time fancying that her

husband intercepts blessings

design'd her by Providence, &

fancies that she sees God & Jesus

Christ in visions, talks of this

sometimes as the effect of a

deluded imagination, at

other times beleives all real.

15. Mrs Stubbs opposite the middle

92. Morefields, raving, & talking very

incoherently, loud in her talk

& abusive to those about her.

with some little inclination to

mischief; very little sleep this

complaint came almost suddenly.

17.   Mrs Wilmot. has been disorder'd for

93.   some years past by the account I

       have had of her, & by her appea:

       :rance I should imagine her head

       to be damag'd beyond repair. She

       would fain have had me convey

       her from Mr Strutton's [Thutton's?] where she

       was confin'd to town in my chariot.

18.   Mrs Webb.⁸⁵ a watchmaker's wife in An:

94   :chor street spital fields, was brought

       to bed on thursday the 9th instant &

       continued very well for 8 or ten days,

       she then began to ramble, was some:

       :times quite raving & obstreperous but

       two days after I first saw her, she

       talk'd nothing but disjointed nonsense

       took very little notice of any thing

C-117

that pass'd, did every thing under her,

grew weaker & weaker, & on wednesday

night or thursday morning died. she

was sister to Mr Fletcher who was my

patient while a boy, & again about

2 years since at Highgate where

he died after an illness of 10 days.

November

4.   Mr Darby a tripe:man in New:

95   :port Market, whom I attended

      about 5 or 6 years ago in the

      same condition which is ge:

      :nerally brought on by drin:
                        frights attended with
      :king. he is in ^ violent tremors &

      convulsive twitchings, & much

much [*sic*] afraid of the Devil, but
it soon gives way to evacuation.

14. Mʳ Rosat. a native of Switzerland.

96 who has been for some time, as a
Merchant in Turkey, from whence
he is just return'd; he was in
a low:spirited way while he
was there, but got over it, he met
with great losses, by putting too
much confidence in a Jew who
deceiv'd him; this affected him
so much that his depression of
spirits return'd to such a degree
that upon his return to England
he eloped from the people, who

were conducting him to his friends, &

was advertis'd,[86] after he was brought

to them he again eloped; & lay out

in the fields, & was again advertis'd.

he appears stupid, & rarely an:

:swers the questions put to him.

but he returns sensible answers

his sister inform'd me that she

observ'd him standing in the

garden yesterday evening for

a full hour staring up at the

moon.—

14.   Mʳ Stanfield a Clergyman

97·   in the County of Huntingdon:

has been ill for a long time.

he told me he knew very well

I was a superior being, & come to

inflict eternal punishment upon

him, went down on his knees, to

beg I would respite him for a

short space, tho he knew it

must come at last. he was

sure he had not died, but

look'd upon himself as in a

state of separation among the

dead, & waiting for the reward

of his evil doings. about 3 weeks after I first saw this Gent.ⁿ he became afraid of ea: :ting & continued obstinate in that point but days before he died wᶜʰ was quite suddenly he eat very hearty & as usual.—

16.   Mʳˢ Holman in Winchester Street has

98   been married about five or six years

was rather disturb'd before her

marriage, fearing the match wᵈ

be broke off, she said if she was not

married to Mr H. she would either hang

or drown herself, however nothing hap:

:pen'd & she was married. after this

upon being brought to bed of 2 girls

about 2 years ago, she was very much

hurried for some time but got

the better of her complaint. she

lay in last July & went thro her

month extremely well, but per:

:ceiv'd herself affected about the

second day she went abroad. She

says she is very happy while she

is sleeping has no dreams to dis:

:turb her, but as soon as she wakes

she is thoroughly unhappy. she does

not care to rise, & when she is per:

suaded, she does not know how to em:

:ploy herself, she quits one room & goes

into another without any intention

cannot settle to work or take any

care of her family. She has been

at Ramsgate[87] but without any

relief.

19.   Mrs Brooke[88] of Malling in Kent has

99   been in a low:spirited way these

six months past, her thoughts are

desponding to the last degree at

some times in the day, & she is

so much afraid of doing mischief

to herself in the night, that be

sides her own maid, a maid of

Mr Duffield's constantly lies in

the room & the doors of the

bedchamber are lock'd & the keys

taken out of them.

23. Mr Heber Long Acre the per:

100 :son who publishes the accounts

of The Horse:races.[89] he had been

under Mr Dale Ingram's[90] care

from some venereal complaint

& whether it proceeded from

the medicines he had taken

or from an accidental fever

that came upon him I know

not but he was feverish &

[end of case book record]

Notes

PREFACE

1. The Monros were exclusively physicians to Bethlem from 1728 until Dr. (later Sir) George Leman Tuthill (1772–1835) was appointed joint physician alongside Edward Thomas Monro in 1816. Thereafter, a Monro continued to act as joint physician until 1853.

2. Jonathan Andrews, Asa Briggs, Roy Porter, Penny Tucker, and Keir Waddington, *The History of Bethlem* (London: Routledge, 1997). For an assessment, see Andrew Scull, "Bethlem Demystified?" *Medical History* 43 (1999), pp. 248–55.

3. For such judgments of Monro as an arch-conservative, see (among others) Richard Hunter and Ida Macalpine, "Introduction," in the facsimile edition of William Battie, *A Treatise on Madness,* and John Monro, *Remarks on Dr Battie's Treatise on Madness* (London: Dawson's, 1962), pp. 7–21; Klaus Doerner, *Madmen and the Bourgeoisie* (Oxford: Blackwell, 1981), pp. 39–46; Roy Porter, *Mind-Forg'd Manacles: A History of Madness in England from the Restoration to the Regency* (London: Athlone, 1987), esp. pp. 128–29, 192–93, 206–8; George Rousseau, "Science," in *The Eighteenth Century,* ed. Pat Rogers (London: Methuen, 1978), pp. 153–207; and Rousseau, "Psychology," *The Ferment of Knowledge,* eds. George Rousseau and Roy Porter (Cambridge: Cambridge University Press, 1980), pp. 143–210. The lone, but persuasive, exception to this scholarly consensus is Akihito Suzuki, "Mind and Its Disease in Enlightenment Medicine" (unpublished Ph.D. diss., University of London, 1992), pp. 221–68. Our own reassessment of John Monro and his place in eighteenth-century mad-doctoring may be found in the companion to the present volume: Jonathan Andrews and Andrew Scull, *Undertaker of the Mind: John Monro and Mad-Doctoring in Eighteenth-Century England* (Berkeley: University of California Press, 2001).

1. CUSTOMERS, PATRONS, AND THEIR MAD-DOCTOR

1. David Ingleby, "Mental Health and the Social Order," *Social Order and the State: Historical and Comparative Essays,* eds. Stanley Cohen and Andrew Scull (Oxford: Basil Blackwell, 1983), p. 142.

2. See, for example, R. A. Houston, *Madness and Society in Eighteenth-Century Scotland* (Oxford: Clarendon, 2000); Roy Porter, *A Social History of Madness: Stories of the Insane* (London: Weidenfeld and Nicolson, 1987); John Walton, "Casting Out and Bringing Back in Victorian England: Pauper Lunatics, 1840–1870," *The Anatomy of Madness: Essays in the History of Psychiatry*, eds. W. F. Bynum, Roy Porter, and Michael Shepherd, vol. 2 (London: Routledge, 1985), pp. 132–46; Richard Adair, Bill Forsythe, and Joseph Melling, "A Danger to the Public? Disposing of Pauper Lunatics in Late-Victorian and Edwardian England," *Medical History* 42 (1998), pp. 1–25; Adair, Melling, and Forsythe, "Migration, Family Structure, and Pauper Lunacy in Victorian England: Admissions to the Devon County Pauper Lunatic Asylum, 1845–1900," *Continuity and Change* 12 (1997), pp. 373–401; Melling, Adair, and Forsythe, "'A Proper Lunatic for Two Years': Pauper Lunatic Children in Victorian and Edwardian England: Child Admissions to the Devon County Asylum," *Journal of Social History* 30 (1997), pp. 371–405; Akihito Suzuki, "The Household and the Care of Lunatics in Eighteenth-Century London," *The Locus of Care: Families, Communities, Institutions, and the Provision of Welfare since Antiquity*, eds. Peregrine Horden and Richard Smith (London: Routledge, 1998), pp. 153–75; and many of the papers in two recent edited collections: *Insanity, Institutions and Society, 1800–1914: A Social History of Madness in Comparative Perspective*, eds. Joseph Melling and Bill Forsythe (London: Routledge, 1999); and *Outside the Walls of the Asylum: The History of Care in the Community, 1750–2000*, eds. Peter Bartlett and David Wright (London: Athlone, 1999).

3. For the historiography, see Andrew Scull, "Somatic Treatments and the Historiography of Psychiatry," *History of Psychiatry* 5 (1994), pp. 1–12; Scull, "Psychiatrists and Historical 'Facts': Part One: The Historiography of Somatic Treatments," *History of Psychiatry* 6 (1995), pp. 225–41; Scull, "Psychiatric Therapeutics and the Historian: Problems and Prospects," *Histoire de la psychiatrie: Nouvelles approches, nouvelles perspectives*, eds. Jacques Gasser and Vincent Barras (Lausanne, Switzerland: Payot, in press). For two splendid recent exceptions to this pattern of neglect, see Joel Braslow, *Mental Ills and Bodily Cures: Psychiatric Treatment in the First Half of the Twentieth Century* (Berkeley: University of California Press, 1997); and David Healy, *The Anti-Depressant Era* (Cambridge, Mass.: Harvard University Press, 1998).

4. "Historians have always found therapeutics an awkward piece of business . . . on the whole, they have responded by ignoring it"; Charles E. Rosenberg, "The Therapeutic Revolution: Medicine, Meaning, and Social Change," *The Therapeutic Revolution*, eds. Morris J. Vogel and Charles E. Rosenberg (Philadelphia: University of Pennsylvania Press, 1976), p. 4. Led by Rosenberg and his students, medical historians, too, have now belatedly turned their attention to the subject, and therapeutics and the processes of therapeutic change have become the focus of some of the best research in the field.

5. Christine Stevenson, "The Architecture of Bethlem at Moorfields," *The History of Bethlem*, eds. Jonathan Andrews et al. (London: Routledge, 1997), p. 230; Stevenson, *Medicine and Magnificence: British Hospital and Asylum Architecture, 1660–1815* (New Haven, Conn.: Yale University Press, 2000);

Stevenson, "Robert Hooke's Bethlem," *Journal of the* [American] *Society of Architectural Historians* 55.3 (Sept. 1996), pp. 254–75.

6. Between 1719 and 1751, seven new hospitals were added to the ancient foundations of St. Thomas's, St. Bartholomew's, and Bethlem. Still others were established in the major provincial cities.

7. For more information on Battie's career and his relations with John Monro, see Andrews and Scull, *Undertaker of the Mind,* chapter 2 *et passim.*

8. Neil McKendrick, John Brewer, and J. H. Plumb, *The Birth of a Consumer Society: The Commercialization of Eighteenth-Century England* (Bloomington: Indiana University Press, 1982).

9. We have explored the similarities between these two stigmatized occupations, undertaking and mad-doctoring, dealing respectively with the corruption and death of body and mind, in the introduction to our companion volume on the eighteenth-century management of lunacy: Jonathan Andrews and Andrew Scull, *Undertaker of the Mind: John Monro and Mad-Doctoring in Eighteenth-Century England* (Berkeley: University of California Press, 2001).

10. In 1727, for £41 per annum, Wright leased a large, white-washed, timber-framed building dating from Elizabethan times, a house variously known as Bethnal House, Kirby's Castle, or the Blind Beggar's House, now rechristened Wright's Madhouse and later called the "White House," scene of some of the worst scandals uncovered by the early-nineteenth-century lunacy reformers. (See, for example, *Minutes of Evidence Taken Before the Select Committee . . . for the Better Regulation of Madhouses in England* [1815], 1st report, pp. 114–15; [1816], 1st report, pp. 1–5, 37–38; *Select Committee on Pauper Lunatics and Lunatic Asylums in the County of Middlesex, 1827,* pp. 17–39, 100–2; J. W. Rogers, *A Statement of the Cruelties, Abuses, and Frauds, Which Are Practised in Mad-houses* [London: For the author, 1816].) It was in an annex to this establishment, known as the Red House, that James Monro treated one Alexander Cruden, a litigious patient who would also come under his son John's care in 1753 (though on the latter occasion Cruden was sent to a madhouse in Little Chelsea).

11. For Cheyne's discussion of this "affliction," see George Cheyne, *The English Malady, or, A Treatise of Nervous Diseases of All Kinds* (London: Printed for G. Strahan and J. Leake, 1733); facsimile ed., reprinted with an introduction by Roy Porter (London and New York: Routledge, 1991).

2. A RARE RESOURCE

1. Alexander Cruden, *The London-Citizen Exceedingly Injured, or a British Inquisition Display'd . . . Addressed to the Legislature, as Plainly Shewing the Absolute Necessity of Regulating Private Madhouses* (London: Cooper and Dodd, 1739); reprinted in *Voices of Madness,* ed. Allan Ingram (Stroud, Gloucestershire: Sutton, 1997), pp. 23–74, quote on p. 69. For more information on Cruden's case, see Andrews and Scull, *Undertaker of the Mind,* chap. 3.

2. Alexander Cruden, *The Adventures of Alexander the Corrector. The Second Part. Giving an Account of a Memorable, or Rather Monstrous, Battle*

Fought, or Rather Not Fought, in Westminster Hall February 20 1754 (London: Printed for the author, 1754), p. 23.

3. For a survey, see Andrew Scull, "Psychiatry and Its Historians," *History of Psychiatry* 2 (1991), pp. 239–50.

4. Our thanks to Joel Braslow for this elegant rendering of this facet of the case book's appeal (personal communication, 3 March 2000).

5. Trevor Turner, personal communication, 25 May 2000. Elaine Murphy, another British psychiatrist, independently reacted along very much the same lines (personal communication, 12 May 2000).

6. Tore Frängsmyr, J. L. Heilbron, and Robin E. Rider, *The Quantifying Spirit in the 18th Century* (Berkeley: University of California Press, 1990).

7. This interpretation of Monro's notations arose in conversation with Paul Weindling, for whose advice on this issue we are grateful.

8. Michel Foucault, *The Birth of the Clinic* (London: Tavistock, 1973; Routledge: reprint, 1993), esp. chap. 6, "Signs and Cases," pp. 88–106; trans. from *Naissance de la clinique* (Presses Universitaires de France, 1963).

9. *The Account Book of Dr Loxham*, Lancashire Record Office, DDPr25/6. Loxham's account book covers the period 1753–92 and records details of over 920 cases. He evidently endeavored to keep his accounts up to date on a monthly basis. Our thanks to Steve King for drawing our attention to the existence of this source and for providing helpful information on its contents.

10. Case book (henceforth CB), pp. C-8, C-55, C-69, C-70, C-91, C-112–13, cases of Mr. [blank] the onanist; AB the servant maid; Mrs. [blank] with Mrs. Blinkhorn, who was so frightened about the consultation that she had refused to see Monro on the appointed day; Mrs. [blank], who was "improperly treated by her nurse"'; Miss [blank] with Mr. Taylor; and Miss [blank] from Chichester, whose friends were averse to accepting that she was mad.

11. CB, pp. C-100–5, "Mr St.—" and "Captn D—n."

12. Other emphases Monro signals in this manner appear more mysterious and closed to interpretation, as when only one or two words are underlined, such as "& hungry" on CB, p. C-88, and "illnesses" on p. C-94.

13. See, for example, CB, pp. C-2, C-29, C-72, C-121.

14. Erwin H. Ackerknecht, "Beitraege zur Geschichte der Medizinalreform von 1848," *Sudhoffs Archiv für Geschichte der Medizin* 25 (1932), pp. 61–109, 113–83; Henry E. Sigerist, "The Social History of Medicine," *Western Journal of Surgery, Obstetrics, and Gynecology* 42 (1940), pp. 715–22; Roy Porter, "The Patient's View: Doing Medical History from Below," *Theory and Society* 14 (1985), pp. 175–98; Paul Weindling, "Medical Practice in Imperial Berlin: The Casebook of Alfred Grotjahn," *Bulletin of the History of Medicine* 61 (1987), pp. 391–410; Guenter B. Risse and John Harley Warner, "Reconstructing Clinical Activities: Patient Records in Medical History," *Social History of Medicine* 5 (1992), pp. 183–205; Steven Noll, "Patient Records as Historical Stories: The Case of Caswell Training School," *Bulletin of the History of Medicine* 68 (1994), pp. 411–28.

15. Gerald A. Gordon, *Role Theory and Illness: A Sociological Perspective* (New Haven, Conn.: College and University Press, 1966).

16. For a classic analysis of the distinction between the study of disease and

the study of illness, and also of the sick role, see, e.g., Arthur Kleinman, *The Illness Narratives: Suffering, Healing and the Human Condition* (New York: Basic Books, 1988). See also James H. Buchanan, *Patient Encounters: The Experience of Disease* (Charlottesville: University Press of Virginia, 1989), and Robert Dingwall, *Aspects of Illness* (London: Martin Robertson, 1976). For a sophisticated and insightful historical analysis of the meaning of illness in early modern England, see Andrew Wear, "The Meaning of Illness in Early Modern England," *History of the Doctor-Patient Relationship: Proceedings of the Fourteenth International Symposium on the Comparative History of Medicine—East and West,* eds. Yosio Kawakita, Shizu Sakai, and Yasuo Otsuka (Tokyo: Ishiyaku EuroAmerica, 1995), pp. 1–29.

17. Lucinda McCray Beier, *Sufferers and Healers: The Experience of Illness in Seventeenth-Century England* (London and New York: Routledge and Kegan Paul, 1987); Roy Porter, ed., *Patients and Practitioners: Lay Perceptions of Medicine in Pre-Industrial Society* (Cambridge: Cambridge University Press, 1985); Roy Porter and Dorothy Porter, *In Sickness and in Health: The English Experience 1650–1850* (London: Fourth Estate, 1988); Roy Porter, *A Social History of Madness;* Porter, ed., *The Faber Book of Madness* (London: Faber and Faber, 1991). See also Christine B. Whittaker, "Chasing the Cure: Irving Fisher's Experience as a Tuberculosis Patient," *Bulletin of the History of Medicine* 48 (1974), pp. 398–415.

18. The paradigmatic example is the extremely subtle use of case book material in Joel Braslow's *Mental Ills and Bodily Cures.* See also Elizabeth Lunbeck, *The Psychiatric Persuasion: Knowledge, Gender, and Power in Modern America* (Princeton, N.J.: Princeton University Press, 1994).

19. For studies of the ways in which the case history has been written, see, e.g., Andrew Cunningham, "Pathology and the Case-History in Giambattista Morgagni's 'On the Seats and Causes of Diseases Investigated Through Anatomy' (1761)," *Medizin, Gesellschaft und Geschichte—Jahrbuch des Instituts für Geschichte der Medizin der Robert Bosch Stiftung. Bd. 14,* ed. Robert Jütte (Stuttgart: F. Steiner, 1991), pp. 37–61; A. Suzuki, "Mind and Its Disease in Enlightenment Medicine," Ph.D. diss., University of London, 1992, Günther B. Risse and John Harley Warner, "Reconstructing Clinical Activities: Patient Records in Medical History," *Social History of Medicine* 5 (1992), pp. 183–205; Trevor Turner, *A Diagnostic Analysis of the Casebooks of Ticehurst House Asylum 1845–1890* (Cambridge: Cambridge University Press, 1992); Turner, "Rich and Mad in Victorian England," *Psychological Medicine* 19 (1989), pp. 22–24; Oeivind Larsen, "Case Histories in Nineteenth-Century Hospitals—What Do They Tell the Historian? Some Methodological Considerations with Special Reference to McKeown's Criticism of Medicine," *Medizin,* pp. 127–48; Frank J. Sulloway, "Reassessing Freud's Case Histories: The Social Construction of Psychoanalysis," *Isis* 82 (1991), pp. 245–75; Mark S. Micale, "Paradigm and Ideology in Psychiatric History Writing: The Case of Psychoanalysis," *Journal of Nervous and Mental Disease* 184 (1996), pp. 146–52; Harriet Nowell-Smith, "Nineteenth-Century Narrative Case Histories: An Inquiry into Stylistics and History," *Canadian Bulletin of Medical History* 12 (1995), pp. 47–67; Rita Charon, "To Build a Case: Medical Histories as Traditions in Conflict," *Litera-*

ture and Medicine 11 (1992), pp. 115–32; Andrea A. Rusnock, "The Weight of Evidence and the Burden of Authority: Case Histories, Medical Statistics and Smallpox Inoculation," *Medicine in the Enlightenment*, ed. Roy Porter (Amsterdam and Atlanta, Ga.: Rodopi, 1995), pp. 289–315; Jonathan Andrews, "Case Notes, Case Histories, and the Patient's Experience of Insanity at Gartnavel Royal Asylum, Glasgow, in the Nineteenth Century," *Social History of Medicine* 11 (1998), pp. 255–81; and Amalie M. Kass, " 'Called to her at three o'clock am': Obstetrical Practice in Physician Case Notes," *Journal of the History of Medicine and Allied Sciences* 50.2 (April 1995), pp. 194–229.

20. Roy Porter, "The Patient's View."

21. For some of the earliest publications of this sort, see, e.g., Charles F. Mullett, "The Lay Outlook on Medicine in England circa 1800–1850," *Bulletin of the History of Medicine* 25 (1951), pp. 169–77; and Gregory Bateson, ed., *Perceval's Narrative: A Patient's Account of His Psychosis, 1830–1832* (Stanford, Calif.: Stanford University Press, 1961). For more recent works, see, e.g., Mary E. Fissell, "The 'Sick and Drooping Poor' in Eighteenth-Century Bristol and Its Region," *Social History of Medicine* 2 (1989), pp. 35–58; Fissell, "The Disappearance of the Patient's Narrative and the Invention of Hospital Medicine," *British Medicine in an Age of Reform*, eds. Roger French and Andrew Wear (London and New York: Routledge, 1991), pp. 91–109; Fissell, "Readers, Texts, and Contexts: Vernacular Medical Works in Early Modern England," *The Popularisation of Medicine, 1650–1850*, ed. Roy Porter (London and New York: Routledge, 1992), pp. 72–96; Fissell, *Patients, Power and the Poor in Eighteenth-Century Bristol* (Cambridge: Cambridge University Press, 1991); Marijke Gijswijt-Hofstra, Hilary Marland, and Hans de Waardt, eds., *Illness and Healing Alternatives in Western Europe* (London: Routledge, 1997); Roy Porter, *Patients and Practitioners*, esp. introduction and chaps. 5, 9, 10; Roy Porter, "Lay Medical Knowledge in the Eighteenth Century: The Evidence of the *Gentleman's Magazine*," *Medical History* 29 (1985), pp. 138–68; Roy Porter and Dorothy Porter, *Patient's Progress: Doctors and Doctoring in Eighteenth-Century England* (Oxford: Polity/Blackwell, 1989); Roy Porter, "Reforming the Patient in the Age of Reform: Thomas Beddoes and Medical Practice," *British Medicine in an Age of Reform*, eds. Roger French and Andrew Wear (London and New York: Routledge, 1991), pp. 9–44; Roy Porter, "The Patient in England, c. 1660–c. 1800," *Medicine in Society: Historical Essays*, ed. Andrew Wear (Cambridge and New York: Cambridge University Press, 1992), pp. 91–118; Roy Porter, ed., *The Faber Book of Madness*; Roy Porter, ed., *The Popularization of Medicine 1650–1850* (London: Routledge, 1992); Vicky Rippere, "The Survival of Traditional Medicine in Lay Medical Views: An Empirical Approach to the History of Medicine," *Medical History* 25 (1981), pp. 411–14; and Ronald C. Sawyer, "Friends or Foes? Doctors and Their Patients in Early Modern England," *History of the Doctor-Patient Relationship*, pp. 31–53.

22. See, e.g., Peter Bartlett, *The Poor Law of Lunacy: The Administration of Pauper Lunatics in Mid-Nineteenth-Century England* (London and Washington, D.C.: Leicester University Press, 1999), esp. pp. 158–72, 278–80; David Wright, "The Certification of Insanity in Nineteenth-Century England and Wales," *History of Psychiatry* 9.3 (Sept. 1998), pp. 267–90; Charlotte MacKen-

zie, *Psychiatry for the Rich: A History of Ticehurst Private Asylum, 1792–1917* (London and New York: Routledge, 1992); and Leonard D. Smith, *Cure, Comfort, and Safe Custody: Public Lunatic Asylums in Early Nineteenth Century England* (London: Leicester University Press, 1999).

23. For individual early modern case histories, see, e.g., J. V. Beckett, "An Eighteenth-Century Case History: Carlisle Spedding 1738," *Medical History* 26 (1982), pp. 303–6; Richard B. Sheridan, "The Doctor and the Buccaneer: Sir Hans Sloane's Case History of Sir Henry Morgan, Jamaica, 1688," *Journal of the History of Medicine and Allied Sciences* 41 (1986), pp. 76–87; and G. M. Longfield-Jones, "The Case History of 'Sir H. M.,'" *Medical History* 32 (1988), pp. 449–60.

24. Elizabeth Allen, J. L. Turk, and Sir Reginald Murley, eds., *The Case Books of John Hunter FRS* (London: Royal Society of Medicine, 1993).

25. For examples of case books and case histories from more recent times, and of medical autobiographies written up loosely in the style of case books, see, e.g., Harold Ellis, *Surgical Case-Histories from the Past* (London and New York: Royal Society of Medicine Press, 1994); Alfred Adler, *Problems of Neurosis: A Book of Case-Histories,* ed. Philippe Mairet (London: Kegan Paul, Trench, Trübner, 1929); Alexander Erskine, *A Hypnotist's Case Book* (London: Rider, 1932); Harry Price, *Leaves from a Psychiatrist's Case-Book* (London: V. Gollancz, 1933); Abraham Groves, *All in the Day's Work: Leaves from a Doctor's Case-Book* (Toronto: Macmillan, 1934); James Harpole, *Leaves from a Surgeon's Case-Book* (New York: Frederick A. Stokes Co., 1938); Charles Berg, *War in the Mind: The Case Book of a Medical Psychologist: An Introduction to the Practical Application of Modern Psychology* (London: Macaulay Press, 1941); Berg, *Clinical Psychology: A Case Book of the Neuroses and Their Treatment* (London: Allen and Unwin, 1948); W. Burns Lingard, *Herbal Prescriptions from a Consultant's Case Book* (London: National Institute of Medical Herbalists, 1958); Eustace Chesser, *Unquiet Minds: Leaves from a Psychologist's Casebook* (London and New York: Rich and Cowan, 1952); Michael J. Goldstein and James O. Palmer, *The Experience of Anxiety: A Casebook* (New York: Oxford University Press, 1963); G. Donald Niswander, Thomas M. Casey, and John A. Humphrey, *A Panorama of Suicide: A Casebook of Psychological Autopsies* (Springfield, Ill.: Charles C. Thomas, 1973); Leonard L. Heston and Renate Heston, *The Medical Casebook of Adolf Hitler: His Illnesses, Doctors, and Drugs* (London: Kimber, 1979); and Alvin E. Rodin and Jack D. Key, *Medical Casebook of Doctor Arthur Conan Doyle: From Practitioner to Sherlock Holmes and Beyond* (Malabar, Fla.: R. E. Krieger, 1984). For eighteenth-century publications highly reliant on case history material, see, e.g., R. W. Stack, *Medical Cases, With Occasional Remarks. To Which is Added an Appendix. Containing the History of a late Extraordinary Case* (Bath: R. Cruttwell, 1784).

26. E.g., Kenneth Dewhurst, ed., *Willis's Oxford Casebook (1650–52)* (Oxford: Sandford Publications, 1981); Jean E. Ward and Joan Yell, eds. and trans., *The Medical Casebook of William Brownrigg, M.D., F.R.S. (1712–1800) of the Town of Whitehaven in Cumberland, Medical History,* Supplement no. 13 (London: Wellcome Institute for the History of Medicine, 1993); Charles F. A. Marmoy, ed., *The Case Book of "La Maison de Charité de Spittlefields" 1739–*

41 (London: Huguenot Society of London, 1981); S. T. Anning, "A Medical Case Book: Leeds, 1781–84," *Medical History* 28 (1984), pp. 420–31; S. Wood, *The Library: Two Further Letters of John Hunter and Notes on Rockingham's Last Illness from Hunter's Case Book* (London: 1949); Jessie Dobson, *Notes from John Hunter's Casebook* (London: 1959; reprinted from the January 1959 issue of the *Journal of the Medical Women's Federation*). For studies of early modern and modern case books, see, e.g., Lucinda McCray Beier, "Seventeenth-Century English Surgery: The Casebook of Joseph Binns," *Medical Theory, Surgical Practice,* ed. Christopher Lawrence (London and New York: Routledge, 1992), pp. 48–84; Amalie M. Kass, "The Obstetrical Casebook of Walter Channing, 1811–1822," *Bulletin of the History of Medicine* 67 (1993), pp. 494–523; Frank M. C. Forster, "Walter Lindesay Richardson, 1826–1879 as Obstetrician: His Case-Book and Midwifery Practice in Early Ballarat," *Festschrift for Kenneth Fitzpatrick Russell, M.B., M.S., D. Litt., F.R.A.C.S., F.R.A.C.P.,* Proceedings of a Symposium Arranged by the Section of Medical History, A.M.A. (Victorian Branch), 25 Feb. 1977 (Carlton, Victoria: Queensberry Hill Press for the Department of Medical History, University of Melbourne, 1978), pp. 142–58; George Wynn, "The Case Book of Dr. Amos A. Evans, Surgeon on the Frigate 'Constitution' in the War of 1812," *Annals of Medical History* 3rd ser. 2 (1940), pp. 70–78; G. J. O. Bridgeman, "An Ophthalmic Case-Book of Eighty Years Ago," *Proceedings of the Royal Society of Medicine Section of the History of Medicine* 48 (1955), pp. 381–84; R. M. Price, "A Case Book of the Philadelphia Almshouse Infirmary: Dr James Rush Attending Physician [8 Oct. 1819 to 10 Feb. 1820]," *Bulletin of the History of Medicine* 59 (1985), pp. 383–89; and Weindling, "Medical Practice in Imperial Berlin." Barbara Duden's *The Woman Beneath the Skin: A Doctor's Patients in Eighteenth-Century Germany* (Cambridge, Mass., and London: Harvard University Press, 1991) is a study of eight books published by Dr. Johannes Pelargius Storch, derived in part from case histories extracted from twenty-one years of entries in his diary.

27. Joan Lane, *John Hall and His Patients: The Medical Practice of Shakespeare's Son-in-Law* (Stratford-upon-Avon: Shakespeare Birthplace Trust in association with Alan Sutton Publishing Ltd., 1996). See also Ward and Yell, *The Medical Casebook of William Brownrigg, M.D., F.R.S.,* which includes a few cases of insanity, melancholy, hypochondria, and nervous illness.

28. Michael MacDonald, *Mystical Bedlam: Madness, Anxiety and Healing in Seventeenth-Century England* (Cambridge: Cambridge University Press, 1981).

29. [Rev.] William Pargeter, *Observations on Maniacal Disorders* (Reading: Printed for the author, 1792); facsimile reprint, ed. Stanley W. Jackson (London and New York: Routledge, 1988).

30. John Haslam, *Illustrations of Madness* (London: Printed by G. Hayden, 1810); facsimile edition, reprinted with an introduction by Roy Porter (London and New York: Routledge, 1988).

31. Cheyne, *The English Malady.* For a biography of the obese diet doctor and soi-disant expert on hypochondria and the vapors, useful though marred by some postmodern posturing, see Anita Guerrini, *Obesity and Depression in the Enlightenment: The Life and Times of George Cheyne* (Norman: University of Oklahoma Press, 2000).

32. Joan Lane, *John Hall and His Patient;* see also the review of this book by Anne Borsay in *Social History of Medicine* 11.2 (Aug. 1998), pp. 315–16.

3. PROFILING PATIENTS AND PATTERNS OF PRACTICE

1. See, however, Akihito Suzuki's fine paper "The Household and the Care of Lunatics" for a subtle examination of some of the available evidence.

2. CB, pp. C-62, C-115.

3. See Andrews and Scull, *Undertaker of the Mind,* chaps. 4 and 6.

4. CB, p. C-8.

5. See, e.g., Lane, *John Hall and His Patients,* as well as Anne Borsay's review of this book in *Social History of Medicine* 11.2 (Aug. 1998), esp. p. 316.

6. Pargeter, *Observations on Maniacal Disorders,* pp. 133–34. For more on this case, in particular with regard to lunar conceptions of epilepsy, see below.

7. While Monro saw only 100 different patients, he made 108 consultations, each of which has been counted in this calculation. If cases seen more than once during 1766 are counted singly, the proportion is 60:39, the sex in one case being unspecified.

8. E.g., CB, pp. C-37, C-63, C-110.

9. CB, pp. C-26–27, C-118.

10. CB, pp. C-15, C-29, C-39, C-42, C-79, C-118.

11. For these cases, see CB, pp. C-25, C-39, C-40, C-45–46, C-56, C-63–64, C-95, C-106, C-118.

12. Anne Digby, *Making a Medical Living: Doctors and Patients in the English Market for Medicine, 1720–1911* (Cambridge: Cambridge University Press, 1994); Irvine Loudon, *Medical Care and the General Practitioner, 1750–1850* (Oxford and New York: Clarendon Press/Oxford University Press, 1986).

13. See H. Temple Phillips, "The History of the Old Private Lunatic Asylum at Fishponds, Bristol, 1740–1859," unpublished M.Sc. thesis, Bristol University, 1973; and Joseph Mason Cox, *Practical Observations on Insanity* (London: Baldwin and Murray, 1804).

14. [Edward Long Fox], *Brislington House: An Asylum for Lunatics Situate Near Bristol, on the Road from Bath* (Bristol: For the author, 1806); A. Fox, "A Short Account of Brislington House, 1804–1906," *Brislington House Quarterly News, Centenary Number* (1906), pp. 4–14. Brislington House remained in the Fox family until it closed its doors in 1951. See also Francis Fox, *History and Present State of Brislington House near Bristol. An Asylum for the Care and Reception of Insane Persons. Established by Edward Long Fox M.D. A.D. 1804. And Now Conducted by Francis and Charles Fox M.D.* (Bristol: Light and Ridler, 1836).

15. Francis Willis Jr., *A Treatise on Mental Derangement* (London: Longman, 1823); Richard Hunter and Ida Macalpine, *George III and the Mad Business* (London: Allen Lane, 1969). On Willis Sr. and George III, see also Andrews and Scull, *Undertaker of the Mind,* chap. 6.

16. MacKenzie, *Psychiatry for the Rich.*

17. William Ll. Parry-Jones, *The Trade in Lunacy: A Study of Private Mad-*

houses in England in the Eighteenth and Nineteenth Centuries (London: Routledge and Kegan Paul, 1972), pp. 77, 116.

18. Ibid., pp. 77, 132–33.

19. The first proprietor, Thomas Bakewell (1761–1835), succeeded his uncle and grandfather, who had also kept a madhouse, and he was succeeded in turn by his son, Samuel Glover Bakewell, M.D. (1811–66). See Parry-Jones, *Trade in Lunacy,* pp. 77, 93; Leonard D. Smith, "To Cure Those Afflicted with the Disease of Insanity: Thomas Bakewell and Spring Vale Asylum," *History of Psychiatry* 4.1 (March 1993), pp. 107–28; and Smith, "Close Confinement in Mighty Prison: Thomas Bakewell and His Campaign against Public Asylums, 1810–1830," *History of Psychiatry* 5.2 (June 1994), pp. 191–214.

20. Parry-Jones, *Trade in Lunacy,* pp. 77–78.

21. CB, pp. C-47, C-73.

22. CB, p. C-92. See also, e.g., cases of Mr. Jones, who "came to me very much confus'd and frighted"; Mr. Bevan, who "called upon me this morning [and] . . . had [also] call'd upon me about a fortnight ago"; an anonymous man who "came to me to relate his case," and a woman who "came to me at home to ask my advice"; CB, pp. C-8, C-29–30, C-70, C-75.

23. E.g., Mrs. Hampson of Hitchin, Herts; Mrs. Alcock of Sussex; Mr. Inge of Tunbridge, Mr. Stanfield of Huntingdon, and Mrs. Brookes of Malling, in Kent; his foreign patients included Mrs. Moreati from Italy, wife of an Italian artist employed in London; and Mr. Rosat of Switzerland, formerly a merchant in Turkey. Miss Hume, born in Antigua, was probably of English descent. See CB, pp. C-13, C-41, C-63, C-80, C-89, C-119, C-120, C-123.

24. Loudon, *Medical Care and the General Practitioner;* Porter, *Patients and Practitioners.*

25. CB, pp. C-120–21.

26. CB, p. C-112 and note.

27. For Scottish cases, see, e.g., CB, pp. C-6, C-43, C-96. The infamous Corrector Alexander Cruden was also, of course, of Scottish extraction (see Andrews and Scull, *Undertaker of the Mind,* chap. 3).

28. E.g., Sir John Sinclair, *Observations on the Scottish Dialect* (London; Edinburgh: Printed for W. Strahan and T. Cadell; W. Creech, 1782); James Anderson, *Present State of the Hebrides* (Edinburgh: Printed for C. Elliot; London: Printed for G. G. J. and J. Robinson, 1785); Samuel Johnson, *A Journey to the Western Isles of Scotland* (London: W. Strahan and T. Cadel, 1775); Donald M'Nichol, *Remarks on Johnson's Journey to the Hebrides* (London: T. Cadell, 1782); Thomas Pennant, *A Tour in Scotland* (1769; London: Chester B. White, 1771); Robert Lindsay, *History of Scotland from 1436 to 1565 . . . ,* ed. R. Freebairn (Edinburgh: Freebairn, 1728); William Robertson, *History of Scotland,* 2 vols. (London: For A. Millar, 1759); Robert Monro, *Expedition with the Worthy Scots Regiment* (London: W. Jones, 1637); Donald Monro, *An Essay on the Dropsy* (London: D. Wilson and T. Durham, 1755); Donald Monro, *Dissertatio medica inauguralis, de hydrope* (Edinburgh: Hamilton, Balfour, and Neil, 1753); Alexander Monro, *Anatomy of the Human Bones and Nerves,* 6th ed. (Edinburgh: G. Hamilton and J. Balfour, 1758); *Edinburgh Medical Essays* (Edinburgh: 1737 and 1747); James Mackenzie, *The History of Health, and the*

Art of Preserving it . . . (Edinburgh and London: Printed and sold by William Gordon . . . , 1758); and Peter Shaw, trans., *Pharmacopoeia Edinburgensis: or, the Dispensatory of the Royal College of Physicians in Edinburgh* . . . (London: W. Innys and J. Richardson, 1753); all these works are itemized in John Monro, *Bibliotheca Elegantissima Monroiana. A Catalogue of the Elegant and Valuable Library of John Monro, M.D. Physician to Bethlehem Hospital, Lately Deceased; which will be Sold by Auction by Leigh & Sotheby* . . . *April 23d, 1792, and the Fourteen Following Days, (Sundays Excepted)* . . . , nos. 367, 645–46, 935, 1034, 1042, 1073–74, 1086, 1101, 1205, 1293, 1301, 1641 (London: For Leigh and Sotheby, 1792). The presence in John Monro's library of a number of books by the Scottish moral philosophers Thomas Reid, D.D. (1710–96), and John Gregory, M.D. (1724–73) (namely, Reid's *An Inquiry into the Human Mind* . . . [London: Printed for T. Cadell, . . . and T. Longman; Edinburgh: For A. Kincaid and J. Bell, 1769] and *Essays on the Intellectual Powers of Man*, nos. 1135 and 1202 [Edinburgh: Printed for John Bell; London: For G. G. J. and J. Robinson, 1785], and Gregory's *A Comparative View of the State and Faculties of Man. With those of the Animal World*, no. 698 [London: Printed for J. Dodsley, 1765]), and of works such as James Usher's *An Introduction to the Theory of the Human Mind*, no. 1334 (London: T. Davis, 1771), makes one wonder how much Monro may have been influenced in his later life by Reid's and Gregory's more psychological approach to human nature and by other ideas of the Scottish Enlightenment. Monro's library also included works by that other famous medico-moral philosopher of the Scottish Enlightenment, Francis Hutcheson, M.D. (1694–1746): e.g., his *Thoughts on Laughter* . . . , no. 863 (Glasgow: Printed by Robert and Andrew Foulis, 1757–58). For more discussion of Monro's library, see Andrews and Scull, *Undertaker of the Mind*, p. 278 n. 122, p. 284 n. 42, page 296 n. 12, p. 300 n. 57, p. 310 n. 8.

29. E.g., see William Murray [Lord Mansfield], *The Thistle; a Dispassionate Examine of the Prejudice of Englishmen in General to the Scotch Nation; and Particularly of a late Arrogant Insult Offered to all Scotchmen, by a Modern English Journalist. In a Letter to the Author of Old England of Dec. 27, 1746*, 2nd ed. (London: H. Carpenter, 1747).

30. CB, pp. C-41–42.

31. For accounts of Dalton, Bartolozzi, Strange, etc., see, e.g., William T. Whitley, *Artists and Their Friends in England 1700–1799* (New York and London: Benjamin Bloom, 1968; originally London and Boston: The Medical Society, 1928), vol. 1, pp. 146, 158–59, 201–2, 227, 229, 307–9; vol. 2, pp. 72, 112, 276–77, 315.

32. Securities (or "bondsmen") were those who signed a bond as security to undertake financial responsibility for another party. In Bethlem's case, the requirement was for two men who were "housekeepers" (i.e., those who owned or paid rent for a house in London or the suburbs) to enter into a bond of £100 to pay for the bedding and clothes during a patient's continuance in the hospital, to remove the patient when discharged, and to pay the charge for burial if the patient died in the hospital. See Jonathan Andrews, "Bedlam Revisited. A History of Bethlem Hospital, c. 1634–1770" (Ph.D. diss., University of London, 1991), appendices 6e, 6f, 6g, and 6h, pp. 566–69.

33. See CB, pp. C-7–8. We are extremely grateful to the archivist Colin Gale, at the Bethlem Royal Hospital Archives, for his hard, if fruitless, work attempting to track down Mrs. Walker for us.

34. For Goupy and Sarah Wright, see *Dictionary of National Biography* (hereafter DNB); Whitley, *Artists,* vol. 1, pp. 8, 44, 68–69, 72–75, 135; vol. 2, p. 72.

35. Goupy's will confirms that he was far from prosperous. He did not expect to die worth much more than £300 and had very little of either liquid assets or personal possessions to dispose of, beyond a debt of £264 owed him by Henry Furness, a sum that he had already gone to Chancery to attest his right to. In the event of Sarah's death the inheritance was to pass to her sister's son, Abraham Purshouse. Possibly the necessary funds for Sarah's maintenance before Goupy's death had come from the proceeds of the sale of his pictures, which we know had taken place in 1765. For Goupy's will, see PCC Prob. 11/949, qn 207, in Family Records Centre, Angel, London.

36. G. S. Rousseau and Roy Porter, eds., *Sexual Underworlds of the Enlightenment,* new ed. (1987; Manchester: Manchester University Press, 1992); Tim Hitchcock, *English Sexualities, 1700–1800* (Basingstoke: Macmillan, 1997); Rosalind Mitchison, *Sexuality and Social Control: Scotland 1660–1780* (Oxford: Basil Blackwell, 1989).

37. See, for instance, G. W. Thornbury, *Life of J. W. M. Turner* (London: Chatto and Windus, 1904); and Thomas Monro, *Dr Thomas Monro (1759–1833) and the Monro Academy, Prints, and Drawing Gallery, February–May 1976* (London: Victoria and Albert Museum, 1976).

38. This diary, like the case book itself, is in the private possession of the Jefferiss family, and, again, we are extremely grateful to them for furnishing us with a Xerox copy of the text.

39. See the discussion of Monro's tenure of this fellowship in Andrews and Scull, *Undertaker of the Mind,* chap. 1.

40. Monro's library (see also note 28, above) included a wide range of books on art, artists, and antiquities, including Lodovico Dolce, *Aretin: A Dialogue on Painting* (Glasgow: Printed for Robert Urie, 1770); William Gilpin, *An Essay on Prints,* 3rd ed. (London: Printed by G. Scott, for R. Blamire; sold by B. Law and R. Faulder, 1781); *Catalogue of Mr Pond'd Etchings and Prints Purchased by Sir E. Astley* (1760); *Catalogue of Uvedden Collection of Prints and Drawings* (1762); Horace Walpole, *Aedes Walpolianae: A Description of the Plates at Houghton Hall,* 2nd ed. (London: Printed by J. Hughs, 1752); Walpole, *Anecdotes of Painting in England . . .* (Twickenham, Strawberry Hill: Thomas Farmer, 1762); Walpole, *Catalogue of Engravers . . . ,* 5 vols. (Strawberry Hill: Thomas Farmer, 1762); James Chelsum, *History of the Art of Engraving in Mezzotinto from its Origins to the Present Time* (Winchester: Printed by J. Robbins; London: Sold by J. and T. Egerton, 1786); and Pierre Monier, *History of Painting, Sculpture, Architecture, Graving . . .* (London: Printed for T. Bennet, D. Midwinter, T. Leigh, and R. Knaplock . . . , 1699). Monro was far from the only contemporary physician to see the social advantages of cultivating a taste in the arts, another notable example being Richard Mead. Monro's collection of books included several of Mead's catalogues: *Catalogue of Dr Mead's Collection of*

Prints and Drawings (undated); *Catalogue of Dr Mead's Pictures* (1764); *Collection of Prints and Drawings* (1755); and *Collection of Gems, Bronzes, Marble and Other Busts* (1755). Monro, *Bibliotheca Elegantissima*, nos. 465–69, 634, 685, 1065, 1072, 1689.

41. See the discussion of this case in Andrews and Scull, *Undertaker of the Mind*, chap. 5.

42. Joseph Strutt, *A Biographical Dictionary; Containing an Historical Account of all the Engravers, from the Earliest Period of the Art of Engraving to the Present Time; and a . . . List of their most Esteemed Works; with the Cyphers, Monograms, and Particular Marks used by each Master . . . To which is Prefixed, an Essay on the Rise and Progress of the Art of Engraving, etc.,* 2 vols. (London: Printed by J. Davis for R. Faulder, 1785); Robert Miller Christy, *Joseph Strutt, Author, Artist, Engraver, and Antiquary, 1749–1802: A Biography* (London: 1912); Joseph Strutt, *A Memoir of the Life of Joseph Strutt, 1749–1802: A Biography* (London: Printed for private circulation, 1896); Thomas Dodd, *A Catalogue of the Extensive and Truly Magnificent Collection of Prints . . . of the French, Flemish, German, and English Engravers . . . also . . . Strutt's Dictionary of Engravers, Illustrated by upwards of 4000 prints, by the Different Artists Therein Mentioned, Arranged in Chronological Order, Forming 24 Volumes . . .* (London: T. Dodd, 1810); Brenda Lilian Hough, "A Consideration of the Antiquarian and Literary Works of Joseph Strutt: With Transcript of a Hitherto Unedited Manuscript Novel," unpublished Ph.D. diss. (Arts), University of London, Queen Mary College, 1984.

43. Samuel Johnson and George Steevens, *The Plays of William Shakespeare: With the Corrections and Illustrations of Various Commentators* (London: Printed for C. Bathurst, 1773). See also George Steevens, *To the Public. Had the last Editor of the Plays of Shakespeare met with the Assistance he had Reason to Expect . . .* (London: 1766); and John Nichols, George Steevens, and George Whetstone, *Six Old Plays, on which Shakespeare Founded his Measure for Measure, Comedy of Errors, Taming the Shrew, King John, King Henry IV and King Henry, King Lear* (London: Printed for S. Leacroft and sold by J. Nichols, 1779).

44. See Bethlem Court of Governors Minutes (henceforth BCGM), 26 Feb. 1752, p. 40, and below, note 66.

45. BCGM, 27 Feb. 1751, p. 484; and 26 Feb. 1752, p. 40.

46. Hogarth was elected a governor less than nine months before James Monro's death and John's appointment as sole physician in his stead, but no record of who nominated him is entered in the governors' minutes. See BCGM, 26 Feb. 1752, p. 40. Mendez had secured his own governorship just before this through the customary £100 charitable donation to the hospitals, which was conveyed to the treasurer by another governor, Alderman Ironside. See BCGM, 1 and 27 Feb. 1751, pp. 480, 483–84.

47. E.g., William Hogarth, *The Analysis of Beauty: Written with a View of Fixing the Fluctuating Ideas of Taste* (London: Printed by J. Reeves for the author, 1753); John Nichols, *Biographical Anecdotes of William Hogarth: With a Catalogue of his Works Chronologically Arranged; and Occasional Remarks,* 2nd ed. (London: Printed by and for J. Nichols, 1782); Monro, *Bibliotheca Elegantissima*, nos. 944, 1085. See notes 28 and 39 above.

48. The evidence is unclear on this point, and it must be acknowledged that the hospital's open access to visitors may have provided Hogarth with all the opportunity he needed. James was also, apparently, the first physician of the family to have his portrait painted by a leading contemporary artist, John Michael Williams (1747). Like that of John Monro, commissioned later, the portrait was donated to the Royal College of Physicians by Henry Monro but is currently on loan to the Bethlem Royal Museum.

49. Bethlem Sub-committee Minutes (henceforth BSCM), 17 May 1783; frontispiece plate in Thomas Bowen, *An Historical Account of the Origin, Progress and Present State of Bethlehem Hospital founded by Henry the Eighth, for the Cure of Lunatics, and Enlarged by Subsequent benefactors, for the Reception and Maintenance of Incurables* (London: For the Governors, 1783). This plate appears to have been engraved by William Sharp (1749–1824), after an original drawing by the famous Royal Academician and prolific (if not monopolistic) illustrator of literary works Thomas Stothard (1755–1834). Stothard's engravings of literary works in the eighteenth century included editions of the Bible, Chaucer, Shakespeare, and Bunyan, and his original designs were also engraved for the 1821 *Caldeonian Muse,* a collection of Scottish poetry, for Cervantes's *Don Quixote,* Richardson's *Clarissa,* Sterne's *Tristram Shandy,* Swift's *Gulliver's Travels,* and for the 1790 edition of Defoe's *Robinson Crusoe* (London: John Stockdale). More pertinently, he also collaborated on Matthew Green's (1696–1737) and John Aikin's (1747–1822) *The Spleen, and other Poems* (London: Printed for T. Cadell, junr. and W. Davies, 1796); on the new edition of (the previously deranged) William Cowper's *Poems* (London: Printed for J. Johnson, etc., 1798); and on a 1799 edition of Somerville's *The Chace* (along with Aikin once again [Dublin: T. Henshall]—see below for quotes on canine madness from this work); and collaborated with Bartolozzi as engraver on Milton's *Paradise Lost* (London: Published by Jeffryes & Co., 1792–95). For biographical details, see DNB; and Shelley M. Bennett, *Thomas Stothard: The Mechanisms of Art Patronage in England circa 1800* (Columbia: University of Missouri Press, 1988). Besides his engraving for Bowen's book, Sharp also did numerous engravings for the *Lady's Magazine,* the East India Company (1792), and the *Copper Plate Magazine* (London: Printed for the proprietors, and sold by G. Kearsly, etc., 1774–77). More interestingly, Sharp was subsequently censured for his prominent involvement in the publication of the prophesies and visions of the putatively deranged Joanna Southcott (1750–1814). See Joanna Southcott [and William Sharp], *Copies and Parts of Copies of Letters and Communications, Written from Joanna Southcott, etc.* (London: 1804); William Sharp, *An Answer to the World: For Putting in Print a Book in 1804, Called Copies and Parts of Copies of Letters and Communications, Written from Joanna Southcott, and Transmitted by Miss Townley to Mr. Sharp in London* (London: Printed by S. Rousseau and sold by E. I. Field, 1806); and Joanna Southcott, *Divine and Spiritual Communications, Written by Joanna Southcott on the Prayers of the Church of England, the Conduct of the Clergy and Calvinistic Methodists, etc.,* with an introduction by W. Sharp (London, 1803).

50. The Royal Academician Joseph Farington (1747–1828) refers repeatedly

to Thomas Monro and his connections with artists such as Turner and Girtin and the art world in general in his diary. He provides considerable details on the doctor's art collection and on his attendance on Cozens and the madness of other artists, as well as on Monro's attendance on George III in 1811–13 and his response to the Madhouses inquiry of 1815. See Farington, *The Farington Diary*, ed. James Greig (London: Hutchison, 1922–28), 8 vols., esp. vol. 1, entries for 26 Jan., 23 Feb., and 2 July 1794, 26 and 27 Nov. 1795, 25 Feb. 1797, 24 Oct. 1798, and 11 April 1801, pp. 37, 43, 57, 113, 115–16, 177, 193, and note 243; vol. 2, 25 Jan., 3, 4, and 5 July, and 28 Oct. 1803, pp. 74, 117, 119, 163; vol. 3, 29 Jan. 1804; vol. 4, 12 Jan. 1807, p. 74; vol. 5, 11 Feb. and 1 March 1808, 5 July 1809, 5 Jan. 1811, pp. 23, 33, 203, 222; vol. 7, 18 Nov. 1811, 29 May and 19 Nov. 1812, 5 Sept. 1813, pp. 61, 85, 113, 203; 7 March 1816, 20 April 1817, 27 July 1820, pp. 59, 122, 256. See also Whitley, *Artists*, vol. 2, p. 325. The diary of Edward Thomas Monro, which catalogues the visits of artists and others to the family home, is in the possession of the Jefferiss family.

51. Dr F. J. G. Jefferiss, "Extracts from a Biography of Dr Thomas Monro," *Dr Thomas Monro (1759–1833) and the Monro Academy, Prints, and Drawing Gallery, February–May 1976* (London: Victoria and Albert Museum, 1976).

52. Thomas Monro, *Catalogue of an Exhibition of Drawings chiefly by Dr. Thomas Monro (Prepared by A. K. Sabin)* (London: 1917); Monro, *Dr Thomas Monro (1759–1833) and the Monro Academy*. See also British Museum catalogue holdings re. Thomas Monro.

53. Farington, *Diary*, vol. 2, 5 July 1803, p. 119.

54. William Schupbach, "John Monro MD and Charles James Fox: Etching by Thomas Rowlandson," *Medical History* 27 (1983), pp. 80–83.

55. E.g., John Mitford, *A Description of the Crimes and Horrors in . . . Warburton's Private Mad-house at Hoxton . . . Called Whitmore House, etc.* (London: Benbow, 1825[?]), pp. 2–3.

56. Ibid. (George III was famous for his habit of thrice repeating isolated words or phrases in the course of his conversation.) As Elaine Murphy has commented (personal communication, 26 April 2000), the general picture of Warburton that emerges from contemporary accounts is of "a vulgarian promoted by luck and cunning," a one-time butcher's apprentice clawing his way to a fortune from the mad-business, ruthlessly speculating in human misery.

57. See Dorothy Stroud, *George Dance, Architect, 1741–1825* (London: Faber and Faber, 1971); George Dance [the Elder] and George Dance [the Younger], *George Dance, the Elder 1695–1768, the Younger 1741–1825: [Catalogue of] the first Exhibition Devoted to these two Distinguished Architects, from 7 July to 30 September 1972 [held at the] Geffrye Museum, Kingsland Road, E.2* (London: Inner London Education Authority, 1972); and George Dance [the Younger], *A Collection of Portraits Sketched from the Life Since the Year 1793 . . . and Engraved in Imitation of the Original Drawings by William Daniell* (London: Longman, Hurst, Rees, Orme, and Brown [etc.], 1809–14).

58. For the Dances' work in connection with St. Luke's, see C. N. French, *The Story of St Luke's Hospital* (London: Heinemann, 1951), pp. 9, 11, 27, 28, 32; and Jonathan Andrews, "Bedlam Revisited: A History of Bethlem Hospital,

c. 1634–1770," unpublished Ph.D. diss., University of London, 1991, appendix 3a(i), p. 559.

59. See Nathaniel Dance and George Dance, *Catalogue of an Exhibition Held at Greater London Council, The Iveagh Bequest . . . 25 June to 4 September, 1977*, introduction by David Goodreau, "Retirement, Comic Drawings by Nathaniel and George Dance the Younger," pp. 54–60 (London: Greater London Council, 1977); and Dance and Dance, *"The Sublime and Beautiful": Portraits and other drawings by Nathaniel Dance and George Dance [catalogue of an exhibition held at the Sabin Galleries, 27 March-18 April 1973]* (London: Sabin Galleries, 1973). Nathaniel Dance seems to have shared Monro's appreciation for Shakespeare, Dance having painted the Bard and this portrait being engraved for Bell's 1774 edition of Shakespeare's works (London: Printed for J. Bell . . . and C. Etherington at York, 1774).

60. See Dance's plans, held at the Corporation of London Record Office, Guildhall, Comp. CL. 114, 126b, 303, dated ca. 1761 and 1790. The first set of plans, which are of the Little Moorgate region, probably relate to Bethlem's application for a lease of this land in 1762; see BCGM, 1 April 1762, pp. 15–16.

61. Farington, *Diary,* vol. 1, 11 April 1801, p. 193, note; diary of Edward Thomas Monro, covering the years ca. 1806–25, in private hands of the Jefferiss family. Sir Charles Dance, a general in the Peninsular War, was also accustomed to visit the Monros.

62. For more extended discussion of these matters, see Andrews and Scull, *Undertaker of the Mind,* chap. 5.

4. THE CRAFT OF CONSULTATION

1. In this respect, they resembled many of their nineteenth- and twentieth-century counterparts, although the ability of the family to contain such problems was more regularly undermined during subsequent centuries, as the public sphere was to play a much larger role in influencing the family's decisions over lunacy. See, e.g., Akihito Suzuki's discussion of the attempts of nineteenth-century families to contain insane family members within the home, as revealed by commission in lunacy legal proceedings, "Enclosing and Disclosing Lunatics in the Family Walls: Domestic Psychiatric Regime and the Public Sphere in Early Nineteenth-Century England," *Outside the Walls of the Asylum: The History of Care in the Community 1750–2000,* eds. Peter Bartlett and David Wright (London: Athlone, 1999), pp. 115–31. For twentieth-century evidence of the reluctance of families to contemplate hospitalization, even in the face of profound disturbance in an intimate, see Marian Radke Yarrow, Charlotte Green Schwartz, Harriet S. Murphy, and Leila Calhoun Deasy, "The Psychological Meaning of Mental Illness in the Family," *Journal of Social Issues* 11 (1955), pp. 12–24; Charlotte Green Schwartz, "Perspectives on Deviance: Wives' Definitions of Their Husbands' Mental Illness," *Psychiatry* 20 (1957), pp. 275–91; and Harold Sampson, Sheldon L. Messinger, and Robert D. Towne, "Family Process and Becoming a Mental Patient," *American Journal of Sociology* 68 (1962), pp. 88–96.

2. Such attitudes did not evaporate with time. A century and a half after

Monro made his entries in his case book, the official organ of a by-now highly organized profession still lamented the persistent public prejudice that infected their practice:

> A large portion of the public, owing to its prejudice against insanity, avoid, until compelled by the direst necessity, any approach to a physician who has experience in treating it. To avoid doing so, they will often resort to the treatment of persons whose knowledge of insanity is practically *nil.* . . . If a medical man is consulted, care is taken, in the large majority of cases, that he is not one whose name is associated with mental diseases; it is only in the last resort, when means are exhausted and the mental breakdown is complete, that an alienist is resorted to. (Anon., "The Disabilities of Alienist Physicians," *Journal of Mental Science* 59 [1913], p. 144, emphasis in the original)

3. CB, pp. C-112–13.

4. John Purcell, *A Treatise of Vapours: or, Hysterick Fits* (London: Newman and Cox, 1702); [Sir] Richard Blackmore, *A Treatise of the Spleen and Vapours: Or, Hypochondriacal and Hysterical Affections. With Three Discourses on the Nature and Cure of the Cholick, Melancholy, and Palsies* (London: Pemberton, 1725); Cheyne, *The English Malady.*

5. For discussion of this issue, see Andrew Scull, *The Most Solitary of Afflictions: Madness and Society in Britain, 1700–1900* (London and New Haven, Conn.: Yale University Press, 1993), pp. 356–61.

6. As late as 1885, Hayes Newington, the proprietor of the English aristocracy's preferred madhouse, Ticehurst Asylum, mournfully acknowledged the reluctance of his potential clientele to use his services:

> Many of the upper classes can and do retain the services of independent specialists and get well without leaving home, or are sent away to medical men's houses. We, therefore, can say that . . . what we . . . get are not infrequently the residue of unsuccessful treatment elsewhere . . . in the case of the wealthy it is well known that an asylum is generally the last thing thought of. (H. F. Hayes Newington, "The Abolition of Private Asylums," *Journal of Mental Science* 31 [1885], p. 143)

7. CB, pp. C-112–13.

8. N. D. Jewson, "Medical Knowledge and the Patronage System in Eighteenth-Century England," *Sociology* 8 (1974), pp. 369–85; Jewson, "The Disappearance of the Sick Man from Medical Cosmology," *Sociology* 10 (1976), pp. 225–44.

9. CB, p. C-9.

10. CB, pp. C-77–78.

11. We are grateful to Trevor Turner for drawing our attention to this point.

12. Our thanks to Steven Shapin for drawing Cheyne's correspondence to our attention.

13. Cheyne to Richardson, July 16, 1739, reprinted in "The Letters of Doctor George Cheyne to Samuel Richardson (1733–1743)," ed. Charles F. Mullett, *University of Missouri Studies,* vol. 18 (Columbia: University of Missouri, 1943), p. 54.

14. On a typical occasion, Cheyne insisted that

> Your Cure . . . Consists:—I. In artificial vomits on great Occasions, and Daily Pumping or Thumb Vomits in the Intervals. II. In little Phlebotomies [bleedings] once a

month or two, to let out the bad Blood and supply with good from Regimen. III. Air and exercise as much as possibly you can take. IV. Perseverance, obstinate and inflexible, in your Milk and Seed Diet . . . V. Chewing a little Rhubarb on Costiveness at Night, and fine Bark in the Day Time . . . You must not think of Jellies; they are Fleshglue, and never digest, but plaster up the concoctive Organs . . . You must lose every *Atom* of the Solids and every *Globule* of the Liquids before you can revive.

And so forth. Cheyne to Richardson, 2 May 1742, *University of Missouri Studies*, vol. 18, pp. 94–95. For further examples among many, see Cheyne to Richardson, 22 June 1738, pp. 37–38; 13 May 1739, pp. 49–50; 20 June 1739, pp. 51–52; 12 Sept. 1739, pp. 56–57; 12 Jan. 1740, pp. 58–59; 12 Feb. 1741, pp. 64–66; 23 Dec. 1741, pp. 76–78.

15. Cheyne to Richardson, 30 Sept. 1738, *University of Missouri Studies*, vol. 18, p. 42.

16. Cheyne to Richardson, 26 April 1742, *University of Missouri Studies*, vol. 18, p. 93.

17. Cheyne to Lady Huntingdon, 19 July 1732, *The Letters of Dr. George Cheyne to the Countess of Huntingdon*, ed. Charles F. Mullett (San Marino, Calif.: Huntington Library, 1940), pp. 4–5.

18. Cheyne to Lady Huntingdon, 29 Dec. 1733, *Letters*, p. 31.

19. Cheyne to Lady Huntingdon, 4 Sept. 1733, *Letters*, pp. 22–23.

20. Cheyne to Lady Huntingdon, 6 Sept. 1735, *Letters*, pp. 50–51.

21. CB, pp. C-57–58.

22. See MacDonald, *Mystical Bedlam*, passim.

23. Again, our thanks to Trevor Turner for the last point.

24. Richard Mead, *A Treatise Concerning the Influence of the Sun and Moon Upon Human Bodies, and the Diseases Thereby Produced . . .* , trans. from the Latin [of the second edition] . . . by T. Stack, etc. (London: Printed for J. Brindley, 1748); originally [*De imperio solis ac lunae in corpora humana, etc.*] *A Discourse Concerning the Action of the Sun and Moon on Animal Bodies; and the Influence Which this May Have in Many Diseases . . . In Two Parts* (London: 1708; 2nd ed., London: Printed for Richard Wellington . . . , 1712). The association of the moon with lunacy provoked endless jibes, couched in lunar metaphors, at the supposed lunatics of the age. See, e.g., Anon., *Pills to Cure Melancholy; or England's Witty and Ingenious Jester: Shewing, no Joke like a True Joke. Containing the Merry Jests of the Earls of Rochester, Pembroke, Warwick, Lord Moon, and Mr. Ogle, the Life Guard Man . . .* (London: Printed for the author, ca. 1750–90), a chapbook that included a skit on John Ogle, a millenarian lifeguardsman who had been admitted to Bethlem under John's father, James Monro. This chapbook was repeatedly reissued in various versions, and there even seems to have been an 1805 edition published in Warrington, entitled *The Diverting Humours of John Ogle*. It was apparently issued originally under a different title: Anon., *Joaks upon Joaks; or, No Joak Like a True Joak: Being the Diverting Humours of John Ogle, Life-Guard-Man. The Merry Pranks of the Lord Mohun, the Earls of Warwick and Pembroke. With the Lord Rochester's Dream; his Maiden's Disappointment* (London: T. Norris, ca. 1720). The date of this source is imprecise, but later editions were, according to the Bodleian and the

British Library, printed and sold in Bow-Church-Yard and other places in the city between ca. 1740 and 1790.

25. Pargeter, *Observations on Maniacal Disorders*, pp. 133–34. Contemporary psychiatrists, mental nurses, and astrologers remain fascinated by this subject, although few modern studies have succeeded in any significant correlation between lunar cycles and mental illness/agitation. See, e.g., Karen Ward, "'Moon Madness': A Study to Investigate the Relationship between Human Behaviour and the Phases of the Moon," unpublished diss. (B. Nur.), University of Nottingham, 1997. During the late 1980s, Robert Howard, a Maudsley Hospital psychiatrist, went so far as to map the timing of patients' escapes from eighteenth-century Bethlem against contemporary lunar cycles and found no confluence of any importance.

26. Tobias George Smollett, *Roderick Random* (Oxford: Oxford University Press, 1981), chap. 63, p. 390.

27. CB, pp. C-2, C-36–37.

28. CB, p. C-87.

29. CB, pp. C-100–105.

30. CB, pp. C-89–90.

31. For discussion, see Andrews and Scull, *Undertaker of the Mind*, chap. 5.

32. Horace Walpole, *Correspondence*, vol. 33 (1954), ed. W. S. Lewis (New Haven, Conn.: Yale University Press, 1937–83), Horace Walpole (henceforth HW) to Horace Mann, 30 July 1783, pp. 423–24. Of course, insanity in a family was invested with its own marital stigma on physical grounds in this period, the threat of passing on a congenital history of madness (which families were also wont to conceal) provoking the breaking off of a good many contemporary engagements. As Walpole himself put it, if "there is madness in the lover's family—how can a parent consent to such an union" (see ibid.). Marrying into madness was generally represented as something of a social anathema among the educated elite, although this itself constituted a recognition of—by way of a persuasion against—the relative frequency of such marriages.

33. Robert Halsband, ed., *The Selected Letters of Lady Mary Wortley Montagu* (Harmondsworth, Middlesex: Penguin, 1970), Mary Wortley Montagu to Lady Bute, 1 March 1752, p. 232. Dismissing the novel, despite weeping over it, as having a subversive tendency to inspire tenderness for deviance and vice, she claimed that "any girl that runs away with a young fellow without intending to marry him should be carried to Bridewell or Bedlam the next day."

34. Reginald Blunt, ed., *Mrs Montagu "Queen of the Blues." Her Letters and Friendships from 1762 to 1800* (London: Constable & Co., 1923), vol. 2, p. 205, letter dated 2 Feb. 1786. See, also, Henry Frederick Thompson, *The Intrigues of a Nabob (R. Barwell): Or, Bengal the Fittest Soil for the Growth of Lust, Injustice and Dishonesty, etc.* (London[?]: Printed for the author, 1780); Warren Hastings, *Original Letters from Warren Hastings, Esq. Sir Eyre Coote, K.B. and Richard Barwell, Esq. to Sir Thomas Rumbold, Bart. and Lord Macartney, K.B.* (London: Printed for J. Debrett, 1787); East India Company Official Documents, *Observations of the Court of Directors on the Conduct of Warren Hastings, Sir J. Clavering, Colonel G. Monson, R. Barwell, and P. Francis, in the Service of the East India Company* (London: East India Company, 1787); Thomas

George Percival Spear, *The Nabobs: A Study of the Social Life of the English in Eighteenth-Century India*, 2nd enlarged ed. (London: Oxford University Press, 1932; 2nd enlarged edition, London [etc.]: Curzon Press, 1980); Michael Edwardes, *Warren Hastings: King of the Nabobs* (London: Hart-Davis, MacGibbon, 1976); and Edwardes, *The Nabobs at Home* (London: Constable, 1991).

35. Thomas Monro [of Magdalen College (1764–1815)], *Essays on Various Subjects . . .* (London: Printed by J. Nichols and sold by C. G. J. and J. Robinson, 1790), p. 165.

36. Nicholas Robinson, *A New System of the Spleen, Vapours, and Hypochondriack Melancholy: Wherein all the Decays of the Nerves, and Lowness of the Spirits, are Mechanically Accounted For* (London: A. Bettesworth, Innys, and Rivington, 1729), pp. 399–400.

37. CB, pp. C-91–92.

38. Typically, George Cheyne cited "an unactive [*sic*], sedentary, or studious life" as a major cause "of the Frequency of nervous Disorders"; *The English Malady*, pp. xx, 52–54. For general background on the long tradition of medical moralizing about the ill effects of solitude and idleness on the mind, see, e.g., Roy Porter, *Mind-Forg'd Manacles*, pp. 60, 88, 93–94, 169.

39. CB, pp. C-44, C-74. Two years after this entry, Tissot's influential treatise, *An Essay on Diseases Incidental to Literary and Sedentary Persons. With Proper Rules for Preventing their Fatal Consequences and Instructions for their Cure* (London: E. and C. Dilly, 1768), received its first English translation. Originally written in Latin under the title *Sermo Inauguralis de Valetudine Litteratorum*, this work was first published in his vernacular French in 1761 under the title *Avis aux Gens de Lettres* (Lausanne: De l'imprimerie de J. Zimmerli, aux depens de François Grasset, 1761). Reprinted as *Avis aux Gens de Lettres et aux Personnes Sedentaires sur leur Santé* (Paris: Chez J. Th. Herissant fils, 1767), from 1768 it was reissued repeatedly under the title *De la Santé des Gens de Lettres*. The book went into a second English edition in 1769 and was reprinted in 1772. Tissot had counseled identically against sedentary and solitary habits in his book *Avis au Peuple sur sa Santé* (Lausanne: De l'imprimerie de J. Zimmerli, aux depens de François Grasset, 1761), which went into numerous reprints and was first published in English in 1765 as *Advice to the People in General, with Regard to their Health* (London: T. Becket and P. A. de Hondt, 1765).

40. CB, pp. C-3–4.

5. DIAGNOSING THE MAD

1. We owe this last point to the psychiatrist and historian Trevor Turner, who asserts that Monro's approach here accords closely with modern British psychiatric practice.

2. CB, pp. C-10–15, C-25–26, C-34–37, C-41–42, C-61, C-96–97.

3. CB, p. C-99.

4. CB, pp. C-21, C-63–64.

5. CB, pp. C-9–10, C-47–48, C-98–99.

6. For a full exploration of the case of Margaret Nicholson, see Andrews and Scull, *Undertaker of the Mind,* pp. 215–53.

7. CB, pp. C-9–10, C-72.

8. CB, pp. C-3, C-29, C-38, C-65, C-73, C-79, C-87, C-90, C-107.

9. CB, pp. C-29, C-35–36.

10. CB, pp. C-7–8.

11. See especially Allan Ingram, *The Madhouse of Language: Writing and Reading Madness in the Eighteenth Century* (London and New York: Routledge, 1991).

12. CB, pp. C-40–41.

13. We owe this suggestion to Trevor Turner.

14. Michael MacDonald, "Insanity and the Realities of History in Early Modern England," *Psychological Medicine* 11 (1981), pp. 11–25, reprinted in *Lectures on the History of Psychiatry. The Squibb Series,* eds. R. M. Murray and T. H. Turner (London: Gaskell, 1990), pp. 60–81; see esp. pp. 67–68. Foucault's emphasis was rather on "delirium" than on "delusion" per se: *Madness and Civilisation: A History of Insanity in the Age of Reason* (London: Tavistock, 1971), trans. and abr. from *Histoire de la folie à l'âge classique* (Paris: Librairie Plon, 1961), chap. 4, pp. 85–116.

15. CB, pp. C-40–41.

16. CB, pp. C-108–9. For the involvement of both James and John Monro in the case of Alexander Cruden, author of a biblical concordance, would-be corrector of morals for the entire kingdom, and recurrent denizen of madhouses, see Andrews and Scull, *Undertaker of the Mind,* chap. 3.

17. CB, pp. C-19–20.

18. Besides the cases of Miss Mombray, Captain Macdonald, and the anonymous woman accompanied by Mrs. Blinkhorn, which are explicitly mentioned here and below, see also the case of Miss Compton, who "hears voices & will some times return answers," and the brother of a tallow chandler who "fancied the Devil had been talking to him"; CB, pp. C-9–10, C-79. Less clear-cut cases of possible auditory hallucinations include Mr. Coltman, who "imagined some of the company had been talking disrespectfully of him"; CB, p. C-24.

19. Most patients, it should be emphasized, appear to have come willingly, although it is often unclear exactly what avenues of referral Monro's cases followed.

20. CB, pp. C-69–70.

21. Philippe Pinel, *A Treatise on Insanity* (New York: Hafner, 1962), trans. from *Traité médico-philosophique sur l'alienation mentale, ou la manie;* facsimile of the 1806 ed. (London); Jean Etienne Esquirol, *Mental Maladies: A Treatise on Insanity,* with an introduction by Raymond de Saussure (New York: Hafner, 1965); facsimile of the 1845 English ed.

22. John Pringle, *Observations on the Nature and Cure of Hospital and Jayl Fevers, in a Letter to Dr Mead . . .* (London: A. Millar and D. Wilson, 1750); Daniel Turner, *Discourse Concerning Fevers . . .* (London: Printed for John Clarke, 1727); John Huxham, *An Essay on Fevers . . . With Dissertations on Slow Nervous Fevers . . . [etc.]* (London: S. Austen, 1750); James Carmichael Smyth, *An Account of the Effects of Swinging, Employed as a Remedy in the Pul-*

monary Consumption and Hectic Fever (London: J. Johnson, 1787). The library also included William Threlfal's *Essay on Epilepsy. In Which a New Theory of that Disease is Attempted, etc.* (London: 1772) and Benjamin Hoadly's *Three Lectures on the Organs of Perspiration . . . the Gulstonian Lectures . . .* (London: Printed for W. Wilkins and sold by J. Roberts, 1740). See Monro, *Bibliotheca Elegantissima*, nos. 662, 868, 943, 1639, 1644.

23. CB, pp. C-1–2. On black slaves in the eighteenth-century metropolis, see Gretchen Gerzina, *Black London: Life before Emancipation* (London: John Murray; New Brunswick, N.J.: Rutgers University Press, 1995).

24. CB, pp. C-40–41.

25. For these hysterical cases, see CB, pp. C-45–46, C-70–71. For the case of hypochondria, see CB, p. C-62.

26. CB, pp. C-70–71.

27. The trial of Lawrence Earl Ferrers before the House of Lords for the murder of his steward was one of the most sensational criminal trials of the eighteenth century. Monro was called as a defense witness by Ferrers, marking the first occasion in Anglo-American jurisprudence that a mad-doctor testified as an expert on the issue of insanity. For a detailed discussion of the crime, the trial, Monro's testimony, and Ferrers's subsequent public execution and dissection, see Andrews and Scull, *Undertaker of the Mind*, chap. 6.

28. CB, pp. C-84–85.

29. CB, p. C-98.

30. CB, pp. C-110–11.

31. CB, p. C-61.

32. CB, pp. C-94–96.

33. CB, pp. C-21–23.

34. CB, pp. C-48–50.

35. Charles Hales, *A Letter Addressed to Caesar Hawkins, Esq; Serjeant Surgeon to His Majesty, Containing New Thoughts and Observations, on the Cure of the Venereal Disease; the Result of Experience, in Long and Extensive Practice. With a few Extraordinary Cases in that Disease: Particularly one of a Servant Belonging to his Majesty's Household; Deemed Entirely a lost Case: Authenticated by the Officers of His Majesty's Mews,* 2nd ed. (London: Printed and sold by J. Wheble et al., 1755, with additions dated 1769), pp. 58–62. To exemplify, Hales referred to a patient of his who was on the verge of marriage and contracted a confirmed pox, with whom he would discourse for an hour at a time on visits. Yet his patient having had a host of medicines, Hales attributed his eventual death to the diffidence of his own judgment and that of others he consulted: "He would leave me to appearance with a tranquil mind and great spirits, fully convinced of his own tormenting misapprehensions, and reconciled to my advice: but soon after he had left me, would retire to his house, and give the utmost latitude to his agitated, and, I suppose, distracted mind" (pp. 62–63). See also Hales, *Salivation not Necessary for the Cure of the Venereal Disease in any Degree Whatever, and all Gleets Curable . . .* , 5th ed. (London: Printed for J. Almon, 1764).

36. CB, pp. C-92–94.

37. CB, pp. C-92–93.

38. See, e.g., Robert James, *A Treatise on Canine Madness* (London: Printed for J. Newbery, 1766). The horrifying, anthropomorphic descriptions of canine madness in medical texts also gravitated to hunting manuals and poems, one typically graphic account describing a mad dog as follows:

> . . . in some dark recess the senseless brute
> Sits sadly pining: deep melancholy,
> And black despair, upon his clouded brow
> Hang low'ring; from his half-op'ning jaws,
> The clammy venom, and infectious froth,
> Distilling fall; and from his lungs inflam'd,
> Malignant vapours taint the ambient air . . .
> Or if outrageous grown, behold alas!
> A yet more dreadful scene; his glaring eyes
> Redden with fury . . .
> This way and that he stares aghast, and starts
> At his own shade . . .
> Raving he runs, and deals destruction round . . .
> Vengeful he bites, and ever'y bite is death.

Later on, an "unhappy youth" merges entirely with the canine identity of the dog that had bitten him, and he is transformed into the (Baskerville-like) quintessence of rabid, bestial madness:

> Now the distended vessels scarce contain
> The wild uproar, but press each weaker part,
> Unable to resist: the tender brain
> And stomach suffer most; convulsions shake
> His trembling nerves, and wand'ring pungent pains
> Pinch sore the sleepless wretch . . .
> The tyrant frenzy reigns . . .
> Raving he foams, and howls and barks, and bates.
> Like agitation in his boiling blood
> Present like species to his troubled mind;
> His nature and his actions all canine . . .
> (William Somerville, *The Chace. A Poem,*
> 5th ed. [London: Printed for W. Bowyer,
> 1767], book 4, pp. 104–5, 110–11,
> ll. 208–36, 319–35)

For examples of rather more sentimental, anthropomorphic views of cats (and their critics), see, e.g., Thomas Gray, *Ode on the Death of a Favorite Cat Drown'd in a Tub of Gold Fishes,* modern ed. (Islip, Oxford: Strawberry Press, 1992); and Tobias George Smollett, *A Sorrowful Ditty; or, The Lady's Lamentation for the Death of her Favorite Cat: A Parody* (London: Printed for J. Tomlinson, 1748). Gray also wrote an ode on the death of a favorite spaniel. For Mrs. Gordon's cat, see CB, pp. C-92–94.

39. Monro's library included, e.g., Robert James, *A New Method of Preventing and Curing the Madness Caused by the Bite of a Mad Dog* (London: T. Osborne, 1743); Jesse Foot, *Essay on the Bite of a Mad Dog: With Observations on John Hunter's Treatment of the Case of Master R—— and also a Recital of the Successful Treatment of Two Cases* (London: Printed for T. Becket, 1788); John Berkenhout, *An Essay on the Bite of a Mad Dog: In Which the Claim to*

Infallibility of the Principal Preservative Remedies Against the Hydrophobia is Examined (London: R. Baldwin, 1783); Joseph Dalby, *The Virtues of Cinnabar and Musk, Against the Bite of a Mad Dog* (Birmingham: By John Baskerville for the author, 1764); and Christopher Nugent, *An Essay on the Hydrophobia: To Which is Prefixed the Case of a Person who was Bit by a Mad Dog; . . . and was Happily Cured* (London: Printed for James Leake and William Frederic, Bath; and sold by M. Cooper, 1753). See Monro, *Bibliotheca Elegantissima,* nos. 1643–44, 1647, 1666.

40. CB, pp. C-90–91.

41. The published exchange between Monro and Battie, the only occasion when the former ventured into print on the subject of insanity, was widely remarked at the time and has since been the focus of much historiographic commentary. See John Monro, *Remarks on Dr. Battie's Treatise on Madness* (London: Printed for Clarke, 1758); and William Battie, *A Treatise on Madness* (London: Whiston and White, 1758). For our perspective on the quarrel, see Andrews and Scull, *Undertaker of the Mind,* chap. 2.

42. CB, pp. C-6–7, C-50, C-56, C-60, C-86, C-114, C-116, C-122.

43. I.e., wider authority granted to medical personnel and institutions. This was a term popularized by French medical reformers and one accorded a growing currency in Britain by campaigners such as the Scottish physician Andrew Duncan.

44. Thomas Monro [of Magdalen College] (1764–1815), "Vicious and foolish people considered insane," in *Essays on Various Subjects* (London: Printed by J. Nichols and Sold by G. G. J. and J. Robinson, 1790), p. 69.

45. Ibid., pp. 69–73.

46. CB, pp. C-81–85.

47. CB, p. C-47.

48. CB, p. C-99.

49. CB, pp. C-66, C-98.

50. Implying uncleanliness in personal hygiene, or possibly incoherence; CB, pp. C-60, C-105.

51. CB, pp. C-47, C-69, C-114.

52. CB, p. C-35.

53. CB, pp. C-10, C-84.

54. CB, p. C-30.

55. CB, p. C-69.

56. CB, pp. C-73–74.

57. CB, p. C-91.

58. CB, p. C-86.

59. CB, pp. C-114, C-123.

60. See George Richardson, *Iconology; or, a Collection of Emblematical Figures, Moral and Instructive; Exhibiting the Images of the Elements and Celestial Bodies . . . Dispositions and Faculties of the Mind, Virtues and Vices . . . Illustrated by a Variety of Authorities from Classical Authors . . . from the most Approved Emblematical Representations of the Ancient Egyptians, Greeks and Romans, and from the Compositions of Cavaliere Cesare Ripa Perugino* (London: Printed for the author, 1779), vol. 2, book 4, plate 41, fig. 352, pp. 109–10:

Melancholy . . . Is a kind of madness, in which the mind is always fixed on one object.* It is characterised by the figure of an aged woman, of a downcast aspect, in a plain dark coloured dress; she is sitting upon flint stones, with her elbow resting on her knee, and her hand supporting her head; and by her side is a withered tree; she is represented aged, because old people are most subject to this malady.** The aspect denotes habitual dejection, and discontented temper. The dark coloured dress indicates gloominess and disorder of mind. Her being seated on the flint stones, signifies obstinacy and depression of spirits, as persons subjected to this disease, have no inclination to speak nor to act. The melancholy and thoughtful attitude, is expressive of fear, heaviness and sorrow. The withered tree denotes that this kind of delirium bereaves a person of all cheerfulness, and impaires the health, as a tree agitated by a storm is stripped of its leaves, withers and decays.

*Black Melancholy sits, and round her throws
A death-like silence, and a dead repose:
Her gloomy presence saddens all the scene,
Shades every flow'r, and darkens ev'ry green;
Deepens the murmur of the falling floods,
And breathes a browner horror on the woods.

** Pallentes habitant morbi, tritisque senectus.

Although Showalter focuses largely on nineteenth-century portrayals of madness as a female malady, she has famously argued for the pervasiveness of the sociomedical construction of the young, Ophelia-like, melancholy madwoman. Elaine Showalter, *The Female Malady: Women, Madness and English Culture 1830–1980* (New York: Pantheon Books, 1985; London: Virago Press, 1987), passim. Similar arguments about hysteria in the nineteenth century have also been much debated.

61. See, e.g., James Boswell, *The Hypochondriack,* 2 vols., ed. Margery Bailey (Stanford, Calif.: Stanford University Press, 1928); Roy Porter, *Mind-Forg'd Manacles*, pp. 88–89, 172–73, 241–46; Roy Porter, " 'The Hunger of Imagination': Approaching Samuel Johnson's Melancholy," *The Anatomy of Madness,* vol. 1, eds. W. F. Bynum, Roy Porter, and Michael Shepherd (London: Tavistock, 1985–88), pp. 63–88.

62. According to this unrelated Thomas Monro and other contemporary critics of the Stoics, anyone who saw "a friend drop into the grave without being compelled . . . to follow him with his tears, may be stiled [*sic*] a philosopher, but cannot have much claim to the title of a man." Meanwhile, "to neither grieve with the miserable, nor rejoice with the fortunate" was to "loosen the bonds by which society is linked together." Indeed, those who attempted to deprive mankind of grief, joy, or the other passions and thus to "emancipate men from nature's imperfection" were themselves guilty of "excessive pride" and "absurdity." Thomas Monro, "The Sway of the Passions over the Human Mind," essay 12, in *Essays on Various Subjects,* pp. 112, 116–18.

63. The debate between Monro and Battie is discussed in Andrews and Scull, *Undertaker of the Mind,* chap. 2.

64. CB, pp. C-2, C-6, C-8, C-16, C-38, C-39, C-64, C-68, C-79, C-119, C-123.

65. Monro, *Remarks,* p. 7. Notably, Malcolm Flemyng's *The Nature of the*

Nervous Fluid; Or, Animal Spirits Demonstrated (London: A. Millar, 1751) was in his library. Monro, *Bibliotheca Elegantissima,* no. 1639.

66. This term is commonly employed by historians of medicine and science to denote more mechanistic notions of physical laws and processes as applied in medicine and science from the late seventeenth century, influenced in particular by the "new" or Newtonian science. The accompanying term "iatrochemical" is used to signify understandings based more concertedly on chemical principles and knowledge.

67. Anon., *An Account of the Progress of an Epidemical Madness. In a Letter to the President and Fellows of the College of Physicians* (London: Printed and sold by J. Roberts, 1735), pp. 19–20.

68. Thomas Monro of Magdalen College, ed., *Olla Podrida, a Periodical Paper, Published at Oxford* (Dublin: Printed by P. Byrne, 1787), no. 1, 17 March 1787, pp. 3–4. Monro goes on to recount how

> in his first fit of poetic phrenzy, he was so considerably elevated and furious, that after having kicked down a whole set of china, the servants were obliged to be called in to hold him. The wet weather still affects him, but he is now less violent, and his domesticks [*sic*] take no other precaution than when they find the glass falling, or the sky clouding over, to remove every thing out of his way. . . .

69. Thomas Monro of Magdalen College, *Essays on Various Subjects,* p. 79.

70. CB, pp. C-28, C-65, C-72.

71. CB, pp. C-18–19.

72. CB, pp. C-34–35, C-114.

73. Miss Graham, e.g., was said to be emaciated and to have "dingy" skin; CB, p. C-43.

74. See Roy Porter, "The Rise of the Physical Examination," *Medicine and the Five Senses,* eds. W. F. Bynum and Roy Porter (Cambridge: Cambridge University Press, 1993), pp. 179–97.

75. CB, pp. C-58, C-79.

76. CB, pp. C-68–69.

77. CB, p. C-45.

78. CB, p. C-52.

79. Pargeter, *Observations on Maniacal Disorders,* p. 135.

80. CB, pp. C-21, C-77.

81. CB, pp. C-32–34.

82. CB, p. C-71. The mention of the milkiness of this woman's urine in conjunction with her "lying in" a year before is suggestive of the gendering of physiological ideas discernible in many other contemporary sources, by which women's reproductive functions were so often seen as profoundly underlying their pathologies.

83. Macalpine and Hunter, *George III and the Mad-Business,* esp. pp. 70, 147, 151, 153, fig. 8.

84. CB, pp. C-11–12, C-27, C-32, C-35.

85. CB, pp. C-32, C-35.

86. CB, pp. C-59–60. For other references to refusals to eat and dietary abnormalities, see CB, pp. C-1–2, C-43, C-78, C-80.

87. "Little is to be said with regard to diet . . ."; Monro, *Remarks,* p. 39. His

library included Thomas Moffet's *Health's Improvement: Or, Rules Comprizing and Discovering the Nature, Method and Manner of Preparing all Sorts of Food Used in this Nation . . . Corrected and Enlarged by Christopher Bennet, . . . To Which is Now Prefix'd, a Short View of the Author's Life and Writings, by Mr. Oldys. And an Introduction, by R. James, M.D.* (London: Printed for T. Osborne, 1746); George Cheyne's *The Natural Method of Curing the Diseases of the Body, and the Disorders of the Mind Depending on the Body. In Three Parts . . .* (London: Printed for Geo. Strahan . . . [etc.], 1742); and James Mackenzie's *The History of Health, and the Art of Preserving it: or, An Account of all that has been Recommended by Physicians and Philosophers, Towards the Preservation of Health . . .* (Edinburgh and London: Printed and sold by William Gordon, etc., 1758), but little else especially concerned with diet. See Monro, *Bibliotheca Elegantissima,* nos. 588, 935, 1068.

88. CB, pp. C-29, C-43, C-66.

89. CB, pp. C-43–44.

90. For sleep disorders, see CB, pp. C-3–4, C-10, C-19, C-32, C-37, C-40, C-42, C-46, C-55, C-57, C-62, C-64, C-68, C-70, C-71, C-78, C-88, C-90, C-91, C-116.

91. CB, pp. C-19, C-46, C-55.

92. CB, pp. C-121–23.

93. CB, p. C-91.

94. CB, p. C-99.

95. Trevor Turner stressed this point to us.

96. Malcolm Nicolson, "The Art of Diagnosis: Medicine and the Five Senses," *Companion Encyclopedia of the History of Medicine,* vol. 2, eds. W. F. Bynum and Roy Porter (London and New York: Routledge, 1993), pp. 801–25.

97. Nigel Walker, *Crime and Insanity in England. Volume One: The Historical Perspective* (Edinburgh: Edinburgh University Press, 1968), p. 62.

6. RELIGION, MADNESS, AND THE CASE BOOK

1. See the extensive discussion in Andrews and Scull, *Undertaker of the Mind,* chap. 3.

2. CB, pp. C-21–23, C-47–48.

3. CB, pp. C-106–8.

4. CB, p. C-65. In early modern England, weavers had a long history as an occupational class of being associated with religious radicalism and enthusiasm.

5. See especially Michael MacDonald, "Religion, Social Change, and Psychological Healing in England, 1600–1800," *The Church and Healing,* ed. W. J. Sheils (Oxford: Blackwell, 1982), pp. 101–25; MacDonald, "Insanity and the Realities of History in Early Modern England"; and MacDonald, *Mystical Bedlam.*

6. For the beginnings of the revolt against enthusiasm, see Henry More, *Enthusiasmus Triumphatus, or, A Discourse of the Nature, Causes, Kinds, and Cure, of Enthusiasme* (London: Morden, 1656). For twentieth-century commentary, see George Williamson, "The Restoration Revolt against Enthusiasm," *Studies in Philology* 2 (1933), pp. 571–603; Thomas Steffan, "The Social Argu-

ment against Enthusiasm (1650–1660)," *Studies in English* 21 (1941), pp. 39–63; Ronald Arbuthnott Knox, *Enthusiasm* (Oxford: Oxford University Press, 1950); and Susie I. Tucker, *Enthusiasm: A Study in Semantic Change* (Cambridge: Cambridge University Press, 1972).

7. Roy Porter, "The Rage of Party: A Glorious Revolution in English Psychiatry?" *Medical History* 27 (1983), p. 40.

8. E.g., Phillip Gretton, *The Insufficiency of Reason, and the Assurance of Revelation . . . a Discourse Preached before the University of Cambridge* (Cambridge: Cambridge University Press, 1732).

9. Nicholas Robinson, *A New System of the Spleen*, p. 250.

10. In the words of William Pargeter, the provincial mad-doctor, "The *doctrines* of the *Methodists* have a greater tendency than those of any other sect to produce the most deplorable effects on the human understanding. The brain is perplexed in the mazes of mystery, and the imagination overpowered by the tremendous description of future torments"; [Rev.] William Pargeter, *Observations on Maniacal Disorders* (Reading: Printed for the author, 1792; facsimile reprint, ed. Stanley W. Jackson, London and New York: Routledge, 1988), p. 31.

11. CB, pp. C-25, C-45.

12. CB, p. C-34.

13. William Perfect, *Select Cases in the Different Species of Insanity, Lunacy, or Madness, with the Modes of Practice as Adopted in the Treatment of Each* (Rochester: Printed and sold by W. Gillman; London: Printed and sold by J. Murray and J. Dew, 1787), pp. 119–20.

14. William Perfect, *Methods of Cure, in some Particular Cases of Insanity* (Rochester: Printed for the author, by T. Fisher, at Rochester; and sold by J. Dodsley and N. Conant [successor to Mr. Whiston], 1777), p. 33. It seems worth noting that Perfect's book was in Monro's library; Monro, *Bibliotheca Elegantissima*, no. 1644.

15. William Perfect, *Select Cases*, p. 122.

16. See, e.g., Hugh Farmer, *An Essay on the Demoniacs of the New Testament* (London: Printed for G. Robinson, 1775); John Moore, *Of Religious Melancholy. A Sermon Preach'd before the Queen at Whitehall* (London: Printed for William Rogers, 1692). Richard Mead's *Medica Sacra* had also included a medical interpretation of the demoniacs.

17. E.g., Leonard Twells, *An Answer to the Enquiry into the Meaning of Demoniacks in the New Testament: Shewing, that the Demons Therein Spoken of were Fallen Angels; and that the Demoniacks were Persons Really Possessed . . .* (London: Printed for R. Gosling, 1737); Twells, *An Answer to the Further Enquiry into the Meaning of Demoniacks in the New Testament . . . In a Second Letter to the Author* (London, 1738); Thomas Newton, *A Dissertation on the Demoniacs in the Gospels* (London: J. and F. Rivington, 1775); John Fell, *Daemoniacs: An Enquiry into the Heathen and the Scripture Doctrine of Daemons, in which the Hypotheses of the Rev. Mr. Farmer, and Others on this Subject, are Particularly Considered* (London: Printed for Charles Dilly, 1779); Nathaniel Lardner, *The Case of the Demoniacs Mentioned in the New Testament: Four Discourses upon Mark v. 19. With an Appendix, etc.* (London, 1758); and Samuel

Pegge, *An Examination of the Enquiry into the Meaning of the Demoniacs in the New Testament. In a Letter to the Author. Wherein it is Shewn, that the Word Demon does not Signify a Departed Soul, either in the Classics or the Scriptures; and Consequently, that the Whole of the Enquiry is Without Foundation* (London, 1739). Notably, rather than medical reinterpretations, most of these works were vindications of the miraculous casting out of demons, although there were conspicuous omissions, such as the works on the demoniacs by Thomas Church (1707–56) and Thomas Hutchinson (1698–1769). See Monro, *Bibliotheca Elegantissima,* nos. 624–25, 658–59, 908, 1099.

18. Smollett, *Roderick Random,* chap. 63, p. 394.

19. This mystic Christian philosophy was based on the writings of Jean Valentin Andreae (1589–1674), telling the tales of one Christian Rosenkreuz. See Frances Amelia Yates, *The Rosicrucian Enlightenment* (1972; London and Boston: Routledge and Kegan Paul, 1999); Christopher Mcintosh, *The Rose Cross and the Age of Reason: Eighteenth-Century Rosicrucianism in Central Europe and Its Relationship to the Enlightenment* (Leiden and New York: E. J. Brill, 1992); Simon Blackburn, *The Oxford Dictionary of Philosophy* (Oxford and New York: Oxford University Press, 1994), p. 332; and Abbé de Villars (Nicolas Pierre Henri), *The Count de Gabalis: Being a Diverting History of the Rosicrucian Doctrine of Spirits, viz. Sylphs, Salamanders, Gnomes, and Dæmons: Shewing their Various Influence upon Human Bodies. Done from the Paris Edition. To which is Prefix'd, Monsieur [Pierre] Bayle's Account of this Work: and of the Sect of the Rosicrucians* (London: Printed for B. Lintott and E. Curll, etc., 1714).

20. CB, p. C-110. Monro employs the phrase "fancies herself" here, which might be taken in contemporary parlance to mean simply "thinks" or "believes herself." Yet the mad-doctor's use of such a term in the context of the putatively deranged nearly always appears to imply that to "fancy" was to wrongly imagine, falsely believe, or delusively think.

21. CB, p. C-79.

22. CB, pp. C-118–19.

23. Smollett, *Roderick Random,* chap. 5, p. 18.

24. Robert Burton's *Anatomy of Melancholy* (London: B. Blake, 1651); facsimile edition, reprinted from 16th ed. (Oxford: Thorntons, 1997), an encyclopedic study and literary compendium of the manifestations, causes, and cures of melancholy, but particularly preoccupied with religious melancholy, was repeatedly reprinted from the time of its initial publication in 1621, and cited again and again in numerous medical and lay writings of the eighteenth century.

25. CB, pp. C-46–47.

26. CB, pp. C-5–6.

27. CB, pp. C-31–34.

28. Michael MacDonald and Terence R. Murphy, *Sleepless Souls: Suicide in Early Modern England* (Oxford and New York: Clarendon/Oxford University Press, 1990); MacDonald, "The Secularisation of Suicide in England 1600–1800," *Past and Present* 111 (1986), pp. 50–97; MacDonald and Murphy, "The Medicalization of Suicide in England: Laymen, Physicians, and Cultural Change, 1500–1870," *Framing Disease: Studies in Cultural History,* eds.

Charles E. Rosenberg and Janet Golden (New Brunswick, N.J.: Rutgers University Press, 1992), pp. 85–103.

29. CB, pp. C-9–10.

30. CB, pp. C-19, C-81.

31. MacDonald, "Religion, Social Change, and Psychological Healing"; J. F. C. Harrison, *The Second Coming: Popular Millenarianism, 1780–1850* (New Brunswick, N.J.: Rutgers University Press, 1979). See also James Obelkevich, *Religion and Rural Society: South Lindsey, 1825–1875* (Oxford: Clarendon Press, 1976), esp. chap. 6.

32. CB, pp. C-115–16.

33. CB, pp. C-120–21.

34. CB, p. C-75.

35. CB, pp. C-2, C-55.

36. CB, pp. C-6–7.

37. Ingram, *The Madhouse of Language*.

38. CB, pp. C-111–12.

39. In Haslam's case, he was so supremely confident "that there existed in the judgement of those who passed for persons of sound mind, a sufficient disrelish for absurdity, to enable them to discriminate the transactions of daylight, from the materials of a dream" (John Haslam, *A Letter to the Governors of Bethlem Hospital, Containing an Account of Their Management of that Institution for the Last Twenty Years* [London: Taylor and Hessey, 1818], p. 31) that he allowed himself to be provoked by one of his patients, James Tilly Matthews, into publishing a volume consisting largely of the latter's writings about his case and his treatment at Bethlem (John Haslam, *Illustrations of Madness* [London: Printed by G. Hayden and sold by Rivingtons, 1810]; facsimile ed., reprinted with an introduction by Roy Porter [London and New York: Routledge, 1988]). Haslam's assumption was that the spectacle of the lunatic protesting his own sanity would instead serve to hold both Matthews and his supporters up to ridicule—that his captive would inadvertently but inevitably condemn himself out of his own mouth, mad speech being a nonsense to be treated as a source of amusement or discarded rather than scrutinized as a source of enlightenment. In this case, at least, the assumption proved to be a disastrous mistake. See Andrew Scull, Charlotte MacKenzie, and Nicholas Hervey, *Masters of Bedlam: The Transformation of the Mad-Doctoring Trade* (Princeton, N.J.: Princeton University Press, 1996), chap. 2.

7. TREATING PATIENTS AND GETTING PAID

1. Compare, for example, Cheyne's famous aphorism: "Vomits are in diseases what bombs are in besieging forts."

2. CB, p. C-26.

3. CB, p. C-119.

4. CB, p. C-63.

5. Monro, *Remarks*, pp. 37–39.

6. CB, pp. C-42–43.

7. CB, p. C-79.

8. Monro, *Remarks*, p. 50: "*Management did more than medicine in this disease.*"

9. E.g., CB, pp. C-10, C-26.

10. E.g., CB, pp. C-78–79.

11. Monro, *Remarks*, pp. 38–39.

12. Ibid., pp. 38–40.

13. Foucault, *Madness and Civilisation*, chaps. 2 and 3; Roy Porter, "Foucault's Great Confinement," *History of the Human Sciences* 3.1 (1990), pp. 47–54; Andrew Scull, "A Failure to Communicate? On the Reception of Foucault's *Histoire de la folie* by Anglo-American Historians," *Rewriting the History of Madness*, eds. Arthur Still and Irving Velody (London: Routledge, 1992), pp. 150–63.

14. See especially Jewson, "Medical Knowledge and the Patronage System."

15. CB, pp. C-86–89.

16. Monro, *Remarks*, p. 59.

17. Nicholas Robinson, *A New System of the Spleen*, esp. pp. 401–2, 406. See also Bryan Robinson, *Observations on the Virtues and Operations of Medicines* (London: J. Nourse, 1752), pp. 145 ff.; and Roy Porter, *Mind-Forg'd Manacles*, pp. 53, 208. Nicholas Robinson was regularly at court and committee meetings during the 1750s and 1760s. For his nomination (by Stephen Hervey Esq.) and election as a governor, when resident at Hatton Garden, see BCGM, 27 March and 6 June 1755, pp. 175, 183–85.

18. "Heroic medicine" is a term applied to the traditional antiphlogistic therapeutics, reflecting the powerful but often painful and debilitating character of many of its central therapeutic weapons: bleeding, purging, vomits, etc.

19. E.g., cases of Mr. Rowley, Mr. Mitchell, and Mr. Stanfield, CB, pp. C-60, C-105, C-121–22.

20. CB, pp. C-2, C-80.

21. Monro, *Remarks*, pp. 38–40, 59; CB, p. C-80.

22. Ibid., p. 38.

23. CB, p. C-65.

24. CB, pp. C-66, C-105.

25. CB, pp. C-86–89.

26. Monro, *Remarks*, p. 6.

27. CB, pp. C-123–24.

28. Monro, *Remarks*, pp. 27–28.

29. CB, p. C-123.

30. See, e.g., Roy Porter, *Health for Sale: Quackery in England 1660–1850* (Manchester and New York: Manchester University Press, 1989); idem, *Quacks* (Stroud: Tempus, 2000).

31. Ibid.; Porter, *Patients and Practitioners*; Porter and Porter, *Patient's Progress*.

32. They were prescribed, for example, in Lord Orford's case; see Andrews and Scull, *Undertaker of the Mind*, chap. 4, note 13.

33. For more on James and Dominiceti, see CB, pp. C-5, C-113, and pp. 153–55, note 8, p. 164, note 47, and pp. 169–71, note 81.

34. According to Hardinge, this was because Battie judged that "the dog had

more brains in him, and more knowledge, than I ever had experienced in our Candidates"; letter of Hardinge to Dr. Edward Barnard, provost of Eton, 9 March 1814, in John Nichols, *Literary Anecdotes of the Eighteenth Century,* vol. 8, part 4 (London: Nichols, Son, and Bentley, 1812–15), pp. 552–53.

35. Ibid., p. 553.

36. CB, pp. C-5, C-113. Thomas Monro of Magdalen College joked about having taken James's Powders when, "at a considerable distance from our Alma Mater," he "was afflicted with a violent fever," elaborating that when the drug "ceased to be of service," a copy of "Jackson," the Oxford newspaper, induced a sweat and the fever abated. Thomas Monro, ed., *Olla Podrida,* no. 17, 7 July 1787, p. 128.

37. William Hawes, *An Account of the late Dr Goldsmith's Illness, so far as Relative to the Exhibition of Dr James's Powder. An Examination of the Rev. Mr John Wesley's Primitive Physic: and an Address to the Public on Premature Death and Premature Internment* (London: Printed for the author by Browne, Dennis, and Wade, 1780), being the 2nd ed. of the work on Wesley, and the 4th of that on Goldsmith's illness, 1st ed. 1774.

38. Monro, *Remarks,* p. 26.

39. CB, p. C-40.

40. Monro, *Remarks,* p. 25.

41. See Andrews and Scull, *Undertaker of the Mind,* chap. 2.

42. See *Journals of Richard Clark, Lord Mayor of London, 1784–5,* Guildhall MS 3385.

43. See Thomas Reeve, *A Cure for the Epidemical Madness of Drinking Tar Water, Lately Imported from Ireland by a Certain R[igh]t R[everen]d Doctor. In a Letter to his L[ordshi]p* (London: Printed for John and Paul Knapton, 1744).

44. See Andrews and Scull, *Undertaker of the Mind,* chap. 1, p. 268, note 26.

45. See Andrews, "A Respectable Mad-Doctor? Richard Hale, F.R.S. (1670–1728)," *Notes and Records of the Royal Society of London* 44 (1990), pp. 169–203.

46. Cruden, *The Adventures of Alexander the Corrector. The Second Part,* pp. 21, 23.

47. Cruden, *The London-Citizen,* p. 35.

48. The Inner Temple is one of the so-called Inns of Court, the London legal societies that possess the exclusive right to admit barristers to the practice of law. A Sergeant-at-law was a judicial officer appointed by the Corporation of London.

49. Margaret Marie Verney, ed., *Verney Letters of the Eighteenth Century from the MSS at Claydon House,* vol. 2 (London: Benn, 1930), p. 202. James's other wealthy clients included Lord Galloway and John Newport (ca. 1720–83), son of the third earl of Bradford and Mrs. Anne Smyth of Chelsea. Newport had inherited an estate worth £12,000–£15,000 per annum from his mother (via the earl), but when he was declared lunatic and placed "under the care of Dr. Munro," the estate passed under trusteeship and reversion to the earl of Bath and a Mr. Herbert. See Walpole, *Correspondence,* vol. 9, p. 148, note 12. This does not appear to be the same Mr. Newport whom John mentions attending as one of his patients at the attorney Williams's in the case book; CB, p. C-81.

50. Alexander Cruden, *The Adventures of Alexander the Corrector, with an Account of the Chelsea Academies, or the Private Places for the Confinement of Such as Are Supposed to be Deprived of the Exercise of their Reason* (London: For the author, 1754), p. 22; Cruden, *The Adventures of Alexander the Corrector. The Second Part,* pp. 21–23.

51. James Carkesse, "The Poetical History of Finnesbury Mad-House," *Lucid Intervalla* (London: The author, 1679), facsimile ed., with an introduction by Michael V. Deporte (Los Angeles: William Andrews Clark Memorial Library, University of California/Augustan Reprint Society, 1979), nos. 195–96, p. 9.

52. William Belcher, *An Address to Humanity, Containing a Letter to Dr. Thomas Monro, A Receipt to Make a Lunatic, and Seize his Estate; and a Sketch of a True Smiling Hyena* (London: The author, 1796). Ironically, Belcher owed his release from many years of confinement in a Hackney madhouse to Thomas Monro.

53. See Ida Hunter and Richard Macalpine, *Three Hundred Years of Psychiatry 1535–1860: A History Presented in Selected English Texts* (Oxford, New York, and Toronto: Oxford University Press, 1963), p. 403. Cf. Andrews, "A Respectable Mad-Doctor?," p. 181.

8. BEING MAD IN EIGHTEENTH-CENTURY ENGLAND

1. Roy Porter, "The Rise of the Physical Examination," *Medicine and the Five Senses,* eds. W. F. Bynum and Roy Porter (Cambridge: Cambridge University Press, 1993), pp. 182–83.

2. See Rosenberg, "The Therapeutic Revolution."

3. CB, pp. C-17–19.

4. CB, pp. C-4–6 (Miss Jefferies), C-9–10 (Miss Compton), C-19 (Miss Greaves), C-55 (AB, a servant maid).

5. Mrs. Hooper, CB, pp. C-109–10.

6. Mr. Walker, CB, pp. C-17–19.

7. Miss Hume, CB, pp. C-13–15.

8. Mr. Whitby, CB, pp. C-63–64.

9. Mr. Sergison, CB, p. C-61.

10. CB, pp. C-89–91.

11. Gill Speak, "An Odd Kind of Melancholy: Reflections on the Glass Delusion in Europe (1440–1680)," *History of Psychiatry* 1.2 (1990), pp. 191–206.

12. CB, pp. C-57, C-80, C-100, C-115.

13. CB, p. C-121.

14. CB, pp. C-71–72, C-85–86.

15. CB, p. C-28.

16. CB, p. C-95.

17. CB, p. C-5.

18. CB, p. C-66.

19. CB, p. C-88.

20. CB, p. C-119.

21. See, e.g., William F. Hixson, *Triumph of the Bankers: Money and Bank-*

ing in the Eighteenth and Nineteenth Centuries (Westport, Conn.: Praeger, 1993); Peter Mathias and John A. Davis, eds., *International Trade and British Economic Growth: From the Eighteenth Century to the Present Day*, The Nature of Industrialization Series, vol. 5 (Oxford: Blackwell, 1996); and S. R. Cope, *The Stock Exchange Revisited: A New Look at the Market in Securities in London in the Eighteenth Century* (London: London School of Economics and Political Science, 1978), reprinted from *Economica* 45 (Feb. 1978). For excellent studies of how this commercial culture also affected the question of authorship, writing, and satire, see Catherine Ingrassia, *Authorship, Commerce, and Gender in Early Eighteenth-Century England: A Culture of Paper Credit* (Cambridge and New York: Cambridge University Press, 1998); and Colin Nicholson, *Writing and the Rise of Finance: Capital Satires of the Early Eighteenth Century*, Cambridge Studies in Eighteenth-Century English Literature and Thought Series (Cambridge and New York: Cambridge University Press, 1994).

    22. See CB, pp. C-3–4 (Mr. Molyneux), pp. C-4–6 (Miss Jefferies), pp. C-10–13 (Mrs. Stone), p. C-63 (Mr. Inge).

    23. CB, pp. C-70, C-72.

    24. See, e.g., CB, pp. C-70, C-124, cases of Heber's illness, where Monro is unsure "whether it proceeded from the medicines he had taken or from an accidental fever that came upon him" and of an anonymous woman who "was improperly treated by her nurse giving her some spirituous liquor during her lying in." See also CB, p. C-7.

    25. CB, p. C-5.

    26. CB, p. C-68.

    27. See CB, pp. C-112–13, the case of Miss — of Chichester, discussed above.

    28. See CB, pp. C-15–16, C-29–31, C-42–43. Monro's advice that he should sleep sitting in his chair seems to have had the desired effect.

    29. CB, pp. C-45–46.

    30. CB, pp. C-70–71.

    31. CB, p. C-55.

    32. CB, pp. C-65–66.

    33. CB, p. C-75.

    34. CB, p. C-8.

    35. CB, pp. C-11–13, C-45.

    36. CB, p. C-65.

    37. CB, p. C-105.

    38. CB, pp. C-61–64.

    39. CB, pp. C-26–27.

    40. E.g., CB, pp. C-6–7 (Mr. Dempster), C-47–48 (Miss Cutter), C-66–67 (Mr. Cawthorne).

    41. CB, p. C-115.

    42. CB, pp. C-71–72.

    43. CB, pp. C-97–98.

    44. Cited in Roy Porter, *Mind-Forg'd Manacles*, p. 2, and Max Byrd, *Visits to Bedlam* (Columbia: University of South Carolina Press, 1974), p. 75.

NOTES TO JOHN MONRO'S 1766 CASE BOOK

1. This was the Hoxton madhouse of John (or Jonathan) Miles (d. 1773), father of Sir Jonathan Miles, to whom he bequeathed the business. See Andrews and Scull, *Undertaker of the Mind*, chap. 5, for more information.

2. Evidently another madhouse, run by a Mr. Dudley at Bloomsbury Square. See Andrews and Scull, *Undertaker of the Mind*, chap. 5.

3. I.e., medicine.

4. Possibly related to Rebecca Molyneux of St. Bartholomew Behind the Exchange, London, admitted to Bethlem 17 June 1769, discharged 16 June 1770 "Incurable & fitt"; securities (see chapter 3, note 32, for an explanation of this term): James Capstack, tailor in Angel Court, Throgmorton Street, and Isaac Wilshire, calender (a "calender," "calenderer," or "calenderman" was a skilled worker who operated a calender machine to press cloth between rollers to smooth and glaze it, or to thin rubber or paper into sheets [*Oxford English Dictionary*]), Buckers Bury; Bethlem Admission Registers (henceforth BAR), p. 290. She was not readmitted to Bethlem as incurable.

5. This may have been the wife of Samuel Whitbread, Esq., the famous brewer and lunacy reformer who resided in Chiswell Street, Moorfields, ca. 1790. See *The Universal British Directory of Trade and Commerce . . .* (London: Printed for the Patentees and sold by C. Stalker and Messrs Brideoake and Fell, 1790). Whitbread himself committed suicide on 6 July 1815 while a member of the 1815–16 Select Committee on Madhouses, depressed and feeling despised by all who knew him.

6. There was an Isaac De Vic who died aged 102 at Chileworth, Romsey, Hampshire, in 1774; *Gentleman's Magazine* (henceforth *GM*) (1774), p. 94.

7. Dr. William Battie, physician to St. Luke's Hospital. See Andrews and Scull, *Undertaker of the Mind*, chap. 2.

8. This was Dr. Robert James's (1705–76) famous Fever Powders, a mixture of mercury and antimony (antimony was composed of regulus, a kind of white arsenic, and sulfur). It was marketed and patented by James as a cure for all kinds of fevers in particular, but also for a host of other major afflictions, including nervous and mental disorders. Some doctors also recommended it for splenetic disorders and for "phrenitis" (literally, brain fever). The way in which this powder was promoted, sold, and prescribed was severely criticized by orthodox medical practitioners from the 1760s to the 1790s. Many regarded it (and with good reason) as of more limited value than James and his supporters claimed, and saw the powder and James himself as tainted with quackery and profiteering. A publication (ca. 1790) by James Adair made no bones about classing James as a nostrum-monger (James M. Adair, *Essays on Fashionable Diseases. The Dangerous Effects of Hot and Crouded Rooms. The Cloathing of Invalids, Lady and Gentlemen Doctors. And on Quacks and Quackery. With the Genuine Patent Prescriptions of Dr. James's Fever Powder, Tickell's Aetherial Spirit, & Godbold's Balsam, taken from the Rolls in Chancery . . . And also the Ingredients and Composition of Many of the most Celebrated Quack Nostrums, As Utilized by several of the best Chemists in Europe . . . With A dedication to Philip Thicknesse . . . Professor of Empiricism and Nostrums, Rape and Murder-Monger to the St.*

James's Chronicle . . . [London: Sold by T. P. Bateman, 1790(?)]). In a gesture of professional loyalty, however, much of the blame from established physicians was diverted away from James himself onto the "ignorant" suppliers and irregular practitioners, who, it was alleged (in a tone that was itself tainted by professional rivalries and gender and class bias), mixed the drug up wrongly or dispensed the drug irresponsibly. (Though he had obtained a patent, James and his powder had a number of imitators.) On the other hand, some of these suppliers had James's personal endorsement. The old woman who had evidently legitimately prepared the powder for many years was said to be "often drunk," rendering the powder inconsistent and untrustworthy in dosage. When James first marketed his "invention," it was attacked as a relabeling exercise rather than a genuine innovation: variants of the same concoction had been around for centuries, and more recently it had been recommended by celebrated authorities such as Paracelsus and Boerhaave. It was alleged that James had stolen the recipe from a Baron Scwanberg, reneging on an original co-partnership agreement. However, James had more or less successfully defended himself against these charges in the 1740s when a lawsuit was brought in Westminster Hall.

The effect produced by a small quantity of James's Powders was considerable: ordinarily, it caused vomiting and purging, and often sweating and salivation; and in excessive doses it brought about unconsciousness or death through poisoning—regrettably, not always a sufficiently compelling reason for physicians to be circumspect in using it. In later years, keen to defend the position he had carved for himself in the medical marketplace, James developed a milder version of the powder (literally, Dr. James's Mild Powder), omitting the mercury additive—but in the process, according to Adair, rendering it less effective in many cases (Adair, *Essays on Fashionable Diseases*, p. 210). The popularity of the powder was at its height in the 1760s despite such considerations. It was not only in heavy demand from patients and regularly prescribed by practitioners but also was being used extensively by the royal navy. The demand was so great from patients themselves that medical men often felt obliged to prescribe the remedy against their better judgment, in situations of considerable risk, as was tragically and sensationally exemplified in the case of Dr. Goldsmith, whose death was attributed by his own doctor and by most contemporary practitioners to his insistence on taking James's Powders. This context helps us to understand why Monro was prepared to try the remedy, even if "in vain," persuaded perhaps by the conviction of his patient's mother that it had worked before. Yet he himself was clearly far from convinced of its utility, and was soon to abandon it in this case.

Attempts were made to counter the adverse publicity surrounding the Goldsmith case by publicizing other successful cases, such as that of Sir Thomas Robinson (e.g., Adair, *Essays on Fashionable Diseases*, p. 21). Advertising, too, stressed the safety of the powder, as the following excerpts from the advertisement inserted in newspapers, magazines, and other publications by the official suppliers of the powder in the 1760s suggest:

> DR JAMES'S POWDER for Fevers, the Small-pox, Measles, Plurisies, Quincies, Acute
> Rheumatisms, Colds, and all Inflammatory Disorders, as well as for those which are
> called Nervous, Hypochondriaca, and Hysteric. Price Two Shillings and Sixpence the

> Paper . . . a safe and certain Cure for the above Disorders, is better prepared for Sea
> Service, (and more convenient) in Bottles, than made up as usual in Marble Paper. . . .
> This Medicine is sold only by J[ames] Newberry, at the Bible and Sun in St Paul's
> Church-yard, and by those who are empowered by him to sell it. . . .
>   Of who may be had,
> DR JAMES'S MILD POWDER . . . so contrived as to have little or no sensible Opera-
> tion, and on that Account is the more proper for Women under certain Circum-
> stances, Infants, and those whose Constitutions are extremely delicate . . .
>   Price 2s 6d.

See *London Evening Post* (henceforth *LEP*), no. 5960 (7–9 Jan. 1766). James also patented and made considerable profit from his "analeptic pills," a purgative for bilious complaints. His first major publication had been his 1743–45 dictionary of medicinal preparations, but he also wrote a 1760 treatise on canine madness. He died at his residence in Bruton Street in 1776; see *GM* (1776), p. 142; and William Munk, *Roll of the Royal College of Physicians of London* (London: Royal College of Physicians, 1878), vol. 2, p. 269. See also J. K. Crellin, "Dr. James's Fever Powder," *Transactions of the British Society for the History of Pharmacy* 1 (1970–77), pp. 136–43. For contemporary critical assessments of James's Powders, see, e.g., Anon., *An Essay On the Power of Nature and Art in Curing Diseases; To Which are Annexed Impartial Reflections on James's Powder* (London: Printed for W. Owen, 1753); Malcolm Flemyng, *A Dissertation on Dr. James's Fever Powder. In which the Different Circumstances, wherein that Remedy may prove Beneficial or Hurtful, are Considered and Distinguished, According to Observation and Reason* (London: Printed for L. Davis and C. Reymers, 1760); William Hawes, *An Account of the late Dr Goldsmith's Illness, so far as relative to the Exhibition of Dr James's Powder. An Examination of the Rev. Mr John Wesley's Primitive Physic: and an Address to the Public on Premature Death and Premature Internment* (London: Printed for the Author by Browne, Dennis and Wade, 1780; being the 2nd ed. of the work on Wesley, and the 4th of that on Goldsmith's illness [1st ed., 1774]); and Adair, *Essays on Fashionable Diseases*, esp. pp. 187–88, 198–99, 207–14. For more positive endorsements, see, e.g., Flemyng, *A Dissertation on Dr James's Fever Powder;* and William White, *Observations on the Use of Dr James's Powder, Emetic Tartar, and Other Antimonial Preparations in Fevers* (London: Printed for T. Cadell, Richardson, and Wallis and T. Wilson, 1774).

    9. Probably the Thomas Southwell who wrote *Medical Essays and Observations; Being an Abridgement of the Useful Medical Papers Contained in the History and Memoirs of the Royal Academy of Sciences at Paris, from their Reestablishment in 1699 to the year 1750, Disposed Under General Heads,* 4 vols. (London: Printed for J. Knox, 1764). For Walker and Goupy, see pp. 35–36.

    10. Peter Inskip ran a madhouse in Little Chelsea, much used by families and parishes from the metropolis and also from the home counties. See Andrews and Scull, *Undertaker of the Mind*, chap. 5, pp. 101, 103, 107–8, 168–69, 363 note 86.

    11. I.e., masturbation. Masturbation, seen not only as a frequent cause or aggravation of mental maladies in the nineteenth century but as actually a distinctive form of insanity in itself, was only beginning to be linked with mental and bodily illness in the eighteenth century. The 1758 publication by the French

physician M. or S. A. D. (Samuel Auguste David) Tissot on the subject was one of the first to emphasize the dangerous effects of the "vice" on health, although it was still the physical and moral consequences with which Tissot was most concerned. Whether either this patient or Monro had read Tissot is unclear, but it seems likely that this new pathologizing of onanism had affected his own, his family's, and his doctor's interpretation of his illness. Tissot's book appears to have been very popular and influential in Europe, going into many editions and also being translated into all the major European languages; the first English translation appeared in 1766 and another in 1781. Thus it played an important part in forming contemporary attitudes toward masturbation. See M. Tissot, *A Treatise on the Crime of Onan; Illustrated with a Variety of Cases, Together with the Method of Cure*, trans. from the third edition of the original (London: Printed for B. Thomas, 1766); and Tissot, *Onanism: or, a Treatise upon the Disorders Produced by Masturbation, or, The Dangerous Effects of Secret and Excessive Venery*, trans. from the last Paris edition by A. Hume (London: Printed for the translator; sold by J. Pridden in Fleet-Street, 1766). For the third French edition, see S. A. D. (Samuel Auguste David) Tissot, *L'onanisme: ou dissertation physique sur les maladies produites par la masturbation. Traduit du latin ... considérablement augmenté par l'auteur* (Lausanne: Marc Chapuis & Co., 1764). It was first published in Latin under the title *Tentamen de Morbis ex Manustupratione in Dissertatio de Febribus Biliosis; seu Historia Epidemiae biliosae Lausannensis, an. 1755* (Lausanne, 1758). Advertisements appeared in the press for Tissot's book throughout 1766, such as that inserted in the *LEP*, no. 5967 (23–25 Jan. 1766), p. 3, col. 3, as follows:

> This Day was publish'd,
> Price 2s sew'd,
> ONANISM; or, A Treatise upon the Disorders produced by Secret and Excessive
> Venery; with the Methods of Cure.
> By M. TISSOT, M.D.
> Fellow of the Royal Society of London, Member of the Medical Physical Society
> of Basle, and of the Oeconomical Society of Berne.
> Translated from the last Paris Edition,
> By A. HUME M.D.
> Propriis extinctum vivere criminibus. Gall.
> Printed for the Translator; and sold by J. Pridden, in Fleet-Street; and all other
> Booksellers in Town and Country.

A letter in the *LEP*, no. 5970 (20–22 Feb. 1766), p. 4, cols. 1 and 2, dated 15 Feb. 1766, refers to a disorder affecting country squires, sportsmen, and others given to venery, some of whom had perished from the addiction, opining "that if Dr Tissot's Onan had been read to them judiciously, they would have all survived."

12. Sir George Robinson (1730–1815) was the eldest son of Sir John Robinson, baronet of Kingsthorpe, Northamptonshire. Baptized in Kingsthorpe on 27 May 1730, George went to school at Oakham, where his tutor was a Mr. Adcock. He was admitted to Trinity College, Cambridge, as a pensioner on 11 April 1749, matriculating there in the same year. He then advanced to the level of Scholar 1750, graduating B.A. 1753, Fellow 1755, and M.A. 1756. He called

upon Monro's assistance in 1766, soon after succeeding his father as the fifth baronet on 31 July 1765. It was in 1766 that his political career was to take off, too, when he became sheriff of Northamptonshire. He was returned as MP for Northampton during 1774–80. His relationship with Sir Francis Chester is not entirely clear to the authors, but it was evidently through marriage, for he had taken as his wife Dorothea Chester, the daughter of John Chester, Esq., of St. Paul's, Covent Garden. He died on 10 Jan./Oct. (sources vary) 1815. See J. and J. A. Venn, *Alumni Cantabridgiensis. A Biographical List of all Known Students, Graduates and Holders of Office at the University of Cambridge, from the Earliest Times to 1900* (Cambridge: Cambridge University Press, 1922–27), vol. 3, p. 469; G. E. Cokayne, *Complete Baronetage,* 5 vols. (Exeter: W. Pollard & Co., 1909); Cokayne, *The Complete Peerage of England, Scotland, Ireland, Great Britain and the United Kingdom, Extant, Extinct or Dormant,* 11 vols. (London: St. Catherine Press, 1910); and *GM* 2 (1815), p. 568.

13. Swithin (or Swithen) Adee (1705–86) was a physician of the old school, whom Monro might well have encountered during his Oxford days. He was educated at Corpus Christi College, Oxford, graduating A.B. 14 June 1721, A.M. 22 Feb. 1724, and M.D. 4 July 1733. After practicing for several years at Guildford and Oxford, in 1762 he moved to London, where he practiced for the next eight years. He became candidate of the College of Physicians 30 Sept. 1762, and fellow 30 Sept. 1763. He was a censor of the college in 1764 and 1770 and delivered the Gulstonian lectures in 1767 and the Harveian Oration in 1769. In 1770 he retired from business and returned to Oxford, spending the remainder of his life among old college friends. He died in Oxford on 12 Aug. 1786, aged eighty-one. He was F.R.S. and F.S.A. and gained recognition for an explanation of the Greek inscription on the Corbridge altar of Astarte. His few publications seem to have been confined to a Latin poem dedicated to Richard Mead— *Meadus: Poema, grati animi testimonium,* published in 1755; a satire on Bolingbroke; and his 1769 Harveian Oration, which likewise contained the poem to Mead. Swithin Adee, *Oratio Anniversaria a Guilelmo Harveio Instituta in Theatro Collegii Medicorum Londinensium Habita Festo Sancti Lucae, 18 Oct. 1769. (Meadus Poema grati animi testimonium, etc.)* (Oxford: Clarendon, 1770); Adee, *The Craftsman's Apology. Being a Vindication of his Conduct and Writings: in Several Letters to the King* [A satire, in verse, on Henry St. John, Viscount Bolingbroke] (London: T. Cooper, 1732). See Munk, *Roll,* vol. 2, p. 256.

14. Possibly Elizabeth Stone of St. Brides, London, admitted to Bethlem 23 March 1771, discharged well 19 Aug. 1771; securities: John Smith, Castile[?] Moorgate, victualer, and John Beeching, London Wall, victualer; BAR, p. 326.

15. Drake and Long were long-established and well-known city merchants, with offices ca. 1776 at 17 Bishopsgate within ("within" indicated it was within the city walls). The partnership appears to have had extensive trading and financial interests. George Drake, Esq., merchant, resided at 34 New Bond Street, and Walter Drake, sugar-broker, at 13 Idol Lane. George Drake was one of the directors of the Bank of England by this date. John Long, merchant, resided at 14 Clement's Inn. There was also a Long and Son, crape and bunting warehouse, at 68 Watling Street. See *The London Directory for the Year 1776,* 9th ed. (London: Printed for T. Lowndes, 1776), pp. 4, 49, and 104. In the 1730s, Roger Drake

(George's father[?]) was director of Royal Exchange Assurance and resided in Crutched Friers, and the merchant company Drake Pennant and Long operated from the same address; see *Directory: Containing an Alphabetical List of the Names and Places of Abode of the Directors of Companies, Persons in Publick Business, Merchants, and Other Eminent Traders in the Cities of London and Westminster, and Borough of Southwark* (London: Printed and sold by Henry Kent, 1736), p. 17.

16. This patient relapses subsequently (see CB, p. C-114), and Monro is called to see him again. He is later admitted to Bethlem. See BAR, p. 294: Thomas Walker of Norton Falgate, Middlesex, admitted 19 Aug. 1769, discharged "Incurable & fitt," 4 Aug. 1770; securities: Luke Reily, gent., Castle Court, Fullwood Rents, Holborn, and William Fern, snuffer maker, Bromlow Street, Holborn. He was not readmitted to Bethlem as incurable. He was possibly related to Joseph Walker, a brewer at Mile End; see *London Directory for the Year 1776*, p. 170.

17. Shoreditch was a major center of the distilling and brewing trade in London at the time.

18. Possibly Mary Greves, Kensington, Middlesex, admitted to Bethlem 13 Nov. 1762, discharged well 21 Sept. 1763; securities: William Simpson, baker at Kensington, and Stephen Leaver, farmer at Brompton, near Kensington; BAR, p. 162.

19. Given that Monro's address was 7 Red Lion Square, Holborn, and that he had taken over a madhouse in Clerkenwell, this presumably would have been one of his more convenient consultations. Miss Lovell was almost certainly related to George Lovell, a glass-cutter resident in Red Lion Street, Bloomsbury, in 1790.

20. This may well have been Thomas Coltman (1747–1826), who married Mary Barlow (1747–86) on 2 Oct. 1769. See Allan Braham, *Wright of Derby; Mr and Mrs Coltman,* National Gallery Exhibition booklet, 1986. He was painted with his wife by Joseph Wright of Derby in 1771, the artist being a friend of Thomas. Thomas lived in St. Werburgh's, Derby, ca. 1771, and Mary was from Astbury, Cheshire. They had no children, and after Mary's death, Thomas remarried in 1789. Thomas was a lover of sports and the country life, as Wright's portrait suggested, depicting him and his wife on horses in the country, flanked by dogs. Coltman leased Gate Burton House in Lincolnshire for some years after his marriage. His seat, however, was Hognaby Priory, near Boston, Lincolnshire, which he inherited in 1768 (it was originally bought by his grandfather in 1715–16). However, the family had been members of the landed gentry for a relatively short period. Braham says that their fortune derived from a coffee house in London, but there is no record of such in Bryant Lillywhite's *London Coffee Houses. A Reference Book of Coffee Houses of the Seventeenth Eighteenth and Nineteenth Centuries* (London: George Allen and Unwin, 1963). Coltman was a friend and correspondent of Sir Joseph Banks, president of the Royal Society; an edition of twenty-two of Banks's letters written during 1791–97 was edited by Warren R. Dawson as *The Banks Letters* (1958). He was deputy lieutenant of Lincolnshire by 1791 and a JP and chairman of the magistrates' bench.

21. The Grecian Coffee House was at No. 19 Devereux Court, or Devereux Court Strand, leading to the Temple. It is mentioned frequently in early-eighteenth-century periodicals and newspapers, including the *Spectator,* the *Tatler,* and the *LEP,* many contributors penning articles and letters from that address. The *LEP* could be bought there, and a number of clubs met there, including a literary club of booksellers composed of people such as Longman, Alderman Cadell, James Dodsley, and Peter Elmsley. It was a popular resort for lawyers because of its proximity to the Temple. See Lillywhite, *London Coffee Houses,* pp. 243–45, no. 494.

22. Possibly related to Samuel Edge, brewer and JP for Westminster; *GM* (1745), p. 109.

23. This was William Macham, advocate and fellow of St. John's College, Oxford, 4 Nov. 1754, having matriculated on 30 June 1741 aged eighteen; B.C.L., 1749; D.C.L., 1754. He had been educated at Merchant Taylor's School and was the only son of Joseph Macham of Collingbourne, Kingston, Co. Wilts, surveyor of the King's Warehouse in the Port of London. Macham had inherited a large fortune, which according to one source "rendered the pursuit of professional emolument unnecessary; and he was not qualified to shine as an advocate." Certainly, he did not practice law, although one wonders if his mental condition also had something to do with his lack of professional attainment. At Doctor's Commons, he was registrar (1765–66), librarian (1771–72), treasurer (1773–74), and president (17 Oct. 1778). He died on 26 Aug. 1789. See Anon. [but attributed to Charles Coote], *Sketches of the Lives and Characters of Eminent English Civilians, with an Historical Introduction Relative to the College of Advocates . . . from the Beginning of the Reign of Henry VIII, to the Close of the Year 1803; by one of the Members of the College* (London: Sold by G. Kearsley, 1804), p. 123; George Drewry Squibb, *A History of the College of Advocates and Doctors of Law* (Oxford: Clarendon, 1977), p. 192; and Joseph Foster, *Alumni Oxonienses: The Members of the University of Oxford, 1500–1714 . . . Being the Matriculation Register of the University* (Oxford: Parker & Co., 1891), vol. 3, p. 893.

24. Possibly Sarah Cookson of Leeds, Yorkshire, admitted to Bethlem 12 May 1764 and discharged "fit" (i.e., fit for readmission as incurable) 10 Nov. 1764; securities: William Dawson, linen draper in Cornhill, and Samuel Whichcote, watchmaker, Fleet Street; BAR, p. 190. She was not readmitted as incurable.

25. I.e., Michael Duffield's Chelsea madhouse. For a discussion of this house, see Andrews and Scull, *Undertaker of the Mind,* chap. 5. For other cases sent or recommended to Duffield's, see CB, pp. C-50–54, C-56–58, C-106–8, C-123–24. According to Hunter and Macalpine, John Martyn (1699–1768), professor of botany at Cambridge University, who introduced the sedative valerian, also attended Duffield's madhouse. In 1743, Duffield charged a patient £4 18s for clothing, plus £25 for three months' lodging and £3 1s 6d for other expenses, making a total of £32 19s 6d; *Three Hundred Years of Psychiatry,* pp. 325, 363, fig. 68.

26. This is almost certainly Sarah Williams of St. James's Westminster, admitted to Bethlem 12 April 1766 and discharged well 26 July 1766; securities: George Price of New Street, St. Martins in the Fields, and David Williams of

Carnaby Street, St. James's, cheesemonger; BAR, p. 228. She may have been related to Hugh and Thomas Williams, who were Carnaby market grocers in 1790. A Mrs. Hester Williams had been one of those cases of alleged false confinement dealt with by the 1763 Madhouses Enquiry, but one in which no evidence of abuse could be found.

27. Elizabeth Moreati, of St. Mary le Bone, Middlesex, admitted to Bethlem 3 May 1766, discharged well 12 Aug. 1766; securities: William Savage of St. Paul's Bakehouse Court, Doctors Commons, gent., and Richard Dalton (1751[?]–91) of Pall Mall, gent.; BAR, p. 229. Her husband was presumably one of a number of Italian artists and craftsmen brought over to England by Dalton in the latter's capacity as Antiquary, Librarian, and Keeper of Drawings, Medals, etc. for George III. Such artists included the famous Venetian engraver Francesco Bartolozzi, who came to England in 1764 to work for Dalton on a salary of £400 per annum, staying with another well-known Italian engraver, Agostino Cipriani. However, Moreati is not mentioned in any of the standard works on Italian engravers in England, not even in Arthur M. Hind's *A History of Engraving and Etching from the Fifteenth Century to the Year 1914*, 3rd rev. ed. of *A Short History of Engraving and Etching* (New York: Dover, 1963), or in Joseph Strutt's *A Biographical Dictionary . . . of all the Engravers, from the Earliest Period of the Art of Engraving to the Present Time . . .*, 2 vols. (London: Printed by J. Davis for Robert Faulder, 1785). He was probably a craftsman rather than an engraver. Unlike Moreati, Bartolozzi left his wife behind in Italy and never saw her again once he settled in England, something for which he has been severely criticized by some art historians. It is possible that the strain of adjustment to life in a foreign country told on the nerves of Mrs. Moreati.

28. Richard Dalton; see note 27, above.

29. Possibly Margery Graham of St. Margaret's Westminster, admitted to Bethlem 4 June 1763 and discharged "fit" 15 Aug. 1764; securities: Gregor Drummond, Esq., James Street, St. Margaret's Westminster, and Archibald Campbell, gent., in Rochester, St. Johns dito; BAR, p. 171. She was not re-admitted as an incurable.

30. Bethnal Green Madhouse was one of the largest madhouses in London. In the early eighteenth century, it appears to have been run by Matthew Wright. Later, it was also run by Robert Cope, gent., who appears regularly, sometimes three or four times a month, in Bethlem's admission registers as a security for patients passed from one house to the other. He also frequently features in London and Middlesex churchwardens and overseers of the poor accounts, receiving payments for patients supported by parishes in Bethnal Green. As yet, we have found no record of a keeper called Mr. Thutton/Strutton.

31. Nicholas Tonkin of St. Andrew Holborn, Middlesex, admitted to Bethlem 9 Aug. 1766, discharged sick and weak 19 Dec. 1767; securities: Thomas Pingo of Kirby Street, engraver, and Thomas Beavor of the Globe, Hatton Garden, victualer; BAR, p. 235.

32. Possibly Elizabeth Worth of Aston Rowant, Oxford, admitted to Bethlem 23 June 1770 and died there of smallpox 31 July 1770; securities: Richard Davis, coffeeman, Mitre Court, Fleet Street, and Robert Mann, shoemaker, Fleet Street; BAR, p. 312. This is a clear indication that Monro had been compiling

case books for the previous years of his practice. See also CB, p. C-55, case of Mr. Frazier.

33. Possibly Margaret Cutter, Ponkisland, Northumberland, admitted to Bethlem 17 March 1764 and discharged "fit" 2 Aug. 1765; securities: William Henry Trent, merchant, Nicholas Lane, near Lombard Street, and Bryan Birkbeck, merchant, 3 King Court, Lombard Street; BAR, p. 188.

34. Possibly (but not likely) George Robinson, St. Giles Cripplegate, London, admitted to Bethlem 3 Nov. 1764 and discharged "fit" 10 Oct. 1766, but not readmitted to the incurables ward; securities: Edward Thornton, victualer, Three Tuns, Red Cross Street, and Richard Jackson, pawnbroker, Barbican; BAR, p. 201.

35. This was Hannah Mackenzie, wife of Peter Mackenzie. For affidavits on this case, see PRO KB1/16/3–4, Trinity 6, Geo. III, nos. 2 and 1, dated 22 May 1766 and 17 June 1766; PRO KB33/20/4. For a full survey of these affidavits, see Elizabeth Foyster, "Wrongful Confinement in Eighteenth-Century England: A Question of Gender?," unpublished paper delivered at University of Wales, Bangor, conference, July 1999, "Social and Medical Representations of the Links between Insanity and Sexuality." For our own discussion of the case, see Andrews and Scull, *Undertaker of the Mind,* chap. 2, p. 70 and note 134; and chap. 5, pp. 168, 171–72.

36. I.e., Peter Day, who kept a madhouse at Paddington, for more on whom see Andrews and Scull, *Undertaker of the Mind,* chap. 5.

37. I.e., John Sherratt, who, according to Foyster, "Wrongful Confinement," was a lawyer and well-known campaigner against private madhouses. See B. Rizzo, "John Sherratt, Negociator," *Bulletin of Research in the Humanities* 86.4 (1985), pp. 413–21.

38. We have been unable to identify this justice of the peace.

39. The King's Bench at Westminster Hall.

40. Possibly Malcolm Fraser of St. Mary Le Bone, Middlesex, admitted to Bethlem 15 Sept. 1770 and discharged well 8 June 1771, having been given a month's leave on 11 May 1771; securities: Richard Powers, carpenter, Sneds Court, Piccadilly, and Alexander Rose, stable keeper, Borlington Gardens; BAR, p. 317.

41. Possibly James Whitehead, St. Mary Magdalen, Bermondsey, admitted to Bethlem 28 March 1760 and discharged "fit" 2 Oct. 1761; securities: Francis Holmes, watchmaker in Rotherhith, and John Lee, bricklayer in Five Foot Lane; BAR, p. 112; or Thomas Whitehead, of Dunham, Nottingham, linen draper at Guildhall, London, declared bankrupt and required to surrender in 1766; *LEP,* no. 5971 (22–25 Feb. 1766), p. 1, col. 4. A John Whitehead, attorney, was resident in Great Queen Street in 1790, but this was a common surname: at least six Whiteheads were mentioned in the London Trade Directory for this year.

42. Dr. William Heberden the elder (1710–1801), one of the most famous physicians of the eighteenth century. Heberden graduated from St. John's College, Cambridge, A.B. 1728, A.M. 1732, M.D. 1739. He practiced medicine and lectured for ten years in Cambridge. At the College of Physicians, he was Candidate (1745), Fellow (1746), Gulstonian Lecturer (1749), Harveian Orator (1750), Croonian Lecturer (1760), Censor (1749, 1755, 1760), Consilarius

(1762), and Elect (1762–81). He was nominated as physician to the Queen in 1761 but declined the post, worried about how his career and reputation might be affected by such a position. His only major publication was evidently *Commentaries on the History and Cure of Diseases,* translated from the Latin by his son, William Heberden, junior (London: T. Payne, 1802). See Munk, *Roll,* vol. 2, pp. 159–64.

43. This patient was possibly the son of Sir William Rowley (1690[?]–1768), Admiral of the Fleet (1762–68) and Lord of the Admiralty (1751–58), who was knighted in 1753. If so, then his mother was Arabella, daughter and heir of Captain George Dawson of County Derry, and he evidently had two brothers, including Joshua (1730[?]–90), a naval officer and later vice-admiral and baronet (1786). (It should be noted, however, that the DNB asserts that Joshua was Rowley's eldest son.)

44. I.e., Sir John Pringle, baronet (1707–82), who was given a baronetcy on 26 May 1766; *LEP,* no. 6019 (27–29 May 1766), p. 3, col. 2. After a rudimentary education at home under a private tutor, Pringle went to St. Andrews University, where he continued his studies under the direction of his uncle, Dr. Francis Pringle. He studied for a year at Edinburgh, and being intended for business in commerce proceeded to Amsterdam. During a casual visit to Leyden, he encountered a lecture by Boerhaave, which made so strong an impression on him that, from Sept. 1728, he decided to devote himself to medicine. He embarked on a medical degree at Leyden in Sept. 1728. Attending a whole course of Boerhaave's and others' lectures, he graduated M.D. Leyden 1730 (his inaugural dissertation was entitled *"De Marcore Senili"*). At Leyden he formed an intimate friendship with van Swieten, the commentator on Boerhaave and later a celebrated professor and practitioner at Vienna. He completed his medical education in Paris, subsequently returning to Edinburgh and commencing practice. In 1734, he was appointed joint professor of moral philosophy, with the right of sole succession, and in 1742 he became personal physician to the earl of Stair, commander of the British army in Flanders. Appointed in charge of the Flanders military hospital, he remained there during the 1744 campaign, his conduct attracting the favorable notice of the duke of Cumberland. He was awarded two commissions (1744) and became physician-general to his Majesty's Forces in the Low Countries, etc., and physician to the Royal Hospitals in the same countries. He resigned his university professorship and accompanied the army to Scotland. Subsequently he remained abroad with the troops and did not return to England until after the Treaty of Aix-la-Chapelle. After taking up residence in London and commencing private practice, in 1749 he was appointed Physician in Ordinary to the Duke of Cumberland. In 1761, he became physician to the Queen's Household, and, in 1763, Physician in Ordinary to the Queen. He was created baronet in 1766 and was gazetted Physician in Ordinary to the King in 1774. He was also physician to the Princess Dowager of Wales. He was LCP (Licentiate of the College of Physicians) (1758), Fellow, *speciali gratia* (1763), and Censor in 1770, but declined to act and paid the fine. His wide national and international contacts saw him become Fellow of College of Physicians of Edinburgh (1735), Foreign Fellow of the Royal Society of Medicine of Paris, and Member of the Royal Society of Gottingen and of the Academy of Sciences at Haarlem and Madrid. He

became F.R.S. in 1745, a member of the Council in 1753, and President of the Royal Society in 1772.

A pioneer of antisepsis, Pringle wrote extensively on the nature and cure of fevers in hospitals, jails, and on board ships, and on diseases of the army and navy; his books on these subjects were in John Monro's collection. Famous as a promoter of experimental investigation, he gave lectures on the annual presentation of the R. S. Copley gold medal for experimental observations. Six of Pringle's lectures edited by Dr. Kippis, mostly on history of natural philosophy, also discussed Captain Cook's methods regarding the preservation of the health of seamen. Pringle was an intimate friend of Cook, and Cook was probably influenced by the former in his hygienic practices on long voyages. These entailed a dietetic code deploying work, rigid attention to cleanliness, and preservation from wet and weather. Injury from a fall and advancing years forced Pringle to resign the Royal Society presidency in 1778, and he retired to Edinburgh in 1781 but was forced back to London by the inclement climate. He died 18 Jan. 1782, aged seventy-five, and was buried at St. James Westminster, and a monument of him by Nollekens was erected in Westminster Abbey. His portrait is by Sir Joshua Reynolds. Besides several contributions to *Philosophical Transactions of the Royal Society,* Pringle's publications include *Observations on the Nature and Cure of Hospital or Jayl Fevers, Observations on the Diseases of the Army* (London: Printed for A. Millar and D. Wilson and T. Payne, 1752), and *A Discourse upon some Late Improvements of the Means for Preserving the Health of Mariners* (London: Printed for the Royal Society, 1776). Pringle was also a member of the Humane Society, established For the Recovery [i.e., resuscitation] of Persons Apparently Drowned. This account is distilled almost verbatim from Munk, *Roll,* vol. 2, pp. 252–56. For more modern assessments of Pringle's work, see, e.g., Sydney Selwyn, "Sir John Pringle; Hospital Reformer, Moral Philosopher and Pioneer of Antiseptics," *Medical History* 10 (1966), pp. 266–74; Charles Gordon, "Sir John Pringle and the Apothecaries," *Pharmaceutical Historian* 19.4 (1989), pp. 5–12.

45. Almost definitely (Sir) Caesar Hawkins (1711–86), who was surgeon to Chelsea Hospital and was appointed sergeant surgeon to the king. Hawkins was an expert on venereal disease. See, e.g., Charles Hales, *A Letter Addressed to Caesar Hawkins . . . Containing New Thoughts and Observations in the Cure of Venereal Disease.* Hawkins inoculated the Prince of Wales, Prince Frederick, and the Bishop of Osnaburgh in 1766. See *LEP,* no. 5980 (27 Feb.–1 Mar. 1766), p. 3, col. 1; no. 5981 (1–4 Mar. 1766), p. 5, col. 3. He was involved in the controversial dismissal of the surgeon Samuel Lee from Chelsea Hospital in the 1750s. See John Ranby and Caesar Hawkins, *The True Account of all the Transactions before . . . the Commissioners for the Officers of Chelsea Hospital, as far as related to the Admission and Dismission of S. Lee, Surgeon . . . To Which is Prefixed a Short Account of the Nature of a Rupture* (London: Printed for John and Paul Knapton, 1754); [Samuel Lee], *A Proper Reply to the Serjeant Surgeons [i.e., J. Ranby & C. Hawkins's] Defence of their Conduct at Chelsea Hospital* (London: W. Owen, 1754).

Possibly, however, this doctor was Charles Hawkins, Esq., surgeon to St. George's Hospital, Pall Mall, London.

46. See note 44, above.

47. Dr. Anthony Relhan (1715–76) was educated at Trinity College, Dublin (A.B., 1735) and studied medicine at Leyden from 1740, returning to Dublin to take his M.D. (1743). He was admitted as fellow (1747) of the College of Physicians in Ireland and made president in 1755. He was physician to Mercers' Hospital but was somewhat ostracized by his colleagues at the college after prescribing James's Powders, subsequently moving to England with James's encouragement. Commencing his practice at Brighton (1759–62/3), Relhan then moved to London. He became candidate of the College of Physicians there on 25 June 1763 and fellow a year later. He was Gulstonian Lecturer in 1765 and gave the Harveian Oration in 1770 (pub. 1771). Relhan, who was a great advocate of natural bathing and of inoculation, published *A Short History of Brighthelmston. With Remarks on its Air, and an Analysis of its Waters, Particularly of an Uncommon Mineral One* (London: Printed for W. Johnston, 1761) and *Refutation of the Reflections Against Inoculation* (London, 1764). See Munk, *Roll*, vol. 2, pp. 257–58. He had been made a fellow of the (English) College of Physicians in 1764, when Monro was a censor. See *Annals/Register of the College of Physicians*, in the Royal College of Physicians Library, London, 25 Jan. 1764, vol. 12, fol. 146.

48. I.e., the famous spa town, where many invalids suffering from mental and nervous (as well as somatic) problems were sent in this period.

49. Possibly related to Jane Sergison of St. Dionis Backchurch, London, admitted to Bethlem 27 May 1769 and discharged well 23 Sept. 1769; securities: Walter Bathurst, upholder, Fenchurch Street, and Henry Gretton, engraver, same place; BAR, p. 289.

50. This was Richard Peers ([?]–1772), alderman of Queenhith Ward (1765–72). His brother, Thomas Peers, had died the year before Richard's appearance in Monro's case book. His son was Sir Richard Peers-Symons, baronet. A Common Councillor for Queenhithe (1746–65), Peers was, like alderman Barlow Trecothick (see CB, p. C-115, note 84), a loyal city politician and a Wilkesite (see below). Both men were prominent governors of Bridewell and Bethlem and attended some of the same court and committee meetings as did John Monro (e.g., BCGM, 18 June, 30 July 1767, 6 Sept. 1770, pp. 176, 183, 310). Peers had been a particularly active subcommittee member during the earlier 1760s (BSCM, 1 Nov. 1760, 2 May 1761, 3 Sept. 1763, 12 and 19 Jan. 1765; Bethlem Grand Committee Minutes, 24 March 1762, 20 Sept. 1763, in BSCM, p. 377). In 1765, he was on a committee that rewarded two patients for helping a basketman (or keeper) retake another patient who had escaped (BSCM, 12 Jan. 1765). Like Trecothick, too, Peers was a clothworker by trade, becoming master of the company in 1763. He became a member of the Committee of City Lands in 1766 and was involved in a number of London charities besides Bethlem (e.g., he was elected one of the stewards of the trustees of the several charity schools of the city and its suburbs in May 1766); *LEP*, no. 5964 (6–8 Feb. 1766), p. 1, col. 2; no. 6011 (8–10 May 1766), p. 3, col. 2. He died on 25 June 1772. See *GM* (1775), p. 539; (1772), p. 343; Alfred B. Beaven, *The Aldermen of the City of London* (London: The Corporation of the City of London; Eden Fisher & Co., 1908), vol. 1, pp. 195, 233; vol. 2, pp. 133, 134, 193, 198, 199, 225, 235.

John Wilkes (1727–97) had created political uproar in the 1760s as a focus of opposition to the Grenville government. Wilkes had been forced into exile in France in 1764, once warrants for his arrest were issued following his publication of material in the *North Briton* (in particular, scandalous gossip about Lord Bute and criticism of the King's Speech). He succeeded in blending issues such as infringements of the freedoms of the press with wider concerns regarding the liberty of the subject and restrictions on free trade (especially with the colonies). Wilkes was expelled from the House of Commons. On his return to England in 1768, with support from smaller city shopkeepers, craftsmen, and tradesmen, Wilkes became the darling of radical urban politics, winning the Middlesex election of that year. However, he was prosecuted for inciting Wilkesite riots and was imprisoned in the King's Bench gaol. See, e.g., Glyn Williams and John Ramsden, *Ruling Britannia: A Political History of Britain 1688–1988* (London: Longman, 1990); and John Brooke and Sir Lewis Namier, *The House of Commons, 1754–1790: Introductory Survey*, History of Parliament Series (London: Her Majesty's Stationery Office, 1964; Oxford: Oxford University Press, 1968), esp. pp. 16–17.

51. Possibly Ann Manley of Hammersmith, Fulham, Middlesex, admitted to Bethlem 23 June 1759 and discharged well 4 Sept. 1760; securities: John Pillips, plumber, Peter Street, Bloomsbury, and John Within, chandler, Bridges Street, Covent Garden; BAR, p. 100.

52. Possibly Robert Cawthorne of Camberwell, whose daughter, Eleanor, with a fortune of £300, married Richard Purchas, "an eminent Scarlet Dyer in Sothwark" on 16 April 1766; *LEP*, no. 5600 (17–19 April 1766), p. 1, col. 2. Possibly related to Jane Cawthorn of Yaxley, Huntingdon, admitted to Bethlem 28 July 1759 and discharged "fit" 28 July 1760; securities: Coles Child, toyman on London Bridge, and Benjamin Silcock, hardwareman, same place; or else to Jane Cawthorne of St. Giles Hanover Square, Middlesex, admitted to Bethlem 22 April 1769 and discharged "Incurable & not fitt" 30 Dec. 1769; securities: John Wilmot, goldsmith, St. Margaret's Hill, and James Showell, whip maker, Oxford Road; BAR, pp. 102, 286. Neither of the patients mentioned in this note was readmitted to the incurables ward. A Joseph Cawthorne, raffia merchant, died at his house in Islington, aged eighty-three, on 25 April 1766; *LEP*, no. 5604 (26–29 April 1766), p. 1, col. 3. A William Cawthorn of St. Peters at Arches, Lincoln, however, was admitted as an incurable 10 June 1769 and died in Bethlem on 10 Dec. 1769; securities: Nathaniel Hardcastle, merchant at Old Swan by Crooked Lane, and Stephen Calley, merchant, same place; Bethlem Incurables Admission Registers, p. 49.

53. I.e., inoculation for smallpox, which was at this time a very controversial, but increasingly popular, medical treatment. See, e.g., *LEP*, no. 6093 (18–20 Nov. 1766), p. 3, col. 3, re. the celebrated Mr. Sutton inoculating six hundred persons in one day at Maidstone and having inoculated near four thousand in Kent, allegedly without losing one. Peter E. Razzell, *The Conquest of Smallpox: The Impact of Inoculation on Smallpox Mortality in Eighteenth-Century Britain* (Firle, Sussex: Caliban Books, 1977); Razzell, *Edward Jenner's Cowpox Vaccine: The History of a Medical Myth*, 2nd ed. (Firle: Caliban Books, 1980).

54. Possibly Hugh Hudson, admitted to Bethlem from the Commissioners for

Sick and Wounded Seamen, 19 June 1756 and discharged well 1 Feb. 1757; BAR, p. 42. By the early nineteenth century, Miles's Hoxton madhouse was being regularly used by the War Office and Admiralty for its lunatics and was spoken of explicitly as a hospital for servicemen. See Andrews and Scull, *Undertaker of the Mind*, chap. 5.

55. Possibly Ann Winter of Seaford Sussex, admitted to Bethlem 31 March 1770 and discharged well 22 Sept. 1770; securities: Cecil Pitt, upholsterer, Moorfields, and Robert Chessey, same place and trade; BAR, p. 307; or perhaps the widow of Mr. Winter, clothworker and presser, who died at his house on Windmill Hill, Moorfields, on 7 May 1766; *LEP*, no. 6011 (8–10 May 1766), p. 3, col. 2.

56. Possibly wife of Thomas Blinkhorn, silk weaver, resident at 3 Wood Street, Spitalfields, of Blinkthorn and Vanes, weavers, in Artillery Lane; see *London Directory for the Year 1766* (London: Printed for T. Lowndes, 1766), p. 17, and *The Universal British Directory of Trade and Commerce . . .* (1790), where Thomas Blinkthorn, a black silk weaver, was now at Raven Row, Spitalfields.

57. This is possibly Kinder of Kinder, Crew, & Co., hosiers, at 4 Fell Street, Wood Street; see *London Directory for the Year 1766*, p. 97.

58. Possibly the wife of James Law, baker, resident in 10 Jewry Street, Aldgate, in 1790.

59. Cow Cross was in West Smithfield, London.

60. Possibly related to William Alcock, son of John of Trotton, cleric, who matriculated from New College Oxford on 5 July 1728, aged nineteen. Alternatively, this patient may have been related to the Oxford physician Nathan Alcock (1707–79) and his brother, Rev. Thomas Alcock of Runcorn, Cheshire, or/and their uncle, John Alcock, vicar of Iver, Bucks. Alternatively/additionally, she may have been related to Mr. Alcock, M.B., organist to the earl of Donegall, vicar-choral of Litchfield, and organist of Sutton-Coldfield, who was unanimously chosen organist of the collegiate church of Tamworth in 1766; *LEP*, no. 5965 (18–21 Jan. 1766), p. 1, col. 3. There was also a Hannah Alcock of Newark-upon-Trent, Nottingham, who was admitted to Bethlem 18 Nov. 1769 and died there 21 April 1770; securities: William Selby, plumber, Green Street, Hanover Square, and John Garston, king's messenger, Whitehall; BAR, p. 299. See also Foster, *Alumni Oxonienses*, vol. 1, p. 13.

61. Probably Elizabeth Wilson, St. George Hanover Square, admitted to Bethlem 14 June 1760 and discharged "fit" 17 Oct. 1761; securities: William Banyar, cheesemonger in Woodstock Street, Hanover Square, and William Tranter, oilman, Cow Lane, near West Smithfield; BAR, p. 115. The admission register includes a crossed-out and evidently mistaken entry about her getting leave for two months on 29 Nov. 1760 and again for two months on 19 Jan. 1761, and being brought back again on 7 March 1761.

62. Possibly related to John Williams of Inner Temple, who died in 1768; *GM* (1768), p. 303.

63. I.e., Hertford. The trial was probably at the Assizes.

64. Possibly the same Mrs. Wilson mentioned earlier (see note 61, above), but this is unlikely as Monro normally specifies a second visit to a patient.

65. Presumably Thomas Reeve (1700–80), who was educated at Emmanuel

College, Cambridge (M.B., 1727; M.D., 1732). He studied at Leyden under Boerhaave and Albinus. He was Candidate (1735), Fellow (1736), Registrar (1739–41), Censor (1741 and 1749), Elect (1750), Consiliarius (1751–3), and President of the College of Physicians (1754–63). Reeve was also physician to St. Thomas's Hospital until his retirement (1740–60) and lived in Throgmorton Street. See Thomas Reeve, *A Cure for the Epidemical Madness of Drinking Tar Water* (London: Printed for John and Paul Knapton . . . , 1744). As president of the college Reeve had thrice chosen Monro as one of the censors. See *Annals/Register of the College of Physicians;* and Munk, *Roll,* vol. 2, pp. 133–34.

66. Possibly Jane Gordon of Rogat, Sussex, admitted to Bethlem (probably after a stay in Bethnal Green madhouse) 18 Aug. 1770 and discharged "Incurable & fitt" 13 July 1771; securities: Robert Cope, gent., Bethnal Green, and Bernard Ellis, innholder, Spurr Inn, Southwark; BAR, p. 316.

67. Possibly wife of James Sheeles (b. 1738), clergyman, who published a sermon on a "day of general fast and humiliation" in 1762 as well as *Threnodia Northumbrica. A Funeral Pindaric Poem Sacred to the Memory of the Right Honourable the Lady Elizabeth Anne Frances Percy* (London: Printed for R. and J. Dodsley; sold by M. Cooper, 1761). Sheeles was also featured in the quondam (mentally deranged) poet Christopher Smart's (1722–71) *Poems on Several Occasions. Viz. Munificence and Modesty. Female Dignity. To Lady Hussey Delaval. Verses from Catullus, after Dining with Mr. Murray. Epitaphs. On the Duchess of Cleveland. On Henry Fielding, Esq. On the Rev. James Sheeles. Epitaph from Demosthenes* (London: Printed for the author, and sold by Mr. Fletcher and Co.; Mr. Davies; Mr. Flexney; Mr. Laurence; and Mr. Almon, 1763).

68. Or Lisham Green, near Paddington.

69. This is possibly Nathaniel Cambden, wine merchant at 14 Dowgate Hill; see *London Directory for the Year 1776,* p. 29. Regarding the word "Snow=hill": the equals sign was the normal way to signify hyphens in eighteenth-century printed materials, but Monro normally abbreviated that in handwriting to a colon—as many contemporary letter-writers and diarists did.

70. This must have been Richard Beecher, or Becher, Esq., who was a director of the East India Company and resident at 25 Portman Square; see *London Directory for the Year 1766,* pp. 6 and 12. He died in Nov. 1782 in Bengal as he was going up the river in a boat for the recovery of his health; see *GM* (1783), p. 541.

71. Clearly this was not an uncommon course of events. A Captain Elliott was married at Whittingham, Northumberland, on 30 Jan. 1766 to Miss Babby Kerr, in that neighborhood, he having "lately returned from the East-Indies, where he acquired a large fortune"; *LEP,* no. 5961 (30 Jan.–1 Feb. 1766), p. 1, col. 1.

72. Possibly "Captain Duncan, of the Wharton Excise yacht," who took "a sloop from Terviere, laden with Holland gin, some teas and china, and carried her into Dunbar in Scotland" in early January 1766; *LEP,* no. 5964 (16–18 Jan. 1766), p. 3, col. 3.

73. I.e., in the service of the East India Company.

74. Possibly John Alwright, glove dyer, of 96 Wood Street, North Street, Westminster, ca. 1790.

75. Monro evidently forgot to enter a word describing the offense done to liberty here.

76. Taverns were commonly used as meeting places by Freemason lodges, and the society's meetings and activities were regularly featured in the newspaper and periodical press of the period. Given the apparent (if exaggerated) pervasiveness of Freemasonry in eighteenth-century society and the suspicion with which this secret society was regarded in many quarters, it does not seem surprising that a number of contemporaries connected their morbid anxieties to it. See, e.g., advertisement in *LEP*, no. 5956 (2–4 Jan. 1766):

FREE-MASONRY
This Day was publish'd, Price 1s 6d
The SIXTH EDITION, corrected, of JACHIN and BOAZ; or, An authentic Key to the Door of Free-Masonry, both Antient [*sic*] and Modern. Calculated not only for the Instruction of every new-made Mason, but also for the Information of all who intend to become Brethren. . . . By a GENTLEMAN belonging to the Jerusalem Lodge. A frequent Visiter [*sic*] at the Queen's-Arms in St Paul's Church-yard, and other eminent Lodges. Printed for W. Nicholl, in St Paul's Church-yard. . . .

77. Israel Pottinger, of St. Faiths, London, admitted to Bethlem 7 Feb. 1767, discharged "at the Request of his wife & Without the Consent of Committee or Doctor," 28 March 1767; securities: Samuel Leach of New Street, Bishopsgate, fishing-tackle maker, and William Lear of Tower Street, printer; BAR, p. 243. This may have been the playwright and poet Israel Pottinger (flourished 1759–1780), who burlesqued the Methodists in 1761 and parodied Sheridan's plays in 1776 and 1780. He wrote, inter alia, *The Methodist: A [Three Act] Comedy: Being a Continuation and Completion of the Plan of The Minor, written by Mr. Foote . . .*, 2nd ed. (London: Printed for I. Pottinger, 1761), completing an earlier work by Samuel Foote. See also Pottinger, *The Humorous Quarrel; or, The Battle of the Greybeards . . .* (London: Printed for I. Pottinger, 1761); Pottinger, *The Duenna: A Comic Opera, in Three Acts . . .* (London: E. Johnson, 1776); Pottinger, *The General Fast: A Lyric Ode: With a Form of Prayer Proper for the Occasion; and a Dedication to the King* (London: 1776); and Pottinger, *The Critic; or a Tragedy Rehearsed: A New Dramatic Piece in Three Acts . . .* (London: S. Bladon, 1780). (Among other thespians who ended up in lunatic hospitals in this period was the well-known actor Samuel Reddish [1735–85], who died in York Asylum but also spent time in St. Luke's, where he was visited by John Taylor, who referred to that hospital as "Bedlam"; John Taylor, *Records Of My Life* [London: Edward Bull, 1832], vol. 1, pp. 48–50; and DNB.) Israel Pottinger was also, possibly, related to Samuel Pottinger of Newbury, Berkshire, admitted to Bethlem on 9 Dec. 1769 and discharged well on 11 May 1771, having "run" (i.e., escaped) on 15 Jan. 1770 and been "Bro[ugh]t agane" (i.e., retaken) on 13 March 1770, and having "run" again on 21 June 1770 and been given "leave [of absence for] 2 months" on 1 Dec. 1770. His securities were Richard Shaw, tallow chandler, Aldersgate Street, and James Bull, carpenter, Bishopsgate Street; BAR, p. 301.

78. Probably Stephen Hooper, a captain from Ramsgate, who died in 1783; *GM* (1783), p. 92.

79. This was Clifford Handeside, evidently a practitioner of man-midwifery. He was identified in the anonymous satirical poem *Iatro-Rhapsodica: OR, a Physical Rhapsody* (London: 1751) as a devotee of the physician and surgeon-midwife John Bamber (1667–1753). See Adrian Wilson, *The Making of Man-Midwifery: Childbirth in England, 1660–1770* (Cambridge, Mass.: Harvard University Press, 1995). Wilson was unsure whether Handeside was a man-midwife, but Monro's notes seem to clinch the matter.

80. Almost certainly William Westbrooke Richardson, who died at Mount Pleasant in Barnet (near Hadley, where the Monros had their country seat) in 1771; *GM* (1771), p. 335.

81. Bartholomew di Dominiceti (flourished 1735–82) was a Venetian physician who had arrived in England in 1753 after being exiled from his native city under somewhat uncertain circumstances and after practicing in Europe for a few years. He seems to have been attracted to England because of its reputation as a land of "liberty," but also presumably because its relatively lightly policed medical marketplace offered him more ample scope for setting up in practice. He moved to Bristol the year following his arrival in England and immediately opened his first bathing apparatus, in March 1755, in Templebeck Street. Ambitious entrepreneur that he was, he erected a larger one in 1757 in Guinea Street and another, similar one on College Green in the same city. Dominiceti claimed to be democratizing medicine by divesting it of scientific phraseology and making it readily and economically available. Yet, in order to publicize, to legitimate, and to gain the sanction of local and medical authorities for his methods, Dominiceti was still at some pains to articulate the scientific basis on which they worked. Thus, when he decided to further expand his business by translating it to London, where he built an even more "commodious apparatus" at Millbank, Westminster, in 1764, he invited both the College of Physicians and the Royal Society to attend and inspect his works. In the following year Dominiceti opened his most "extensive apparatus at Chelsea," extending a further invitation to "the faculty, and learned in particular"; Dominiceti, *A Plan for Extending the Use of Artificial Water-Baths, Pumps, Vapours, and Dry-Baths, Fumigations, and Frictions; By the Mode and Means Invented and Directed by Dr Bartholomew di Dominiceti* (London: The author, 1771), p. 9.

The Chelsea apparatus was situated in the grounds of his own house in Cheyne Walk, a fashionable area of Chelsea next to China Walk and King's Road, and it was this apparatus that Monro's patient had evidently attended. It was described by Dominiceti as follows:

> This apparatus consists of a variety of Water-Baths and Pumps, each of which is placed in a neat and convenient room, warmed as the weather and necessity require, medicated with ten different sorts of vegetable, or mineral substances, and all differently heated, or cooled gradually, or instantaneously; according to the disorders, constitutions, and other circumstances that occur. . . .

Dominiceti, *Plan for Extending*, pp. 9–10. In fact, there were five types of oper-

ations on offer: a water bath, pumps, dry and vaporous baths, moist or dry fumigations, and "sleous, spirituous or dry frictions"; pp. 12–13. Contiguous to
every water bath in a separate apartment was a vaporous and a dry bath, the former warmed by the vapors of boiling water, and medicated as previously speci-
fied. The apparatus was impressively large, two hundred twenty feet long, thirty
feet broad, and two stories high, and contained thirty-six sweating and seven
fumigating bed chambers, with separate waiting rooms for ladies and gentlemen;
six water baths with pumps; twelve vapor and dry baths, all also segregated by
sex and class; drying apartments for garments and blankets, and a large, thirty-
foot-square room for the amusement of the convalescent.

The baths were supposed to operate in a "natural," cleansing way, wholly in
accord with humoral theory reconstituted by mechanism. By opening the pores
and "admitting" healing vapors "into the muscular and nervous fibres of the
whole animal system" and by circulating in the blood, these baths, purportedly,
"without any force . . . disperse the most remote, obstinate obstructions, [and]
draw from the pores of the skin the adhesive scorbutic humours" and restore
"excretory, secretory and circulatory equilibrium"; p. 11.

Although there were charitable dispensations on admission to the less well off
or deserving sections of society, nonetheless profit was clearly the dominant
motivation behind Dominiceti's business activities. With tickets at Chelsea variously priced and scaled at five guineas for twenty visits, or twenty guineas for one
hundred and twenty visits, the apparatus was primarily aimed at the respectable,
the genteel, and the wealthy, conceived of as "an ASYLUM OF HEALTH, for
the Superior Orders of the community," Dominiceti, *An Address from Dr.
Dominiceti of Chelsea. Humbly Submitted to the Consideration of the Commons
of Great Britain, Individually, Introducing a Petition, which is Proposed to be
Presented to that Honourable House in Parliament Assembled . . . Introductory
to a Petition [Praying the Grant of Letters Patent for his Machine called the
Economist]* (London: The author, 1782), p. 21.

By 1771, Dominiceti claimed to have treated over twelve thousand patients.
Yet his activities had aroused considerable ire and censure from other rival and
unsympathetic practitioners in both Bristol and London. Many believed him a
quack and his techniques seriously flawed, if not wholly ineffective. Some
accused him of marketing old medicine as if it were a novelty; some berated him
as a profiteer and criticized his high fees, and others resented him mainly
because he was an Italian and a "Papist" who had successfully intruded onto
their patch and damaged their own livelihoods. The famous surgeon and
anatomist John Hunter totally deplored the efforts of "Signior Dominiceti" on
behalf of one of his patients, a Mr. Padmore, a gardener who had become para-
lyzed after a fall from a horse. Dominiceti

> saw him, and assured him of a cure in a fortnight: he began by bathing him in warm
> water in which herbs had been boiled. He was sensibly worse from this practice, and
> the Doctor got him removed to his warm baths at Chelsea but he died in four days.
> N.B. He was in perfect health in all other respects when the Doctor took him in hand.

See Elizabeth Allen, J. L. Turk, and Sir Reginald Murley, eds., *The Case Books of
John Hunter* (London: Royal Society of Medicine, 1993), no. 302, pp. 207–8.

Dominiceti promoted his "invention" and countered such charges in a vigorous but typical eighteenth-century way. He ventured repeatedly into print, endorsing his baths and attacking his critics. He sent addresses to the Houses of Commons and Lords, and in 1766 he gained a royal patent and the patronage of H.R.H. the Duke of York and his family. He emphasized the backing for bathing in the texts of a host of classical and modern medical authorities, from Hippocrates and Galen to Floyer, Baynard, and Cheyne. Additionally, during the 1750s and 1760s, he obtained and published testimonials and endorsements from a legion of the eminent and the respectable, clergy, lawyers, surgeons, apothecaries, and chemists among them, testifying to his humanity and skill in medicine, chemistry, and anatomy. His attacks on other available medicines as themselves nugatory, if not "nauseous" and damaging to health, seem to have further raised the hackles of some practitioners, but his patients voted with their feet and attended his baths in droves. Keen to protect his business from the opportunism of imitators, Dominiceti also took measures to repulse the efforts of other "pseudo" practitioners, such as an Irishman in Chelsea who had styled himself "Achmet" and had sought his support for a similar scheme in Ireland. However, Dominiceti generally seems to have failed in his attempts to prevent such imitations. Most conspicuously, he failed during 1773 when he took legal means to block the patent application of a rival practitioner called John Irvine, whose method of distilling fresh water from salt water the Italian alleged to have been intellectual theft from his own system.

He was assisted in his practice by his son, for whom he had helped to build another establishment at Panton Street, Haymarket, which opened on 4 March 1779. Rhodomonte was almost as dedicated a publicist as his father had been and presumably inherited the entire business on the latter's death. See, e.g., Rhodomonte Dominiceti, *A Dissertation on the Artificial Medicated Water Baths . . . Together with a Description of the Apparatus, Erected in Panton-Square, Hay-Market*, 2nd ed. (London: Printed for the Author, 1782; 3rd ed., 1794). For Bartholomew di Dominiceti and his baths, see Bartholomew di Dominiceti, *A Short and Calm Apology of Bartholomew di Dominiceti, &c. from Venice, Physician, Surgeon, and Chymist, in Regard to the many Injuries and Repeated Affronts he has, Uncall'd for, met with during the 6 years he has been in Bristol, etc.* (Bristol: Printed for S. Farley, 1762); Dominiceti, *Begin. To the Public, etc.* [extracts from an address to the Royal Society and College of Physicians, on his baths, with remarks by Justus] (London: J. Towers, 1764); Dominiceti, *A Plan for Extending*; Dominiceti, *Medical Anecdotes of the Last Thirty Years, Illustrated with Medical Truths, and Addressed to the Medical Faculty; but in an Especial Manner, to the People at Large. With an Appendix, and Copious Index* (London: L. Davis, 1781); and Dominiceti, *An Address*. Mary Fissell, *Patients, Power and the Poor in Eighteenth-Century Bristol*, unfortunately fails to mention Dominiceti.

82. See CB, p. C-17, for earlier reference to Mr. Walker.

83. Earlier referred to as "Mr Devic"; see CB, p. C-4.

84. This was probably the wife of Barlow Trecothick (1718[?]–75), alderman of Vintry Ward (1764–74). She died three years after appearing in the case book, on 31 July 1769; GM (1769), p. 414. Trecothick himself was a leading

London tradesman and politician. A clothworker by trade, he did military service in Colonel White's regiment during 1770–75 and was treasurer (1773) and vice president (1773–75) of the Honourable Artillery Company. A London MP during 1768–74, he was a loyal city Whig and an ally of Wilkes, repeatedly voting with Peers and the opposition on the side of Wilkes and his supporters in the heady political climate of the 1760s and 1770s. He became a sheriff of London in 1766. Canvases and thanks he addressed to the London liverymen for votes for him to be returned as an MP in 1768 are held at the Bodleian Library, Oxford. Peers's and Trecothick's voting patterns in city politics closely resembled those of other prominent aldermen who were also governors of Bridewell and Bethlem and regularly attended the hospital's court meetings in the 1760s: men such as Sir Robert Ladbroke, Brass Crosby (musician, then goldsmith; Alderman of Bread-Street Ward), and John Sawbridge. Peers and Trecothick voted together on the Wilkesite side in the issue of the election of Sir Matthew Blakiston, another notable Bethlem governor. Trecothick was one of a group of opposition aldermen elected during 1768–78 out of their turns. He succeeded William Beckford as Lord Mayor on the latter's death on 21 June 1770. Trecothick died on 28 May 1775. See BCGM, e.g., 1 and 8 April 1762, 13 Feb., 24 April, 25 July 1765, 18 June, 30 July 1767, 28 July 1768, pp. 11, 18, 98, 111, 124, 142, 176, 180, 229; GM (1775), p. 304; LEP, nos. 5997 and 5999, 10–12 and 12–15 April, p. 3, col. 2, and p. 4, col. 2; Beaven, Aldermen of the City of London, vol. 1, pp. 214, 233, 280, 292, 320, 325, 349; vol. 2, pp. xxvi, xliv, xlvi, xlix, lviii, 132, 135, 139, 235; Brooke and Namier, The House of Commons, 1754–1790: Introductory Survey; and Brooke and Namier, The House of Commons 1754–1790 (London: Published for the History of Parliament Trust by Secker and Warburg, 1985). Trecothick was probably involved in or connected to Trecothick and Apthorp, merchants, of 26 Bucklerbury, later called Trecothick, Twaites and Co; London Directory for the Year 1776, p. 165; The Universal British Directory of Trade and Commerce . . . (1790).

85. Possibly the wife of Benjamin Webb, watchmaker, resident at 21 St. John's Square, Clerkenwell, by 1790.

86. I.e., an advertisement for him as missing and absconded from home was placed in the papers, a relatively customary and increasing practice during this period, although the more genteel families were less likely to take advantage of so public a medium for displaying their private woes. These advertisements tended to go into tremendous detail in order to facilitate identification. See, e.g., LEP, no. 3821 (14–16 April 1752), where an advertisement appears requesting any information as to the whereabouts of Lawrence Lodge, who "went off from" Starbotton West Riding, Yorkshire, and had spoken of traveling by sea. His friends appealed for "no Master of any Vessel to take him, he not being able to take Care of him[self], and being of good Family." Lodge was described in the advertisement as "disorder'd in Mind," aged about fifty, "very strong black complexion'd," and five feet ten inches in height, with a "fresh mole" on his left cheek and black curly hair. His clothing was also described.

87. I.e., to the baths (or, possibly, the sea bathing) at Ramsgate. See, e.g., Anon., The New Margate and Ramsgate Guide in Letters to a Friend Describing the Accomodations & Amusements of those Delightful Watering Places in Prose

& *Verse* (London: Printed for H. Turpin, & T. Wilkins, ca. 1780); and George Saville Carey, *The Balnea, or, An Impartial Description of all the Popular Watering Places in England: Interspersed with Original Sketches and Incidental Anecdotes, in Excursions to Margate, Ramsgate [etc.] . . . with Observations on Several Ancient and Respectable Towns and Cities Leading to the above Remarkable Places* (London: Printed by J. W. Myers, for W. West . . . [etc.], 1799).

88. Brooke was a very common name among people in Kent in the eighteenth century. E.g., there was Samuel Brooke of Birchington, who died in 1774; Robert Brooke of Margate who died in 1767; and Captain Robert Brooke of Margate, whose relative died in 1784. See *GM* (1767), p. 524; (1774), p. 287; (1784), p. 475.

89. I.e., Reginald Heber (d. 1769) of Chancery Lane. Heber published *An Historical List of Horse-Matches Run; and of Plates and Prizes Run for in Great Britain and Ireland, in . . . 1751 (–1768). With a list of the Principal Cockmatches of the Year,* 18 vols. (London: Printed by E. Owen, M. Witts and Samuel Chandler, 1752–69). See also John B. Podeschi, *Books on the Horse and Horsemanship: Riding, Hunting, Breeding and Racing 1400–1941. A Catalogue* (London: The Tate Gallery Publications Department, 1981), p. 383. Notices by Heber about horses, races, and prizes were regularly inserted in newspapers such as the *LEP* during this period, although, interestingly, they disappear from the newspaper during the latter part of October and throughout November 1766, when Heber falls ill and appears in the case book. Just months before this, Heber had offered a reward in the same paper for any information leading to the apprehension of a malicious graffiti writer (an angry creditor?) who had defaced the gates to his country house with some rather anti-Semitic threats. (For background on attitudes toward Jews at this time, see Todd M. Endelman, *The Jews of Georgian England, 1714–1830* [Philadelphia: Jewish Publication Society of America, 1979].) This may not have helped his mental state, but the episode provides a good indication that Heber was a nouveau riche and one of the better off and better connected among Monro's clientele, evidently being an acquaintance of the famous magistrate Sir John Fielding.

Hadley 24 March 1766

WHEREAS, about three Months ago, the following Words were written on the Gates of Mr. REGINALD HEBER's House, at Hadley, near Barnet, in the County of Middlesex, viz.

Mr Heber notwithstanding your high New Gates and great Dog we are determined to shoot you, or fire your House if you do not [pay]—£600

———

for by God we will.

And whereas, on the 14th of this Instant, March, there were also written on the same Gates the following Words, viz.

Mr Hebrew you are sure of I will set your House on fire.

Now, for the better Discovery of the Person or Persons guilty of writing the above Incendiary Words, the said Mr HEBER hereby promises a Reward of Five Guineas, to any Person or Persons who will discover the Offender or Offenders who wrote the said Incendiary Words, or either of the said Sentences, to be paid upon Conviction of any one or more of such Offenders, by Sir JOHN FIELDING at his House in Bow-Street, Covent-Garden.

R. HEBER

See *LEP*, no. 5990 (22–25 March 1766). Having succeeded John Chenny in 1742 in compiling the horse race listings, Heber was himself succeeded after his death in 1769 by William Tuting and Thomas Fawconer. For other anti-Semitic commentary, see CB, p. C-119, case of Mr. Rosat, who "met with great losses, by putting too much confidence in a Jew who deceiv'd him."

90. A John Ingram had kept Mile End madhouse at Dog Row, Mile End New Town, Stepney, in the early eighteenth century, another establishment much used by metropolitan parishes. The accounts of metropolitan parish officers include payments to him for their lunatic members throughout the early 1700s. Five patients were sent to Ingram, for example, by St. Botolph Bishopsgate during 1715–19, at a cost of 4s per week per patient. Although John Ingram was referred to as a doctor in parish records, he was no specialist, being paid for a host of medical services to local parishioners. Most conspicuously, his nurse was paid for taking poor parishioners in to be fluxed or salivated. However, the Ingram mentioned here is probably Dale Ingram (1710–93), son of John, who may have inherited a concern in the same madhouse. He was a man-midwife, professor of anatomy and surgery and surgeon to Christ's Hospital, and a major contemporary entrepreneur in the treatment of nervous disorders. Ingram was also the patentee of oriental balsam, a drug advertised in the press as follows:

> BOSEM, or ORIENTAL BALSAM. THIS CORDIAL MEDICINE the Chinese, Arabians, &c. for Ages used to preserve Health, being the richest known: It prolongs Life, relieves the Sleepy Affection, Palsy, Apoplexy, Disorders of the Liver and Spleen, Nervous Fits, Hysterical and Hypochondriacal Affections, Headachs, Languor of Spirits, Infirmities of Age, and all Disorders arising from the Balsam of the Blood impaired. This is carefully prepared under the Inspection of D. INGRAM, in Arundel-Street in the Strand, Man Midwife, Professor of Anatomy and Surgery, and Surgeon on Xchrist's Hospital; where it may be had. Also at Messrs. Fletcher's . . . etc. Ask for the BOSEM, or LADIES BALSAM.

See *LEP*, no. 5999 (12–15 April 1766), p. 4, col. 3.

Ingram, a trained surgeon, was a prolific author on medical subjects. See Dale Ingram, *An Essay on the Cause and Seat of the Gout: In Which the Opinions of Several Authors are Consider'd, and Some External Operations Recommended* (Reading: J. Newbery & C. Micklewright; London: J. Robinson, 1743); Ingram, *Practical Cases and Observations in Surgery* (London: J. Clarke, 1751); Ingram, *An Historical Account of the Several Plagues that have Appeared in the World. With an Enquiry into the Present Prevailing Opinion, that the Plague is a Contagious Distemper . . . To Which are Added a Particular Account of the Yellow Fever, etc.* (London: R. Baldwin and J. Clark, 1755); Ingram, *An Enquiry into the Origin and Nature of Magnesia Alba, and the Properties of Epsom Waters. Demonstrating that Magnesia made with those Waters Exceeds all Others* (London: W. Owen, 1767); Ingram, *The Blow, or, An Inquiry into the Causes of the late Mr. Clarke's Death: Supposed to have been Killed at Brentford. Humbly Inscribed to the Public* (London: Printed for Messrs. Richardson and Urquhart, 1769); Ingram, *A Strict and Impartial Enquiry into the Cause and Death of the late William Scawen, Esq; of Woodcote-Lodge, in Surrey: Ascertaining, from the Medical Evidences Against Jane Butterfield, the Impossibility of Poison having been given him. To which is Added, an Account of Accidental Poisons, to which*

Families are Exposed, with their Antidotes (London: Printed for T. Cadell, 1777); Ingram, *The Art of Farriery both in Theory and Practice, Containing the Causes, Symptoms, and Cure of all Diseases Incident to Horses . . . The Whole Revised, Corrected, and Enlarged by a Physician. To Which is Added, a New Method of Curing a Strain in the Back Sinews, and the Anatomy of a Horse's Leg, with some Observations on Shoeing, also an Appendix, Containing . . . Observations on the Late Epidemical Distemper Amoung Horses . . . By an Eminent Surgeon,* 4th ed. (London: Printed for Carnan and Newbery, S. Crowder, and B. Collins, 1778); Ingram, *The Dissection or an Examination of Mr. Ingram's Blow, (Relative to the Death of the late Mr. Clarke,) in which are Contained some Pertinent Cases from Morgagni and Mr. Pott; with some Remarks on Mr. Bromfield's Vindication of Himself; and a Brief Account of his Behaviour Towards Mr. Aylett, Surgeon, at Windsor* (London: Printed for the author; and sold by S. Bladon, C. Parker and F. Blyth, 1769); and Anon., *A Letter to Mr. Dale Ingram. In which the Arguments he has Advanced in his Enquiry into the Cause of Mr. Clark's Death are Confuted* (London: J. Murray, 1769).

Bibliography

PRIMARY SOURCES

ARCHIVAL SOURCES

Bethlem Royal Hospital Archives, Beckenham, Kent. Bethlem Admission Registers (BAR).
———. Bridewell and Bethlem Committee and Sub-committeee Minutes (BSCM).
———. Bridewell and Bethlem Court of Governors Minutes (BCGM).
College of Physicians, London, Annals/Register of the College of Physicians.
Corporation of London Record Office, Guildhall, Comp. CL. 114, 126b, 303, George Dance's plans of Bedlam at London Wall and Little Moorgate, dated ca. 1761 and 1790.
Family Records Centre, Angel, London (Goupy's will), PCC Prob. 11/949, qn 207.

OFFICIAL PUBLICATIONS

Minutes of Evidence Taken Before the Select Committee . . . for the Better Regulation of Madhouses in England. Reports 1–4. London: House of Commons, 1815–1816.
Select Committee on Pauper Lunatics and Lunatic Asylums in the County of Middlesex, 1827. London: House of Commons, 1827.

REFERENCE WORKS

Brooke, John, and Sir Lewis Namier. *The House of Commons, 1754–1790: Introductory Survey.* London: Her Majesty's Stationery Office, 1964.
———. *The House of Commons 1754–1790.* London: Published for the History of Parliament Trust by Secker and Warburg, 1985.
Cokayne, G. E. *Complete Baronetage.* 5 vols. Exeter: W. Pollard & Co., 1909.
———, ed. *The Complete Peerage of England, Scotland, Ireland, Great Britain and the United Kingdom, Extant, Extinct or Dormant.* 11 vols. London: St. Catherine Press, 1910.

Dictionary of National Biography. Oxford: Oxford University Press, 1995. CD ROM version.

Foster, Joseph. *Alumni Oxonienses: The Members of the University of Oxford, 1500–1714 . . . Being the Matriculation Register of the University.* 4 vols. Oxford: Parker & Co., 1891.

————. *Alumni Oxonienses: The Members of the University of Oxford, 1715– 1886 . . . Being the Matriculation Register of the University.* 4 vols. Oxford: Parker & Co., 1891–2.

Lillywhite, Bryant. *London Coffee Houses. A Reference Book of Coffee Houses of the Seventeenth Eighteenth and Nineteenth Centuries.* London: George Allen and Unwin, 1963.

Munk, William. *The Roll of the Royal College of Physicians of London.* . . . 2nd ed., rev. and enl. 3 vols. London: Royal College of Physicians, 1878.

Venn, John, and J. A. Venn. *Alumni Cantabridgiensis. A Biographical List of all Known Students, Graduates and Holders of Office at the University of Cambridge, from the Earliest Times to 1900.* 4 vols. Cambridge: Cambridge University Press, 1922–27.

MAGAZINES, NEWSPAPERS, AND DIRECTORIES

Directory: Containing an Alphabetical List of the Names and Places of Abode of the Directors of Companies, Persons in Publick Business, merchants, and other Eminent Traders in the Cities of London and Westminster, and Borough of Southwark. London: Printed and sold by Henry Kent, 1736.

The Gentleman's Magazine.

The London Directory for the Year 1766. London: Printed for T. Lowndes, 1766.

The London Directory for the Year 1776. London: Printed by T. Lowndes, 1776.

The London Evening Post (LEP).

The Universal British Directory of Trade and Commerce. . . . London: Printed for the Patentees and sold by C. Stalker and Messrs Brideoake and Fell, 1790.

BOOKS AND ARTICLES

Adair, James M. *Essays on Fashionable Diseases. The Dangerous Effects of Hot and Crouded Rooms. The Cloathing of Invalids, Lady and Gentlemen Doctors. And on Quacks and Quackery. With the Genuine Patent Prescriptions of Dr. James's Fever Powder, Tickell's Aetherial Spirit, & Godbold's Balsam, taken from the Rolls in Chancery . . . And also the Ingredients and Composition of Many of the most Celebrated Quack Nostrums, As Utilized by Several of the best Chemists in Europe . . . With a dedication to Philip Thicknesse . . . Professor of Empiricism and Nostrums, Rape and Murder-Monger to the St. James's Chronicle.* . . . London: Sold by T. P. Bateman, 1790[?].

Adee, Swithin. *The Craftsman's Apology. Being a Vindication of his Conduct and Writings: in Several Letters to the King* [A satire, in verse, on Henry St. John, Viscount Bolingbroke]. London: T. Cooper, 1732.

————. *Oratio Anniversaria a Guilelmo Harveio Instituta in Theatro Collegii*

Medicorum Londinensium Habita Festo Sancti Lucae, 18 Oct. 1769.
(Meadus Poema grati animi testimonium, etc.). Oxford: Clarendon, 1770.

Aikin, John. *The Spleen, and Other Poems.* London: Printed for T. Cadell, junr.
and W. Davies, 1796.

Anderson, James. *Present State of the Hebrides.* Edinburgh: Printed for C. Elliot.
London: Printed for G. G. J. and J. Robinson, 1785.

Anon. *An Account of the Progress of an Epidemical Madness. In a Letter to the
President and Fellows of the College of Physicians.* London: Printed and sold
by J. Roberts, 1735.

Anon. *An Essay On the Power of Nature and Art in Curing Diseases; To Which
are Annexed Impartial Reflections on James's Powder.* London: Printed for
W. Owen, 1753.

Anon. *A Letter to Mr. Dale Ingram. In which the Arguments he has Advanced
in his Enquiry into the Cause of Mr. Clark's Death are Confuted.* London: J.
Murray, 1769.

Anon. *The New Margate and Ramsgate Guide in Letters to a Friend Describing
the Accomodations & Amusements of those Delightful Watering Places in
Prose & Verse.* London: Printed for H. Turpin and T. Wilkins, ca. 1780.

Anon. "The Disabilities of Alienist Physicians." *Journal of Mental Science* 59
(1913): 144.

Battie, William. *A Treatise on Madness.* London: Printed for J. Whiston and B.
White, 1758; facsimile ed., reprinted with an introduction by Richard
Hunter and Ida Macalpine. London: Dawson's, 1962.

Belcher, William. *An Address to Humanity, Containing a Letter to Dr. Thomas
Monro, A Receipt to Make A Lunatic, and Seize his Estate; and a Sketch of
a True Smiling Hyena.* London: The author, 1796.

Berkenhout, John. *An Essay on the Bite of a Mad Dog: In Which the Claim to
Infallibility of the Principal Preservative Remedies Against the Hydrophobia
is Examined.* London: R. Baldwin, 1783.

Blackmore, [Sir] Richard. *A Treatise of the Spleen and Vapours: Or, Hypochondriacal and Hysterical Affections. With Three Discourses on the Nature and
Cure of the Cholick, Melancholy, and Palsies.* London: Pemberton, 1725.

Boswell, James. *The Hypochondriack.* 2 vols. Ed. Margery Bailey. Stanford,
Calif.: Stanford University Press, 1928.

Bowen, Thomas. *An Historical Account of the Origin, Progress and Present State
of Bethlehem Hospital founded by Henry the Eighth, for the Cure of
Lunatics, and Enlarged by Subsequent Benefactors, for the Reception and
Maintenance of Incurables.* London: For the Governors, 1783.

Burton, Robert. *The Anatomy of Melancholy.* London: B. Blake, 1651; facsimile edition, reprinted from 16th ed. Oxford: Thorntons, 1997.

Carey, George Saville. *The Balnea, or, An Impartial Description of all the Pop-
ular Watering Places in England: Interspersed with Original Sketches and
Incidental Anecdotes, in Excursions to Margate, Ramsgate [etc.] . . . with
Observations on Several Ancient and Respectable Towns and Cities Leading
to the above Remarkable Places.* London: Printed by J. W. Myers, for W.
West . . . (etc.), 1799.

Carkesse, James. *Lucida Intervalla.* London: The Author, 1679; facsimile ed., with an introduction by Michael V. Deporte. Los Angeles: William Andrews Clark Memorial Library, University of California/Augustan Reprint Society, 1979, nos. 195–96.

Chelsum, James. *History of the Art of Engraving in Mezzotinto from its Origins to the Present Time.* Winchester: Printed by J. Robbins; London: Sold by J. and T. Egerton, 1786.

Cheyne, George. *The Natural Method of Curing the Diseases of the Body, and the Disorders of the Mind Depending on the Body. In Three Parts.* . . . London: Printed for Geo. Strahan . . . (etc.), 1742.

———. *The Letters of Dr. George Cheyne to the Countess of Huntingdon.* Ed. Charles F. Mullett. San Marino, Calif.: Huntington Library, 1940.

———. "The Letters of Doctor George Cheyne to Samuel Richardson (1733–1743)." *University of Missouri Studies.* Vol. 18. Ed. Charles F. Mullett. Columbia: University of Missouri, 1943.

———. *The English Malady, or, A Treatise of Nervous Diseases of All Kinds.* London: Printed for G. Strahan and J. Leake, 1733; facsimile ed., reprinted with an introduction by Roy Porter. London and New York: Routledge, 1991.

[Coote, Charles]. *Sketches of the Lives and Characters of Eminent English Civilians, with an Historical Introduction Relative to the College of Advocates . . . from the Beginning of the Reign of Henry VIII, to the Close of the Year 1803; by one of the Members of the College.* London: Sold by G. Kearsley, 1804.

Cowper, William. *Poems.* London: Printed for J. Johnson, etc., 1798.

Cox, Joseph Mason. *Practical Observations on Insanity.* London: Baldwin and Murray, 1804.

Cruden, Alexander. *The London-Citizen Exceedingly Injured, or a British Inquisition Display'd . . . Addressed to the Legislature, as Plainly Shewing the Absolute Necessity of Regulating Private Madhouses.* London: Cooper and Dodd, 1739; reprinted in *Voices of Madness.* Ed. Allan Ingram. Stroud, Gloucestershire: Sutton, 1997. 23–74.

———. *The Adventures of Alexander the Corrector, with an Account of the Chelsea Academies, or the Private Places for the Confinement of Such as Are Supposed to Be Deprived of the Exercise of their Reason.* London: For the author, 1754.

———. *The Adventures of Alexander the Corrector. The Second Part. Giving an Account of a Memorable, or Rather Monstrous, Battle Fought, or Rather Not Fought, in Westminster Hall February 20 1754.* London: Printed for the author, 1754.

———. *The Adventures of Alexander the Corector. The Third Part. Giving an Account of his Wonderful Escape from an Academy at Bethnal Green.* London: Printed for the author, 1755.

Dalby, Joseph. *The Virtues of Cinnabar and Musk, Against the Bite of a Mad Dog.* Birmingham: By John Baskerville for the author, 1764.

Dance, George [the Elder], and George Dance [the Younger]. *George Dance, the Elder 1695–1768, the Younger 1741–1825: [Catalogue of] the first Exhibition Devoted to these two Distinguished Architects, from 7 July to 30 September 1972 [held at the] Geffrye Museum, Kingsland Road, E.2.* London: Inner London Education Authority, 1972.

Dance, George [the Younger]. *A Collection of Portraits Sketched from the Life Since the Year 1793 . . . and Engraved in Imitation of the Original Drawings by William Daniell.* London: Longman, Hurst, Rees, Orme, and Brown, etc., 1809–14.

Dodd, Thomas. *A Catalogue of the Extensive and Truly Magnificent Collection of Prints . . . of the French, Flemish, German, and English Engravers . . . also . . . Strutt's Dictionary of Engravers, Illustrated by upwards of 4000 prints, by the Different Artists Therein Mentioned, Arranged in Chronological Order, Forming 24 Volumes. . . .* London: T. Dodd, 1810.

Dolce, Lodovico. *Aretin: A Dialogue on Painting.* Glasgow: Printed for Robert Urie, 1770.

Dominiceti, Bartholomew di. *A Short and Calm Apology of Bartholomew di Dominiceti, &c. from Venice, Physician, Surgeon, and Chymist, in Regard to the many Injuries and Repeated Affronts he has, Uncall'd for, met with during the 6 years he has been in Bristol, etc.* Bristol: Printed for S. Farley, 1762.

———. *Begin. To the Public, etc.* [extracts from an address to the Royal Society and College of Physicians, on his baths, with remarks by Justus]. London: J. Towers, 1764.

———. *A Plan for Extending the Use of Artificial Water-Baths, Pumps, Vapours, and Dry-Baths, Fumigations, and Frictions; By the Mode and Means Invented and Directed by Dr Bartholomew di Dominiceti.* London: The author, 1771.

———. *Medical Anecdotes of the Last Thirty Years, Illustrated with Medical Truths, and Addressed to the Medical Faculty; but in an Especial Manner, to the People at Large. With an Appendix, and Copious Index.* London: L. Davis, 1781.

———. *An Address from Dr. Dominiceti of Chelsea. Humbly Submitted to the Consideration of the Commons of Great Britain, Individually, Introducing a Petition, which is Proposed to be presented to that Honourable House in Parliament Assembled . . . Introductory to a Petition [praying the Grant of Letters Patent for his Machine called the Economist].* London: The author, 1782.

Dominiceti, Rhodomonte. *A Dissertation on the Artificial Medicated Water Baths . . . Together with a Description of the Apparatus, Erected in Panton-Square, Hay-Market.* 2nd ed. London: Printed for the author, 1782. 3rd ed. 1794.

East India Company Official Documents. *Observations of the Court of Directors on the Conduct of Warren Hastings, Sir J. Clavering, Colonel G. Monson, R. Barwell, and P. Francis, in the Service of the East India Company.* London: East India Company, 1787.

Esquirol, Jean Etienne. *Mental Maladies: A Treatise on Insanity.* With an introduction by Raymond de Saussure; facsimile of the English edition of 1845. New York: Hafner, 1965.

Farington, Joseph. *The Farington Diary.* Ed. James Greig. 8 vols. London: Hutchison, 1922–28.

Farmer, Hugh. *An Essay on the Demoniacs of the New Testament.* London: Printed for G. Robinson, 1775.

Fell, John. *Daemoniacs: An Enquiry into the Heathen and the Scripture Doctrine of Daemons, in which the Hypotheses of the Rev. Mr. Farmer, and Others on this Subject, are Particularly Considered.* London: Printed for Charles Dilly, 1779.

Flemyng, Malcolm. *The Nature of the Nervous Fluid; Or, Animal Spirits Demonstrated.* London: A. Millar, 1751.

———. *A Dissertation on Dr. James's Fever Powder. In which the Different Circumstances, Wherein that Remedy May Prove Beneficial or Hurtful, are Considered and Distinguished, According to Observation and Reason.* London: Printed for L. Davis and C. Reymers, 1760.

Foot, Jesse. *Essay on the Bite of a Mad Dog: With Observations on John Hunter's Treatment of the Case of Master R—— and also a Recital of the Successful Treatment of Two Cases.* London: Printed for T. Becket, 1788.

[Fox, Edward Long.] *Brislington House: An Asylum for Lunatics Situate Near Bristol, on the Road from Bath.* Bristol: For the author, 1806.

Fox, Francis. *History and Present State of Brislington House near Bristol. An Asylum for the Care and Reception of Insane Persons. Established by Edward Long Fox M.D. A.D. 1804. And Now Conducted by Francis and Charles Fox M.D.* Bristol: Light and Ridler, 1836.

Gilpin, William. *An Essay on Prints.* 3rd ed. London: Printed by G. Scott, for R. Blamire; sold by B. Law and R. Faulder, 1781.

Gray, Thomas. *Ode on the Death of a Favorite Cat Drown'd in a Tub of Gold Fishes.* Modern ed. Islip, Oxford: Strawberry Press, 1992.

Gregory, John. *A Comparative View of the State and Faculties of Man. With those of the Animal World.* London: Printed for J. Dodsley, 1765.

Gretton, Phillip. *The Insufficiency of Reason, and the Assurance of Revelation . . . a Discourse Preached before the University of Cambridge.* Cambridge: Cambridge University Press, 1732.

Hales, Charles. *A Letter Addressed to Caesar Hawkins, Esq; Serjeant Surgeon to His Majesty, Containing New Thoughts and Observations, on the Cure of the Venereal Disease; the Result of Experience, in Long and Extensive Practice. With a few Extraordinary Cases in that Disease: Particularly one of a Servant Belonging to his Majesty's Household; Deemed Entirely a lost Case: Authenticated by the Officers of His Majesty's Mews.* 2nd ed. London: Printed and sold by J. Wheble et al., 1755 (with additions dated 1769).

———. *Salivation not Necessary for the Cure of the Venereal Disease in any Degree Whatever, and all Gleets Curable. . . .* 5th ed. London: Printed for J. Almon, 1764.

Haslam, John. *Illustrations of Madness.* London: Printed by G. Hayden and sold by Rivingtons, 1810; facsimile ed., reprinted with an introduction by Roy Porter. London and New York: Routledge, 1988.

———. *A Letter to the Governors of Bethlem Hospital, Containing an Account of Their Management of that Institution for the Last Twenty Years.* London: Taylor and Hessey, 1818.

Hastings, Warren. *Original Letters from Warren Hastings, Esq. Sir Eyre Coote, K.B. and Richard Barwell, Esq. to Sir Thomas Rumbold, Bart. and Lord Macartney, K.B.* London: Printed for J. Debrett, 1787.

Hawes, William. *An Account of the late Dr Goldsmith's Illness, so far as relative to the Exhibition of Dr James's Powder. An Examination of the Rev. Mr John Wesley's Primitive Physic: and an Address to the Public on Premature Death and Premature Internment.* London: Printed for the author by Browne, Dennis, and Wade, 1780; being the 2nd ed. of the work on Wesley, and the 4th of that on Goldsmith's illness; 1st ed., 1774.

Heber, Reginald. *An Historical List of Horse-Matches Run; and of Plates and Prizes Run for in Great Britain and Ireland, in . . . 1751 (−1768). With a list of the Principal Cockmatches of the Year.* 18 vols. London: Printed by E. Owen, M. Witts, and Samuel Chandler, 1752–69.

Heberden, William (the elder). *Commentaries on the History and Cure of Diseases,* translated from the Latin by William Heberden (junior). London: T. Payne, 1802.

Hind, Arthur M. *A History of Engraving and Etching from the Fifteenth Century to the Year 1914.* 3rd rev. ed. of *A Short History of Engraving and Etching.* New York: Dover, 1963.

Hoadly, Benjamin. *Three Lectures on the Organs of Perspiration . . . the Gulstonian Lectures. . . .* London: Printed for W. Wilkins and sold by J. Roberts, 1740.

Hogarth, William. *The Analysis of Beauty: Written with a View of Fixing the Fluctuating Ideas of Taste.* London: Printed by J. Reeves for the author, 1753.

Hutcheson, Francis. *Thoughts on Laughter. . . .* Glasgow: Printed by Robert and Andrew Foulis, 1757–58.

Huxham, John. *An Essay on Fevers . . . With Dissertations on Slow Nervous Fevers. . . .* London: S. Austen, 1750.

Ingram, Dale. *An Essay on the Cause and Seat of the Gout: In Which the Opinions of Several Authors are Consider'd, and Some External Operations Recommended.* Reading: J. Newbery and C. Micklewright. London: J. Robinson, 1743.

———. *Practical Cases and Observations in Surgery.* London: J. Clarke, 1751.

———. *An Historical Account of the Several Plagues that have Appeared in the World. With an Enquiry into the Present Prevailing Opinion, that the Plague is a Contagious Distemper . . . To Which are Added a Particular Account of the Yellow Fever, etc.* London: R. Baldwin and J. Clark, 1755.

———. *An Enquiry into the Origin and Nature of Magnesia Alba, and the Properties of Epsom Waters. Demonstrating that Magnesia made with those Waters Exceeds all Others.* London: W. Owen, 1767.

———. *The Blow, or, An Inquiry into the Causes of the late Mr. Clarke's Death: Supposed to have been Killed at Brentford. Humbly Inscribed to the Public.* London: Printed for Messrs. Richardson and Urquhart, 1769.

———. *The Dissection or an Examination of Mr. Ingram's Blow, (Relative to the Death of the late Mr. Clarke,) in which are Contained some Pertinent Cases from Morgagni and Mr. Pott; with some Remarks on Mr. Bromfield's Vindication of Himself; and a Brief Account of his Behaviour Towards Mr. Aylett, Surgeon, at Windsor.* London: Printed for the author; and sold by S. Bladon, C. Parker and F. Blyth, 1769.

————. *A Strict and Impartial Enquiry into the Cause and Death of the late William Scawen, Esq; of Woodcote-Lodge, in Surrey: Ascertaining, from the Medical Evidences Against Jane Butterfield, the Impossibility of Poison having been given him. To which is Added, an Account of Accidental Poisons, to which Families are Exposed, with their Antidotes.* London: Printed for T. Cadell, 1777.

————. *The Art of Farriery both in Theory and Practice, Containing the Causes, Symptoms, and Cure of all Diseases Incident to Horses . . . The Whole Revised, Corrected, and Enlarged by a Physician. To Which is Added, a New Method of Curing a Strain in the Back Sinews, and the Anatomy of a Horse's Leg, with some Observations on Shoeing, also an Appendix, Containing . . . Observations on the Late Epidemical Distemper Amoung Horses . . . By an Eminent Surgeon.* 4th ed. London: Printed for Carnan and Newbery, S. Crowder, and B. Collins, 1778.

James, Robert. *A New Method of Preventing and Curing the Madness Caused by the Bite of a Mad Dog.* London: T. Osborne, 1743.

————. *A Treatise on Canine Madness.* London: Printed for J. Newbery, 1766.

Johnson, Samuel. *A Journey to the Western Isles of Scotland.* London: W. Strahan and T. Cadel, 1775.

Johnson, Samuel, and George Steevens. *The Plays of William Shakespeare: With the Corrections and Illustrations of Various Commentators.* London: Printed for C. Bathurst, 1773.

Lardner, Nathaniel. *The Case of the Demoniacs Mentioned in the New Testament: Four Discourses upon Mark v. 19. With an Appendix, etc.* London, 1758.

[Lee, Samuel]. *A Proper Reply to the Serjeant Surgeons [i.e., J. Ranby & C. Hawkins's] Defence of their Conduct at Chelsea Hospital.* London: W. Owen, 1754.

Lindsay, Robert. *History of Scotland from 1436 to 1565. . . .* Ed. R. Freebairn. Edinburgh: Freebairn, 1728.

Mackenzie, James. *The History of Health, and the Art of Preserving it: or, An Account of all that has been Recommended by Physicians and Philosophers, Towards the Preservation of Health. . . .* Edinburgh and London: Printed and sold by William Gordon, etc., 1758.

Mead, Richard. *A Treatise Concerning the Influence of the Sun and Moon Upon Human Bodies, and the Diseases Thereby Produced. . . .* Trans. from the Latin [of the 2nd ed.] . . . by T. Stack, etc. London: Printed for J. Brindley, 1748; originally *[De imperio solis ac lunae in corpora humana, etc.] A Discourse Concerning the Action of the Sun and Moon on Animal Bodies; and the Influence Which this May Have in Many Diseases . . . In Two Parts.* London, 1708. London: Printed for Richard Wellington . . . , 1712.

Milton, John. *Paradise Lost.* London: Published by Jeffryes & Co., 1792–95.

Mitford, John. *A Description of the Crimes and Horrors in . . . Warburton's Private Mad-house at Hoxton . . . Called Whitmore House, etc.* London: Benbow, 1825[?].

M'Nichol, Donald. *Remarks on Johnson's Journey to the Hebrides.* London: T. Cadell, 1782.

Moffet, Thomas. *Health's Improvement: Or, Rules Comprizing and Discovering the Nature, Method and Manner of Preparing all Sorts of Food Used in this Nation . . . Corrected and Enlarged by Christopher Bennet, . . . To Which is Now Prefix'd, a Short View of the Author's Life and Writings, by Mr. Oldys. And an Introduction, by R. James, M.D.* London: Printed for T. Osborne, 1746.

Monier, Pierre. *History of Painting, Sculpture, Architecture, Graving. . . .* London: Printed for T. Bennet, D. Midwinter, T. Leigh, and R. Knaplock . . . , 1699.

Monro, Alexander. *Anatomy of the Human Bones and Nerves.* 6th ed. Edinburgh: G. Hamilton and J. Balfour, 1758.

Monro, Donald. *Dissertatio medica inauguralis, de hydrope.* Edinburgh: Hamilton, Balfour, and Neil, 1753.

———. *An Essay on the Dropsy.* London: D. Wilson and T. Durham, 1755.

Monro, John. *Remarks on Dr. Battie's Treatise on Madness.* London: Printed for John Clarke . . . , 1758; facsimile ed., reprinted with an introduction by Richard Hunter and Ida Macalpine. London: Dawson's, 1962.

———. *Bibliotheca Elegantissima Monroiana. A Catalogue of the Elegant and Valuable Library of John Monro, M.D. Physician to Bethlehem Hospital, Lately Deceased; which will be Sold by Auction by Leigh & Sotheby . . . April 23d, 1792, and the Fourteen Following Days, (Sundays Excepted). . . .* London: For Leigh and Sotheby, 1792.

Monro, Robert. *Expedition with the Worthy Scots Regiment.* London: W. Jones, 1637.

Monro, Thomas [of Magdalen College], ed. *Olla Podrida, a Periodical Paper, Published at Oxford.* Dublin: Printed by P. Byrne, 1787.

———. *Essays on Various Subjects.* London: Printed by J. Nichols and Sold by G. G. J. and J. Robinson, 1790.

Moore, John. *Of Religious Melancholy. A Sermon Preach'd before the Queen at Whitehall.* London: Printed for William Rogers, 1692.

More, Henry. *Enthusiasmus Triumphatus, or, A Discourse of the Nature, Causes, Kinds, and Cure, of Enthusiasme.* London: Morden, 1656.

Murray, William [Lord Mansfield]. *The Thistle; a Dispassionate Examine of the Prejudice of Englishmen in General to the Scotch Nation; and Particularly of a late Arrogant Insult Offered to all Scotchmen, by a Modern English Journalist. In a Letter to the Author of Old England of Dec. 27, 1746.* 2nd ed. London: H. Carpenter, 1747.

Newington, H. F. Hayes. "The Abolition of Private Asylums." *Journal of Mental Science* 31 (1885): 143.

Newton, Thomas. *A Dissertation on the Demoniacs in the Gospels.* London: J. and F. Rivington, 1775.

Nichols, John. *Biographical Anecdotes of William Hogarth: With a Catalogue of his Works Chronologically Arranged; and Occasional Remarks,* 2nd ed. London: Printed by and for J. Nichols, 1782.

———. *Literary Anecdotes of the Eighteenth Century. . . .* 9 vols. London: Nichols, Son, and Bentley, 1812–15.

Nichols, John, George Steevens, and George Whetstone. *Six Old Plays, on which Shakespeare Founded his Measure for Measure, Comedy of Errors, Taming the Shrew, King John, King Henry IV and King Henry, King Lear.* London: Printed for S. Leacroft and sold by J. Nichols, 1779.

Nugent, Christopher. *An Essay on the Hydrophobia: To Which is Prefixed the Case of a Person who was Bit by a Mad Dog; . . . and was Happily Cured.* London: Printed for James Leake and William Frederic, Bath, and sold by M. Cooper, 1753.

Ogle, John. *The Diverting Humours of John Ogle.* Warrington, 1805.

———— [Anon.]. *Joaks upon Joaks; or, No Joak Like a True Joak: Being the Diverting Humours of John Ogle, Life-Guard-Man. The Merry Pranks of the Lord Mohun, the Earls of Warwick and Pembroke. With the Lord Rochester's Dream; his Maiden's Disappointment.* London: T. Norris, ca. 1720.

———— [Anon.]. *Pills to Cure Melancholy; or England's Witty and Ingenious Jester: Shewing, no Joke like a True Joke. Containing the Merry Jests of the Earls of Rochester, Pembroke, Warwick, Lord Moon, and Mr. Ogle, the Life Guard Man. . . .* London: Printed for the author, ca. 1750–90.

Pargeter, [Rev.] William. *Observations on Maniacal Disorders.* Reading: Printed for the author, 1792; facsimile reprint, ed. Stanley W. Jackson. London and New York: Routledge, 1988.

Pegge, Samuel. *An Examination of the Enquiry into the Meaning of the Demoniacs in the New Testament. In a Letter to the Author. Wherein it is Shewn, that the Word Demon does not Signify a Departed Soul, either in the Classics or the Scriptures; and Consequently, that the Whole of the Enquiry is Without Foundation.* London: Printed for Fletcher Gyles, 1739.

Pennant, Thomas. *A Tour in Scotland.* 1769. London: Chester B. White, 1771.

[Perceval, John]. *A Narrative of the Treatment Experienced by a Gentleman, During a State of Mental Derangement. . . .* London: E. Wilson, 1838; in modern ed. by Gregory Bateson, retitled *Perceval's Narrative: A Patient's Account of His Psychosis, 1830–1832.* Stanford, Calif.: Stanford University Press, 1961.

Perfect, William. *Methods of Cure, in some Particular Cases of Insanity.* Rochester: Printed for the author, by T. Fisher, at Rochester; and sold by J. Dodsley and N. Conant (successor to Mr. Whiston); London, 1777.

————. *Select Cases in the Different Species of Insanity, Lunacy, or Madness, with the Modes of Practice as Adopted in the Treatment of Each.* Rochester: Printed and sold by W. Gillman; London: Printed and sold by J. Murray and J. Dew, 1787.

Pinel, Philippe. *A Treatise on Insanity.* Trans. from *Traité medico-philosophique sur l'alienation mentale, ou la manie;* facsimile of the London 1806 ed. New York: Hafner, 1962.

Pottinger, Israel. *The Humorous Quarrel; or, The Battle of the Greybeards. . . .* London: Printed for I. Pottinger, 1761.

————. *The Methodist: A [Three Act] Comedy: Being a Continuation and Completion of the Plan of The Minor, written by Mr. Foote. . . .* 2nd ed. London: Printed for I. Pottinger, 1761.

————. *The Duenna: A Comic Opera, in Three Acts. . . .* London: E. Johnson, 1776.

———. *The General Fast: A Lyric Ode: With a Form of Prayer Proper for the Occasion; and a Dedication to the King.* London, 1776.

———. *The Critic; or a Tragedy Rehearsed: A New Dramatic Piece in Three Acts. . . .* London: S. Bladon, 1780.

Pringle, John. *Observations on the Nature and Cure of Hospital or Jayl Fevers, in a Letter to Dr Mead. . . .* London: Printed for A. Millar and D. Wilson, 1750.

———. *Observations on the Diseases of the Army.* London: Printed for A. Millar and D. Wilson and T. Payne, 1752.

———. *A Discourse upon some Late Improvements of the Means for Preserving the Health of Mariners.* London: Printed for the Royal Society, 1776.

Purcell, John. *A Treatise of Vapours, or, Hysterick Fits.* London: Newman and Cox, 1702.

Ranby, John, and [Sir] Caesar Hawkins. *The True Account of all the Transactions before . . . the Commissioners for the Officers of Chelsea Hospital, as far as Related to the Admission and Dismission of S. Lee, Surgeon . . . To Which is Prefixed a Short Account of the Nature of a Rupture.* London: Printed for John and Paul Knapton, 1754.

Reeve, Thomas. *A Cure for the Epidemical Madness of Drinking Tar Water, Lately Imported from Ireland by a Certain R[igh]t R[everen]d Doctor. In a Letter to his L[ordshi]p.* London: Printed for John and Paul Knapton, 1744.

Reid, Thomas. *An Inquiry into the Human Mind. . . .* London: Printed for T. Cadell . . . and T. Longman; Edinburgh: For A. Kincaid and J. Bell, 1769.

———. *Essays on the Intellectual Powers of Man.* Edinburgh: Printed for John Bell; London: For G. G. J. and J. Robinson, 1785.

Relhan, Anthony. *A Short History of Brighthelmston. With Remarks on its Air, and an Analysis of its Waters, Particularly of an Uncommon Mineral One.* London: Printed for W. Johnston, 1761.

———. *Refutation of the Reflections Against Inoculation.* London, 1764.

Richardson, George. *Iconology; or, a Collection of Emblematical Figures, Moral and Instructive; Exhibiting the Images of the Elements and Celestial Bodies . . . Dispositions and Faculties of the Mind, Virtues and Vices . . . Illustrated by a Variety of Authorities from Classical Authors . . . from the most Approved Emblematical Representations of the Ancient Egyptians, Greeks and Romans, and from the Compositions of Cavaliere Cesare Ripa Perugino.* 2 vols. London: Printed for the author, 1779.

Robertson, William. *History of Scotland.* 2 vols. London: For A. Millar, 1759.

Robinson, Bryan. *Observations on the Virtues and Operations of Medicines.* London: J. Nourse, 1752.

Robinson, Nicholas. *A New System of the Spleen, Vapours, and Hypochondriack Melancholy: Wherein all the Decays of the Nerves, and Lowness of the Spirits, are Mechanically Accounted For.* London: A. Bettesworth, Innys, and Rivington, 1729.

Rogers, J. W. *A Statement of the Cruelties, Abuses, and Frauds, Which Are Practised in Mad-houses.* London: For the author, 1816.

Shakespeare, William. *Works.* London: Printed for J. Bell . . . and C. Etherington at York, 1774.

Sharp, William. *An Answer to the World: For Putting in Print a Book in 1804, Called Copies and Parts of Copies of Letters and Communications, Written from Joanna Southcott, and Transmitted by Miss Townley to Mr. Sharp in London*. London: Printed by S. Rousseau and sold by E. I. Field, 1806.

Shaw, Peter, trans. *Pharmacopoeia Edinburgensis: or, the Dispensatory of the Royal College of Physicians in Edinburgh.* . . . London: W. Innys and J. Richardson, 1753.

Sheeles, James. *Threnodia Northumbrica. A Funeral Pindaric Poem Sacred to the Memory of the Right Honourable the Lady Elizabeth Anne Frances Percy.* London: Printed for R. and J. Dodsley; sold by M. Cooper, 1761.

Sinclair, [Sir] John. *Observations on the Scottish Dialect.* London and Edinburgh: Printed for W. Strahan and T. Cadell; W. Creech, 1782.

Smart, Christopher. *Poems on Several Occasions. Viz. Munificence and Modesty. Female Dignity. To Lady Hussey Delaval. Verses from Catullus, after Dining with Mr. Murray. Epitaphs. On the Duchess of Cleveland. On Henry Fielding, Esq. On the Rev. James Sheeles. Epitaph from Demosthenes.* London: Printed for the author and sold by Mr. Fletcher & Co.; Mr. Davies; Mr. Flexney; Mr. Laurence; & Mr. Almon, 1763.

Smollett, Tobias George. *A Sorrowful Ditty; or, the Lady's Lamentation for the Death of her Favourite Cat, a Parody.* London: Printed for J. Tomlinson, 1748.

———. *Roderick Random.* Oxford: Oxford University Press, 1981.

Smyth, James Carmichael. *An Account of the Effects of Swinging, Employed as a Remedy in the Pulmonary Consumption and Hectic Fever.* London: J. Johnson, 1787.

Somerville, William. *The Chace. A Poem.* 5th ed. London: Printed for W. Bowyer, 1767.

Southcott, Joanna. *Divine and Spiritual Communications, Written by Joanna Southcott on the Prayers of the Church of England, the Conduct of the Clergy and Calvinistic Methodists, etc.,* with an introduction by W. Sharp. London, 1803.

Southcott, Joanna [and William Sharp]. *Copies and Parts of Copies of Letters and Communications, Written from Joanna Southcott, etc.* London, 1804.

Southwell, Thomas. *Medical Essays and Observations; Being an Abridgement of the Useful Medical Papers Contained in the History and Memoirs of the Royal Academy of Sciences at Paris, from their Re-establishment in 1699 to the year 1750, Disposed Under General Heads.* 4 vols. London: Printed for J. Knox, 1764.

Steevens, George. *To the Public. Had the last Editor of the Plays of Shakespeare met with the Assistance he had Reason to Expect.* . . . London, 1766.

Strutt, Joseph. *A Biographical Dictionary; Containing an Historical Account of all the Engravers, from the Earliest Period of the Art of Engraving to the Present Time; and a . . . List of their most Esteemed Works; with the Cyphers, Monograms, and Particular Marks used by each Master . . . To which is Prefixed, an Essay on the Rise and Progress of the Art of Engraving, etc.* 2 vols. London: Printed by J. Davis for R. Faulder, 1785.

Taylor, John. *Records of My Life.* 2 vols. London: Edward Bull, 1832.

Thompson, Henry Frederick. *The Intrigues of a Nabob (R. Barwell): Or, Bengal the Fittest Soil for the Growth of Lust, Injustice and Dishonesty, etc.* London[?]: Printed for the author, 1780.

Threlfal, William. *Essay on Epilepsy. In Which a New Theory of that Disease is Attempted, etc.* London, 1772.

Tissot, M., or S. A. D. [David, Samuel Auguste]. *L'onanisme: ou dissertation physique sur les maladies produites par la masturbation. Traduit du latin . . . considérablement augmenté par l'auteur.* Lausanne: Marc Chapuis, 1764.

———. *Advice to the People in General, with Regard to their Health.* London: T. Becket and P. A. de Hondt, 1765.

———. *Onanism: or, A Treatise upon the Disorders Produced by Masturbation, or, The Dangerous Effects of Secret and Excessive Venery.* Trans. from the last Paris ed. by A. Hume. London: Printed for the translator; sold by J. Pridden in Fleet-Street, 1766.

———. *A Treatise on the Crime of Onan; Illustrated with a Variety of Cases, Together with the Method of Cure.* Trans. from the 3rd ed. of the original. London: Printed for B. Thomas, 1766.

———. *An Essay on Diseases Incidental to Literary and Sedentary Persons. With Proper Rules for Preventing their Fatal Consequences and Instructions for their Cure.* London: E. and C. Dilly, 1768.

Turner, Daniel. *Discourse Concerning Fevers. . . .* London: Printed for John Clarke, 1727.

Twells, Leonard. *An Answer to the Enquiry into the Meaning of Demoniacks in the New Testament: Shewing, that the Demons Therein Spoken of were Fallen Angels; and that the Demoniacks were Persons Really Possessed. . . .* London: Printed for R. Gosling, 1737.

———. *An Answer to the Further Enquiry into the Meaning of Demoniacks in the New Testament . . . In a Second Letter to the Author.* London, 1738.

Usher, James. *An Introduction to the Theory of the Human Mind.* London: T. Davis, 1771.

Verney, Margaret Marie, ed. *Verney Letters of the Eighteenth Century from the MSS at Claydon House.* London: Benn, 1930.

Villars, Abbé de [Henri, Nicolas Pierre]. *The Count de Gabalis: Being a Diverting History of the Rosicrucian Doctrine of Spirits, viz. Sylphs, Salamanders, Gnomes, and Dæmons: Shewing their Various Influence upon Human Bodies. Done from the Paris Edition. To which is Prefix'd, Monsieur [Pierre] Bayle's Account of this Work: and of the Sect of the Rosicrucians.* London: Printed for B. Lintott and E. Curll, etc., 1714.

Walpole, Horace. *Aedes Walpolianae: A Description of the Plates at Houghton Hall.* 2nd. ed. London: Printed by J. Hughs, 1752.

———. *Anecdotes of Painting in England. . . .* Twickenham, Strawberry Hill: Thomas Farmer, 1762.

———. *Catalogue of Engravers. . . .* 5 vols. Twickenham, Strawberry Hill: n.p., 1762.

———. *Correspondence.* Ed. W. S. Lewis. 48 vols. New Haven, Conn.: Yale University Press, 1937–83.

White, William. *Observations on the Use of Dr James's Powder, Emetic Tartar, and Other Antimonial Preparations in Fevers.* London: Printed for T. Cadell, Richardson, and Wallis and T. Wilson, 1774.

Willis, Francis Jr. *A Treatise on Mental Derangement.* London: Longman, 1823.

CASE BOOKS

Adler, Alfred. *Problems of Neurosis: A Book of Case-Histories.* Ed. Philippe Mairet. London: Kegan Paul, Trench, Trübner, 1929.

Allen, Elizabeth, J. L. Turk, and Sir Reginald Murley, eds. *The Case Books of John Hunter FRS.* London: Royal Society of Medicine, 1993.

Anning, S. T. "A Medical Case Book: Leeds, 1781–84." *Medical History* 28 (1984): 420–31.

Dewhurst, Kenneth, ed. *Willis's Oxford Casebook (1650–52).* Oxford: Sandford Publications, 1981.

Dobson, Jessie. *Notes from John Hunter's Casebook.* London, 1959; reprinted from the January 1959 issue of the *Journal of the Medical Women's Federation.*

Loxham, Richard. *The Account Book of Dr Loxham,* Lancashire Record Office, DDPr25/6.

Marmoy, Charles F. A., ed. *The Case Book of "La Maison de Charite de Spittlefields" 1739–41.* London: Huguenot Society of London, 1981.

Rodin, Alvin E., and Jack D. Key. *Medical Casebook of Doctor Arthur Conan Doyle: From Practitioner to Sherlock Holmes and Beyond.* Malabar, Fla.: R. E. Krieger, 1984.

Stack, R. W. *Medical Cases, With Occasional Remarks. To Which is Added an Appendix. Containing the History of a late Extraordinary Case.* Bath: R. Cruttwell, 1784.

Ward, Jean E., and Joan Yell, eds. and trans. *The Medical Casebook of William Brownrigg, M.D., F.R.S. (1712–1800) of the Town of Whitehaven in Cumberland, Medical History.* Supplement no. 13. London: Wellcome Institute for the History of Medicine, 1993.

Wood, S., ed. *The Library: Two Further Letters of John Hunter and Notes on Rockingham's Last Illness from Hunter's Case Book.* London, 1949.

SECONDARY SOURCES

BOOKS, ARTICLES, AND CHAPTERS

Ackerknecht, Erwin H. "Beitraege zur Geschichte der Medizinalreform von 1848." *Sudhoffs Archiv für Geschichte der Medizin* 25 (1932): 61–109, 113–83.

Adair, Richard, Bill Forsythe, and Joseph Melling. "Migration, Family Structure, and Pauper Lunacy in Victorian England: Admissions to the Devon County Pauper Lunatic Asylum, 1845–1900." *Continuity and Change* 12 (1997): 373–401.

———. "A Danger to the Public? Disposing of Pauper Lunatics in Late-Victorian and Edwardian England." *Medical History* 42 (1998): 1–25.

Andrews, Jonathan. "The Lot of the 'Incurably' Insane in Enlightenment England." *Eighteenth Century Life* 12.1 (1988): 1–18.

———. "'In her Vapours . . . [or] Indeed in her Madness'? Mrs Clerke's Case: An Early Eighteenth Century Psychiatric Controversy." *History of Psychiatry* 1.1 (1990): 125–44.

———. "A Respectable Mad-Doctor? Richard Hale, F.R.S. (1670–1728)." *Notes and Records of the Royal Society of London* 44 (1990): 169–203.

———. "'Hardly a Hospital, but a Charity for Pauper Lunatics'? Therapeutics at Bethlem in the Seventeenth and Eighteenth Centuries." *Medicine and Charity before the Welfare State.* Eds. Jonathan Barry and Colin Jones. London and New York: Routledge, 1991. 63–82.

———. "The Politics of Committal to Bethlem." *Medicine and the Enlightenment.* Ed. Roy Porter. Amsterdam: Rodopi, 1995. 6–63.

———. "Case Notes, Case Histories, and the Patient's Experience of Insanity at Gartnavel Royal Asylum, Glasgow, in the Nineteenth Century." *Social History of Medicine* 11 (1998): 255–81.

Andrews, Jonathan, Asa Briggs, Roy Porter, Penny Tucker, and Keir Waddington. *The History of Bethlem.* London: Routledge, 1997.

Andrews, Jonathan, and Andrew Scull. *Undertaker of the Mind: John Monro and Mad-Doctoring in Eighteenth-Century England.* Berkeley: University of California Press, 2001.

Bartlett, Peter. *The Poor Law of Lunacy: The Administration of Pauper Lunatics in Mid-Nineteenth-Century England.* London and Washington: Leicester University Press, 1999.

Bartlett, Peter, and David Wright, eds. *Outside the Walls of the Asylum: The History of Care in the Community, 1750–2000.* London: Athlone, 1999.

Beaven, Alfred B. *The Aldermen of the City of London.* 2 vols. London: The Corporation of the City of London; Eden Fisher & Co., 1908.

Beckett, J. V. "An Eighteenth-Century Case History: Carlisle Spedding 1738." *Medical History* 26 (1982): 303–6.

Beier, Lucinda McCray. *Sufferers and Healers: The Experience of Illness in Seventeenth-Century England.* London and New York: Routledge and Kegan Paul, 1987.

———. "Seventeenth-Century English Surgery: The Casebook of Joseph Binns." *Medical Theory, Surgical Practice.* Ed. Christopher Lawrence. London and New York: Routledge, 1992. 48–84.

Bennett, Shelley M. *Thomas Stothard: The Mechanisms of Art Patronage in England circa 1800.* Columbia: University of Missouri Press, 1988.

Berg, Charles. *War in the Mind: The Case Book of a Medical Psychologist: An Introduction to the Practical Application of Modern Psychology.* London: Macaulay Press, 1941.

———. *Clinical Psychology: A Case Book of the Neuroses and Their Treatment.* London: Allen and Unwin, 1948.

Blackburn, Simon. *The Oxford Dictionary of Philosophy.* Oxford and New York: Oxford University Press, 1994.

Blunt, Reginald, ed. *Mrs Montagu "Queen of the Blues." Her Letters and Friendships from 1762 to 1800.* 2 vols. London: Constable & Co., 1923.

Borsay, Anne. Rev. of *John Hall and His Patients: The Medical Practice of Shakespeare's Son-in-Law,* by Joan Lane. *Social History of Medicine* 11.2 (Aug. 1998): 315–16.

Braham, Allan. *Wright of Derby; Mr and Mrs Coltman.* National Gallery Exhibition booklet, 1986.

Braslow, Joel. *Mental Ills and Bodily Cures: Psychiatric Treatment in the First Half of the Twentieth Century.* Berkeley: University of California Press, 1997.

Bridgeman, G. J. O. "An Ophthalmic Case-Book of Eighty Years Ago." *Proceedings of the Royal Society of Medicine Section of the History of Medicine* 48 (1955): 381–84.

Buchanan, James H. *Patient Encounters: The Experience of Disease.* Charlottesville: University Press of Virginia, 1989.

Byrd, Max. *Visits to Bedlam.* Columbia: University of South Carolina Press, 1974.

Charon, Rita. "To Build a Case: Medical Histories as Traditions in Conflict." *Literature and Medicine* 11 (1992): 115–32.

Chesser, Eustace. *Unquiet Minds: Leaves from a Psychologist's Casebook.* London and New York: Rich and Cowan, 1952.

Christy, Robert Miller. *Joseph Strutt, Author, Artist, Engraver, and Antiquary, 1749–1802: A Biography.* London, 1912.

Cope, S. R. *The Stock Exchange Revisited: A New Look at the Market in Securities in London in the Eighteenth Century.* Reprinted from *Economica* 45 (Feb. 1978). London: London School of Economics and Political Science, 1978.

Crellin, J. K. "Dr. James's Fever Powder." *Transactions of the British Society for the History of Pharmacy* 1 (1970–77): 136–43.

Cunningham, Andrew. "Pathology and the Case-History in Giambattista Morgagni's 'On the Seats and Causes of Diseases Investigated Through Anatomy' (1761)." *Medizin, Gesellschaft und Geschichte—Jahrbuch des Instituts für Geschichte der Medizin der Robert Bosch Stiftung. Bd. 14.* Ed. Robert Jütte. Stuttgart: F. Steiner, 1991. 37–61.

Dance, Nathaniel, and George Dance. *"The Sublime and Beautiful": Portraits and Other Drawings by Nathaniel Dance and George Dance [catalogue of an exhibition held at the Sabin Galleries, 27 March–18 April 1973].* London: Sabin Galleries, 1973.

———. *Catalogue of an Exhibition Held at Greater London Council, The Iveagh Bequest . . . 25 June to 4 September, 1977,* with an introduction by David Goodreau, "Retirement, Comic Drawings by Nathaniel and George Dance the Younger." London: Greater London Council, 1977. 54–60.

Digby, Anne. *Making a Medical Living: Doctors and Patients in the English Market for Medicine, 1720–1911.* Cambridge: Cambridge University Press, 1994.

Dingwall, Robert. *Aspects of Illness.* London: Martin Robertson, 1976.

Doerner, Klaus. *Madmen and the Bourgeoisie.* Oxford: Blackwell, 1981.

Duden, Barbara. *The Woman Beneath the Skin: A Doctor's Patients in Eighteenth-Century Germany.* Cambridge, Mass., and London: Harvard University Press, 1991.

Edwardes, Michael. *Warren Hastings: King of the Nabobs*. London: Hart-Davis, MacGibbon, 1976.

———. *The Nabobs at Home*. London: Constable, 1991.

Ellis, Harold. *Surgical Case-Histories from the Past*. London and New York: Royal Society of Medicine Press, 1994.

Endelman, Todd M. *The Jews of Georgian England, 1714–1830*. Philadelphia: Jewish Publication Society of America, 1979.

Erskine, Alexander. *A Hypnotist's Case Book*. London: Rider, 1932.

Fissell, Mary E. "The 'Sick and Drooping Poor' in Eighteenth-Century Bristol and Its Region." *Social History of Medicine* 2 (1989): 35–58.

———. "The Disappearance of the Patient's Narrative and the Invention of Hospital Medicine." *British Medicine in an Age of Reform*. Eds. Roger French and Andrew Wear. London and New York: Routledge, 1991. 91–109.

———. *Patients, Power and the Poor in Eighteenth-Century Bristol*. Cambridge: Cambridge University Press, 1991.

———. "Readers, Texts, and Contexts: Vernacular Medical Works in Early Modern England." *The Popularisation of Medicine, 1650–1850*. Ed. Roy Porter. London and New York: Routledge, 1992. 72–96.

Forster, Frank M. C. "Walter Lindesay Richardson, 1826–1879 as Obstetrician: His Case-Book and Midwifery Practice in Early Ballarat." *Festschrift for Kenneth Fitzpatrick Russell, M.B., M.S., D. Litt., F.R.A.C.S., F.R.A.C.P.* Proceedings of a Symposium Arranged by the Section of Medical History, A.M.A. (Victorian Branch), 25 Feb. 1977; Carlton, Victoria: Queensberry Hill Press for the Department of Medical History, University of Melbourne, 1978. 142–58.

Foucault, Michel. *Madness and Civilisation: A History of Insanity in the Age of Reason*. London: Tavistock, 1971. Trans. and abr. from *Histoire de la folie à l'âge classique*. Paris: Librairie Plon, 1961.

———. *The Birth of the Clinic*. London: Tavistock, 1973; Routledge: reprint, 1993. Trans. from *Naissance de la clinique*. Presses Universitaires de France, 1963.

Fox, A. "A Short Account of Brislington House, 1804–1906." *Brislington House Quarterly News, Centenary Number* (1906): 4–14.

Foyster, Elizabeth. "Wrongful Confinement in Eighteenth-Century England: A Question of Gender?" Unpublished paper delivered at University of Wales, Bangor, conference, July 1999, "Social and Medical Representations of the Links between Insanity and Sexuality."

Frängsmyr, Tore, J. L. Heilbron, and Robin E. Rider. *The Quantifying Spirit in the Eighteenth Century*. Berkeley: University of California Press, 1990.

French, C. N. *The Story of St Luke's Hospital*. London: Heinemann, 1951.

Gerzina, Gretchen. *Black London: Life before Emancipation*. London: John Murray; New Brunswick, N.J.: Rutgers University Press, 1995.

Gijswijt-Hofstra, Marijke, Hilary Marland, and Hans de Waardt, eds. *Illness and Healing Alternatives in Western Europe*. London: Routledge, 1997.

Goldstein, Michael J., and James O. Palmer. *The Experience of Anxiety: A Casebook*. New York: Oxford University Press, 1963.

Gordon, Charles. "Sir John Pringle and the Apothecaries." *Pharmaceutical Historian* 19.4 (1989): 5–12.

Gordon, Gerald A. *Role Theory and Illness: A Sociological Perspective.* New Haven, Conn.: College and University Press, 1966.

Groves, Abraham. *All in the Day's Work: Leaves from a Doctor's Case-Book.* Toronto: Macmillan, 1934.

Guerrini, Anita. *Obesity and Depression in the Enlightenment: The Life and Times of George Cheyne.* Norman: University of Oklahoma Press, 2000.

Halsband, Robert, ed. *The Selected Letters of Lady Mary Wortley Montagu.* Harmondsworth, Middlesex: Penguin, 1970.

Harpole, James. *Leaves from a Surgeon's Case-Book.* New York: Frederick A. Stokes Co., 1938.

Harrison, J. F. C. *The Second Coming: Popular Millenarianism, 1780–1850.* New Brunswick, N.J.: Rutgers University Press, 1979.

Healy, David. *The Anti-Depressant Era.* Cambridge, Mass.: Harvard University Press, 1998.

Heston, Leonard L., and Renate Heston. *The Medical Casebook of Adolf Hitler: His Illnesses, Doctors, and Drugs.* London: Kimber, 1979.

Hitchcock, Tim. *English Sexualities, 1700–1800.* Basingstoke: Macmillan, 1997.

Hixson, William F. *Triumph of the Bankers: Money and Banking in the Eighteenth and Nineteenth Centuries.* Westport, Conn.: Praeger, 1993.

Houston, R. A. *Madness and Society in Eighteenth-Century Scotland.* Oxford: Clarendon, 2000.

Hunter, Richard, and Ida Macalpine. Introduction to the facsimile edition of William Battie, *A Treatise on Madness,* and John Monro, *Remarks on Dr. Battie's Treatise on Madness.* London: Dawson's, 1962. 7–21.

———. *Three Hundred Years of Psychiatry 1535–1860: A History Presented in Selected English Texts.* Oxford, New York, and Toronto: Oxford University Press, 1963.

Ingleby, David. "Mental Health and the Social Order." *Social Order and the State: Historical and Comparative Essays.* Eds. Stanley Cohen and Andrew Scull. Oxford: Basil Blackwell, 1983. 141–88.

Ingram, Allan. *The Madhouse of Language: Writing and Reading Madness in the Eighteenth Century.* London and New York: Routledge, 1991.

———, ed. *Voices of Madness.* Stroud, Gloucestershire: Sutton, 1997.

Ingrassia, Catherine. *Authorship, Commerce, and Gender in Early Eighteenth-Century England: A Culture of Paper Credit.* Cambridge; New York: Cambridge University Press, 1998.

Jefferiss, [Dr.] F. J. G. "Extracts from a Biography of Dr Thomas Monro." *Dr Thomas Monro (1759–1833) and the Monro Academy, Prints, and Drawing Gallery, February–May 1976.* London: Victoria and Albert Museum, 1976.

Jewson, N. D. "Medical Knowledge and the Patronage System in Eighteenth-Century England." *Sociology* 8 (1974): 369–85.

———. "The Disappearance of the Sick Man from Medical Cosmology." *Sociology* 10 (1976): 225–44.

Jütte, Robert, ed. *Medizin, Gesellschaft und Geschichte—Jahrbuch des Instituts für Geschichte der Medizin der Robert Bosch Stiftung. Bd. 14.* Stuttgart: F. Steiner, 1991.

Kass, Amalie M. "The Obstetrical Casebook of Walter Channing, 1811–1822." *Bulletin of the History of Medicine* 67 (1993): 494–523.

———. "'Called to her at three o'clock am': Obstetrical Practice in Physician Case Notes." *Journal of the History of Medicine and Allied Sciences* 50.2 (April 1995): 194–229.

Kleinman, Arthur. *The Illness Narratives: Suffering, Healing and the Human Condition.* New York: Basic Books, 1988.

Knox, Ronald Arbuthnott. *Enthusiasm.* Oxford: Oxford University Press, 1950.

Lane, Joan. *John Hall and His Patients: The Medical Practice of Shakespeare's Son-in-Law.* Stratford-upon-Avon: Shakespeare Birthplace Trust in association with Alan Sutton Publishing Ltd., 1996.

Larsen, Oeivind. "Case Histories in Nineteenth-Century Hospitals—What Do They Tell the Historian? Some Methodological Considerations with Special Reference to McKeown's Criticism of Medicine." *Medizin, Gesellschaft und Geschichte—Jahrbuch des Instituts für Geschichte der Medizin der Robert Bosch Stiftung. Bd. 14.* Ed. Robert Jütte. Stuttgart: F. Steiner, 1991. 127–48.

Lingard, W. Burns. *Herbal Prescriptions from a Consultant's Case Book.* London: National Institute of Medical Herbalists, 1958.

Longfield-Jones, G. M. "The Case History of 'Sir H. M.'" *Medical History* 32 (1988): 449–60.

Loudon, Irvine. *Medical Care and the General Practitioner, 1750–1850.* Oxford and New York: Clarendon/Oxford University Press, 1986.

Lunbeck, Elizabeth. *The Psychiatric Persuasion: Knowledge, Gender, and Power in Modern America.* Princeton, N.J.: Princeton University Press, 1994.

Macalpine, Ida, and Richard Hunter. *George III and the Mad-Business.* London: Allen Lane/Penguin Press, 1969; Pimlico, 1991.

MacDonald, Michael. *Mystical Bedlam: Madness, Anxiety and Healing in Seventeenth-Century England.* Cambridge: Cambridge University Press, 1981.

———. "Religion, Social Change, and Psychological Healing in England, 1600–1800." *The Church and Healing.* Ed. W. J. Sheils. Oxford: Blackwell, 1982. 101–25.

———. "The Secularisation of Suicide in England 1600–1800." *Past and Present* 111 (1986): 50–97.

———. "Insanity and the Realities of History in Early Modern England." *Psychological Medicine* 11 (1981): 11–25; reprinted in *Lectures on the History of Psychiatry.* Eds. R. M. Murray and T. H. Turner. The Squibb Series. London: Gaskell, 1990. 60–81.

———. "The Medicalization of Suicide in England: Laymen, Physicians, and Cultural Change, 1500–1870." *Framing Disease: Studies in Cultural History.* Eds. Charles E. Rosenberg and Janet Golden. New Brunswick, N.J.: Rutgers University Press, 1992. 85–103.

MacDonald, Michael, and Terence R. Murphy. *Sleepless Souls: Suicide in Early Modern England.* Oxford and New York: Clarendon/Oxford University Press, 1990.

MacKenzie, Charlotte. *Psychiatry for the Rich: A History of Ticehurst Private Asylum, 1792–1917.* London and New York: Routledge, 1992.

Mathias, Peter, and John A. Davis, eds. *International Trade and British Economic Growth: From the Eighteenth Century to the Present Day.* The Nature of Industrialization Series. Vol. 5. Oxford: Blackwell, 1996.

Mcintosh, Christopher. *The Rose Cross and the Age of Reason: Eighteenth-Century Rosicrucianism in Central Europe and Its Relationship to the Enlightenment.* Leiden and New York: E. J. Brill, 1992.

McKendrick, Neil, John Brewer, and J. H. Plumb. *The Birth of a Consumer Society: The Commercialization of Eighteenth Century England.* London: Europa, 1982.

Melling, Joseph, with Richard Adair and Bill Forsythe. " 'A Proper Lunatic for Two Years': Pauper Lunatic Children in Victorian and Edwardian England: Child Admissions to the Devon County Asylum." *Journal of Social History* 30 (1997): 371–405.

Melling, Joseph, and Bill Forsythe, eds. *Insanity, Institutions and Society, 1800–1914: A Social History of Madness in Comparative Perspective.* London: Routledge, 1999.

Micale, Mark S. "Paradigm and Ideology in Psychiatric History Writing: The Case of Psychoanalysis." *Journal of Nervous and Mental Disease* 184 (1996): 146–52.

Mitchison, Rosalind. *Sexuality and Social Control: Scotland 1660–1780.* Oxford: Basil Blackwell, 1989.

Monro, Thomas. *Catalogue of an Exhibition of Drawings chiefly by Dr. Thomas Monro (Prepared by A. K. Sabin).* London, 1917.

———. *Dr Thomas Monro (1759–1833) and the Monro Academy, Prints, and Drawing Gallery, February–May 1976.* London: Victorian and Albert Museum, 1976.

Mullett, Charles F. "The Lay Outlook on Medicine in England circa 1800–1850." *Bulletin of the History of Medicine* 25 (1951): 169–75.

Nicholson, Colin. *Writing and the Rise of Finance: Capital Satires of the Early Eighteenth Century.* Series: Cambridge Studies in Eighteenth-Century English Literature and Thought. Cambridge and New York: Cambridge University Press, 1994.

Nicolson, Malcolm. "The Art of Diagnosis: Medicine and the Five Senses." *Companion Encyclopedia of the History of Medicine.* Eds. W. F. Bynum and Roy Porter. Vol. 2. London and New York: Routledge, 1993. 801–25.

Niswander, G. Donald, Thomas M. Casey, and John A. Humphrey. *A Panorama of Suicide: A Casebook of Psychological Autopsies.* Springfield, Ill.: Charles C. Thomas, 1973.

Noll, Steven. "Patient Records as Historical Stories: The Case of Caswell Training School." *Bulletin of the History of Medicine* 68 (1994): 411–28.

Nowell-Smith, Harriet. "Nineteenth-Century Narrative Case Histories: An Inquiry into Stylistics and History." *Canadian Bulletin of Medical History* 12 (1995): 47–67.

Obelkevich, James. *Religion and Rural Society: South Lindsey, 1825–1875.* Oxford: Clarendon Press, 1976.

Parry-Jones, William Ll. *The Trade in Lunacy: A Study of Private Madhouses in England in the Eighteenth and Nineteenth Centuries*. London: Routledge and Kegan Paul, 1972.

Podeschi, John B. *Books on the Horse and Horsemanship: Riding, Hunting, Breeding and Racing 1400–1941. A Catalogue*. London: Tate Gallery Publications Department, 1981.

Porter, Roy. "The Rage of Party: A Glorious Revolution in English Psychiatry?" *Medical History* 27 (1983): 35–50.

———. " 'The Hunger of Imagination': Approaching Samuel Johnson's Melancholy." *The Anatomy of Madness*. Vol. 1. Eds. W. F. Bynum, Roy Porter, and Michael Shepherd. London: Tavistock, 1985. 63–88.

———. "Lay Medical Knowledge in the Eighteenth Century: The Evidence of the *Gentleman's Magazine*." *Medical History* 29 (1985): 138–68.

———, ed. *Patients and Practitioners: Lay Perceptions of Medicine in Pre-industrial Society*. Cambridge and New York: Cambridge University Press, 1985.

———. "The Patient's View: Doing Medical History from Below." *Theory and Society* 14 (1985): 175–98.

———. *Mind-Forg'd Manacles. A History of Madness in England from the Restoration to the Regency*. London: Athlone, 1987.

———. *A Social History of Madness: Stories of the Insane*. London: Weidenfeld and Nicolson, 1987.

———. *Health for Sale: Quackery in England 1660–1850*. Manchester and New York: Manchester University Press, 1989.

———. "Foucault's Great Confinement." *History of the Human Sciences* 3.1 (1990): 47–54.

———, ed. *The Faber Book of Madness*. London: Faber and Faber, 1991.

———. "Reforming the Patient in the Age of Reform: Thomas Beddoes and Medical Practice." *British Medicine in an Age of Reform*. Eds. Roger French and Andrew Wear. London and New York: Routledge, 1991. 9–44.

———. "The Patient in England, c. 1660–c. 1800." *Medicine in Society: Historical Essays*. Ed. Andrew Wear. Cambridge and New York: Cambridge University Press, 1992. 91–118.

———, ed. *The Popularization of Medicine 1650–1850*. London: Routledge, 1992.

———. "The Rise of the Physical Examination." *Medicine and the Five Senses*. Eds. W. F. Bynum and Roy Porter. Cambridge: Cambridge University Press, 1993. 179–97.

———. *Quacks: Fakers and Charlatans in English Medicine*. Stroud: Tempus, 2000.

Porter, Roy, and Dorothy Porter. *In Sickness and in Health: The English Experience 1650–1850*. London: Fourth Estate, 1988.

———. *Patient's Progress: Doctors and Doctoring in Eighteenth-Century England*. Oxford: Polity/Blackwell, 1989.

Price, Harry. *Leaves from a Psychiatrist's Case-Book*. London: V. Gollancz, 1933.

Price, R. M. "A Case Book of the Philadelphia Almshouse Infirmary: Dr James

Rush Attending Physician [8 October 1819 to 10 February 1820]." *Bulletin of the History of Medicine* 59 (1985): 383–89.

Razzell, Peter E. *The Conquest of Smallpox: The Impact of Inoculation on Smallpox Mortality in Eighteenth-Century Britain.* Firle, Sussex: Caliban Books, 1977.

———. *Edward Jenner's Cowpox Vaccine: The History of a Medical Myth.* 2nd ed. Firle, Sussex: Caliban Books, 1980.

Rippere, Vicky. "The Survival of Traditional Medicine in Lay Medical Views: An Empirical Approach to the History of Medicine." *Medical History* 25 (1981): 411–14.

Risse, Guenter B., and John Harley Warner. "Reconstructing Clinical Activities: Patient Records in Medical History." *Social History of Medicine* 5 (1992): 183–205.

Rizzo, B. "John Sherratt, Negociator." *Bulletin of Research in the Humanities* 86.4 (1985): 413–21.

Rosenberg, Charles E. "The Therapeutic Revolution: Medicine, Meaning, and Social Change in Nineteenth-Century America." *The Therapeutic Revolution.* Eds. Morris J. Vogel and Charles E. Rosenberg. Philadelphia: University of Pennsylvania Press, 1979. 3–25.

Rousseau, George S. "Science." *The Eighteenth Century.* Ed. Pat Rogers. London: Methuen, 1978. 153–207.

———. "Psychology." *The Ferment of Knowledge.* Eds. George Rousseau and Roy Porter. Cambridge: Cambridge University Press, 1980. 143–210.

Rousseau, George S., and Roy Porter, eds. *Sexual Underworlds of the Enlightenment.* 1987. Manchester: Manchester University Press, 1992.

Rusnock, Andrea A. "The Weight of Evidence and the Burden of Authority: Case Histories, Medical Statistics and Smallpox Inoculation." *Medicine in the Enlightenment.* Ed. Roy Porter. Amsterdam and Atlanta: Rodopi, 1995. 289–315.

Sampson, Harold, Sheldon L. Messinger, and Robert D. Towne. "Family Process and Becoming a Mental Patient." *American Journal of Sociology* 68 (1962): 88–96.

Sawyer, Ronald C. "Friends or Foes? Doctors and their Patients in Early Modern England." *History of the Doctor-Patient Relationship: Proceedings of the Fourteenth International Symposium on the Comparative History of Medicine—East and West.* Eds. Yosio Kawakita, Shizu Sakai, and Yasuo Otsuka. Tokyo: Ishiyaku EuroAmerica, 1995. 31–53.

Schupbach, William. "John Monro MD and Charles James Fox: Etching by Thomas Rowlandson." *Medical History* 27 (1983): 80–83.

Schwartz, Charlotte Green. "Perspectives on Deviance: Wives' Definitions of Their Husbands' Mental Illness." *Psychiatry* 20 (1957): 275–91.

Scull, Andrew. "Psychiatry and Its Historians." *History of Psychiatry* 2 (1991): 239–50.

———. "A Failure to Communicate? On the Reception of Foucault's *Histoire de la folie* by Anglo-American Historians." *Rewriting the History of Madness.* Eds. Arthur Still and Irving Velody. London: Routledge, 1992. 150–63.

————. *The Most Solitary of Afflictions: Madness and Society in Britain, 1700–1900*. London and New Haven, Conn.: Yale University Press, 1993.

————. "Somatic Treatments and the Historiography of Psychiatry." *History of Psychiatry* 5 (1994): 1–12.

————. "Psychiatrists and Historical 'Facts': Part 1: The Historiography of Somatic Treatments." *History of Psychiatry* 6 (1995): 225–41.

————. "Bethlem Demystified?" *Medical History* 43 (1999): 248–55.

————. "Psychiatric Therapeutics and the Historian: Problems and Prospects." *Histoire de la psychiatrie: Nouvelles approches, nouvelles perspectives*. Eds. Jacques Gasser and Vincent Barras. Lausanne, Switzerland: Payot, in press.

Scull, Andrew, Charlotte MacKenzie, and Nicholas Hervey. *Masters of Bedlam: The Transformation of the Mad-Doctoring Trade*. Princeton, N.J.: Princeton University Press, 1996.

Selwyn, Sydney. "Sir John Pringle; Hospital Reformer, Moral Philosopher and Pioneer of Antiseptics." *Medical History* 10 (1966): 266–74.

Sheridan, Richard B. "The Doctor and the Buccaneer: Sir Hans Sloane's Case History of Sir Henry Morgan, Jamaica, 1688." *Journal of the History of Medicine and Allied Sciences* 41 (1986): 76–87.

Showalter, Elaine. *The Female Malady: Women, Madness and English Culture 1830–1980*. New York: Pantheon Books, 1985; London: Virago Press, 1987.

Sigerist, Henry E. "The Social History of Medicine." *Western Journal of Surgery, Obstetrics, and Gynecology* 42 (1940): 715–22.

Smith, Leonard D. "To Cure Those Afflicted with the Disease of Insanity: Thomas Bakewell and Spring Vale Asylum." *History of Psychiatry* 4.1 (March 1993): 107–28.

————. "Close Confinement in Mighty Prison: Thomas Bakewell and His Campaign against Public Asylums, 1810–1830." *History of Psychiatry* 5.2 (June 1994): 191–214.

————. *Cure, Comfort, and Safe Custody: Public Lunatic Asylums in Early Nineteenth Century England*. London: Leicester University Press, 1999.

Speak, Gill. "An Odd Kind of Melancholy: Reflections on the Glass Delusion in Europe (1440–1680)." *History of Psychiatry* 1 (1990): 191–206.

Spear, Thomas George Percival. *The Nabobs: A Study of the Social Life of the English in Eighteenth-Century India*. 2nd enlarged ed. Oxford: Oxford University Press, 1932; London [etc.]: Curzon Press, 1980.

Squibb, George Drewry. *Doctors' Commons: A History of the College of Advocates and Doctors of Law*. Oxford: Clarendon, 1977.

Steffan, Thomas. "The Social Argument against Enthusiasm (1650–1660)." *Studies in English* 21 (1941): 39–63.

Stevenson, Christine. "Robert Hooke's Bethlem." *Journal of the [American] Society of Architectural Historians* 55.3 (Sept. 1996): 254–75.

————. "The Architecture of Bethlem at Moorfields." *The History of Bethlem*. Jonathan Andrews, Asa Briggs, Roy Porter, Penny Tucker, and Keir Waddington. London: Routledge, 1997. 230–59.

————. *Medicine and Magnificence: British Hospital and Asylum Architecture, 1660–1815*. New Haven, Conn.: Yale University Press, 2000.

Stroud, Dorothy. *George Dance, Architect, 1741–1825.* London: Faber and Faber, 1971.

Strutt, Joseph. *A Memoir of the Life of Joseph Strutt, 1749–1802.* London: Printed for private circulation, 1896.

Sulloway, Frank J. "Reassessing Freud's Case Histories: The Social Construction of Psychoanalysis." *Isis* 82 (1991): 245–75.

Suzuki, Akihito. "The Household and the Care of Lunatics in Eighteenth-Century London." *The Locus of Care: Families, Communities, Institutions, and the Provision of Welfare since Antiquity.* Eds. Peregrine Horden and Richard Smith. London: Routledge, 1998. 153–75.

———. "Enclosing and Disclosing Lunatics in the Family Walls: Domestic Psychiatric Regime and the Public Sphere in Early Nineteenth-Century England." *Outside the Walls of the Asylum: The History of Care in the Community 1750–2000.* Eds. Peter Bartlett and David Wright. London: Athlone, 1999. 115–31.

Thornbury, G. W. *Life of J. W. M. Turner.* London: Chatto and Windus, 1904.

Tucker, Susie I. *Enthusiasm: A Study in Semantic Change.* Cambridge: Cambridge University Press, 1972.

Turner, Trevor. "Rich and Mad in Victorian England." *Psychological Medicine* 19 (1989): 29–44.

———. *A Diagnostic Analysis of the Casebooks of Ticehurst House Asylum 1845–1890.* Cambridge: Cambridge University Press, 1992.

Walker, Nigel. *Crime and Insanity in England. Volume 1: The Historical Perspective.* Edinburgh: Edinburgh University Press, 1968.

Walton, John. "Casting Out and Bringing Back in Victorian England: Pauper Lunatics, 1840–1870." *The Anatomy of Madness: Essays in the History of Psychiatry.* Vol. 2. Eds. W. F. Bynum, Roy Porter, and Michael Shepherd. London: Routledge, 1985. 132–46.

Wear, Andrew. "The Meaning of Illness in Early Modern England." *History of the Doctor-Patient Relationship: Proceedings of the Fourteenth International Symposium on the Comparative History of Medicine—East and West.* Eds. Yosio Kawakita, Shizu Sakai, and Yasuo Otsuka. Tokyo: Ishiyaku Euro-America, 1995. 1–29.

Weindling, Paul. "Medical Practice in Imperial Berlin: The Casebook of Alfred Grotjahn." *Bulletin of the History of Medicine* 61 (1987): 391–410.

Whitley, William T. *Artists and Their Friends in England 1700–1799.* 2 vols. New York and London: Benjamin Bloom, 1968; originally London and Boston: The Medical Society, 1928.

Whittaker, Christine B. "Chasing the Cure: Irving Fisher's Experience as a Tuberculosis Patient." *Bulletin of the History of Medicine* 48 (1974): 398–415.

Williams, Glyn, and John Ramsden. *Ruling Britannia: A Political History of Britain 1688–1988.* London: Longman, 1990.

Williamson, George. "The Restoration Revolt against Enthusiasm." *Studies in Philology* 2 (1933): 571–603.

Wright, David. "The Certification of Insanity in Nineteenth-Century England and Wales." *History of Psychiatry* 9.3 (Sept. 1998): 267–90.

Wynn, George. "The Case Book of Dr. Amos A. Evans, Surgeon on the Frigate 'Constitution' in the War of 1812." *Annals of Medical History* 3rd ser. 2 (1940): 70–78.

Yarrow, Marian Radke, Charlotte Green Schwartz, Harriet S. Murphy, and Leila Calhoun Deasy. "The Psychological Meaning of Mental Illness in the Family." *Journal of Social Issues* 11 (1955): 12–24.

Yates, Frances Amelia. *The Rosicrucian Enlightenment.* 1972; London and Boston: Routledge and Kegan Paul, 1999.

UNPUBLISHED DISSERTATIONS

Andrews, Jonathan. "Bedlam Revisited. A History of Bethlem Hospital, c. 1634–1770." Ph.D. diss. University of London, 1991.

Hough, Brenda Lilian. "A Consideration of the Antiquarian and Literary Works of Joseph Strutt: With Transcript of a Hitherto Unedited Manuscript Novel." Ph.D. diss. (Arts). University of London, Queen Mary College, 1984.

Phillips, H. Temple. "The History of the Old Private Lunatic Asylum at Fishponds, Bristol, 1740–1859." M.Sc. thesis. Bristol University, 1973.

Suzuki, Akihito. "Mind and Its Disease in Enlightenment Medicine." Ph.D. diss. University of London, 1992.

Ward, Karen. "'Moon Madness': A Study to Investigate the Relationship between Human Behaviour and the Phases of the Moon." Diss. (B. Nur.). University of Nottingham, 1997.

Index

Page numbers in italics indicate figures. Page numbers beginning with C- indicate pages of the case book transcription.

Ackerknecht, Erwin, 23
Act for Regulating Madhouses (1774), 43
Addington, Anthony, 43
Adee, Swithin, 104, C-9, 157*n*13
Alcock, Mrs., 97, 110, C-80
alcoholism. *See* drink
Allen, Thomas, 105
Allwright, Mr., C-105
Anatomy of Melancholy (Burton), 147*n*24
Anchor Street, C-117
Andrews, Jonathan, xi, xii
Anglicans, 83, 84
animals: mad, 32, 65–66, C-91–93, 141*n*38; spirits of, 75
Anther, Miss, 59, C-38
Antigua, C-13
antimony, 3
aphasia, 60
apoplexy, 60, C-29
aristocracy: and madness, 9, 29, 135*n*6; and medical profession, 49–50; and Methodism, 82; and Ticehurst Asylum, 32, 135*n*6
Arnold, Thomas, 32
Aspridge, Mr., 90, 97, C-2
astrology, 52, 113
asylums. *See* madhouses

Bakewell family, 32
Barnet, 33
Bartolozzi, Francesco, 34, 35
Barwell, Mrs., 55
Barwell, Richard, 55
Bath, C-59
bathing, 100, 101
Battie, William, 9, 20, 32, 66, 75, 77, 79, 101, 105, 106, 112, C-5, C-50, C-51, C-52, 142*n*41

beating, 97–98
Bedlam. *See* Bethlem
Beecher, Mr., C-102
Beier, Lucinda, 23
Belcher, William, 105
Belle Grove Asylum, 32
Bennett, John, 36, 44
Bethlem, xi, 14, 26, 30, 31, 35, 37, 38, 41, 51, 52, 61, 67, 91, 104, 105, C-63, C-66, C-80, 119*n*1; admission to, 35, 61; architecture of, 8; governors of, 9, 14, 37, 56, 96; history of, xiii, 6–7; and Hogarth, 37; incurables' ward at, *40*; inmates of, 7; museum at, 7, 132*n*48; and restraint, 98; and securities for admission, 129*n*32
Bethnal Green, 9, *10*, 43, C-43
Bethnal Green madhouse, *10*, 41, 104, 160*n*30
Bevan, Mr., 29, 31, 69, 93, 103, 113, C-15, C-29, C-30, C-39, C-42
Bishopsgate, 7, 8
Blackmore, Sir Richard, 45, 76
bleeding, 55, 92, C-26
Blinkhorn, Mrs., 21, 62, C-69
Bloomsbury, 43, C-1
Boswell, James, 72
Bowen, Thomas, 37, *39*
Bridewell, 14, 37
Brislington House, 32
Bristol, 101
Bromfield, Mrs., 89, C-80
Brooke, Mrs., 99
Brooke House, 43–44, 106
Buckley, Mr., C-20

Calcutta, 55
Campden, Miss, 59, 63, 68, 69, C-98

Carkesse, James, 105
Carnaby Street, C-38
case book, John Monro's, xiii, 61, 62,
  69, 72, 107, 112, 113; characteristics
  of, 16–17, 21–22; discovery of, xi–xii;
  and historians, 13, 14–15, 23, 24–25;
  and outcomes, 102–3; and publishers,
  24–26; and religion, 82, 83; and therapeutics, 92–93, 100; uses of, 16–20,
  26–27, 28, 102, 109; and women, 71
case books: and eighteenth-century medicine, 16, 18, 28; evolution of, 23–24;
  of John Hall, 25, 27; and historians,
  23–24; of John Hunter, 25; of Richard
  Loxham, 18–19, 21, 122n9; value of,
  24–25
Castle Yard, C-81
Catholicism, 85
Cawthorne, Mr., C-66
chains, 99
Chelsea, 9, 43, 100, 101, C-7, C-113
Chester, Sir Francis, 28, 48, 94, C-8
Cheyne, George, 11, 19, 26, 46, 47, 49,
  50–51, 79, 135n14
Chichester, 33, 46, 47, C-112
Child, Lady Dorothy, 106
children, and madness, 30
Cibber, Caius Gabriel, 37, 39
Clapton, 106
Clarissa (Fielding), 54
Clarke, William, 43
Clarke's madhouse, C-6, C-80
Clerkenwell, 106, C-21
Clerkenwell madhouse, 106
cold bathing, 50
Coltman, Mr., 31, C-23, 158n20
Compton, Miss, 59, 69, 80, 88–89, C-9
confinement, 5, 9, 42, 45–47, 61, 67, 68,
  83, 95, 96, 99, 100, 114, 115, C-51,
  C-52, C-68, C-106, C-107
constipation, 78, C-96
consumers, and the marketplace, 9
Cookson, Mrs., 78, 79, 80, 88, C-31
Cox, Joseph Mason, 32
Cozens, John Robert, 38, 41
Cross Lane, C-100
Crowther, Richard, 104
Cruden, Alexander, 14, 61, 83, 89, 104,
  105, 115, 121n10
Cullen, William, 32
Cutter, Miss, 59, 83, C-47

Dalton, Richard, 34, C-41, 160n27
Dance, George, the Elder, 41
Dance, George, the Younger, 41
Dance, Nathaniel, 7, 41
Darby, Mr., 93, C-118

Day's madhouse, C-53
delirium, 62, 101
delirium tremens, 60
delusions, 48, 60, 61, 62, 64, 66, 76, 89,
  93, 110, 114, 115
dementia, 60
Dempster, Mr., C-6
depression, 70, 75, 87, 91, 111, C-4,
  C-6. See also melancholy
Devic's madhouse, C-4
Devil, the, 85, 86, 87, 93, 109, 113,
  C-17, C-25, C-45, C-75, C-79, C-119
Devy, Mr., C-115
diagnosis, 13, 21, 24, 45–47, 62, 77–79,
  107–9; by correspondence, 49, 50;
  patient history's role in, 107
Dibsdale, Mrs., 69, 97, 114, C-65
dietetics, 26, 55, 79, 93
Diggers, 84
Distress'd Orphan, or Love in a Mad-
  house (Haywood), 54
doctor-patient relationship, 49
Dominiceti, Bartholomew di, 101, 102,
  C-113, 169n81
drink, and insanity, 56, 60–61, 78, 87,
  103, C-4, C-24, C-40, C-77
Drury Lane, C-81
Dudley's madhouse, C-1, 159n25
Duffield, Michael, 9, 43, 99, 104, C-57,
  C-124
Duffield's madhouse, 99, C-31, C-51,
  C-52, C-56, C-106
Duncan, Mrs., 58, 60, 69, 77, 79, 85,
  C-34

East India Company, 55
economy, in eighteenth century, 111–12;
  of London, 9
Edge, Mrs., 58, 85, 94, C-25
Edmonton, C-111
Elder, Mrs., 58, 92, 114, C-96, C-97
emotional disturbance, 69, 73, 113–14
English Malady, the, 11, 26
engraving, 34, 35, 36
Enlightenment, the, 52, 73; and superstition, 86
epilepsy, 29, 52, 60, 86, C-79
Esquirol, J. E. D., 62
extravagance, 70

false confinement, 96
families and mental illness, 5, 9, 45–47,
  51, 58, 61, 68–69, 70–71, 85, 94, 95,
  96, 110, 111, 112, 113, 134n1; and
  compulsion, 97, 98, 100; and demand
  for madhouses, 99
fancy, 64, 86, 89, 147n20

Farington, Joseph, 38, 132*n*50
Farnham, C-114
Fermanagh, Lord, 105
Ferrers, Earl, 28, 63, 81, 140*n*27
fever, 62, C-2, C-11, C-64, C-80, C-124
Fifth Monarchists, 84
Finch, William, 32
Finch family, 32
Finsbury madhouse, 105
Fishponds Asylum, 32
Fitzgerald, Mr., 80, 95–96, 98, 111, C-86
Fleet Market, C-75
Fletcher, Mr., 31, C-118
Flora (patient), 62, C-1–2
Fludger, Mrs., 110, 114–15, C-115
Foote, Samuel, 82
force-feeding, 96–97
Foucault, Michel, 61, 95
Fox, Charles James, 39–40, *40*
Fox family, 32
Frazer, Mr., C-55
frenzy, C-35, C-40, C-67

gender: and madness, 30, 53–55, 59–60, 70–71; and physiology, 144*n*82
general paralysis of the insane, 60
George III, 34, 35, 79, 133*n*56; and Thomas Warburton, 41; and Francis Willis, 32
Gilchrist, Miss, 21, 53–54, 110, C-100
Girdler, Joseph, 104, 105
Girtin, Thomas, 37
glass delusion, 110
Glocester Street, C-94
Godwin, Mrs., 31, 113, C-45
Goldsmith, Dr., 101, 154*n*8
Gordon, Mrs., 32, 65–66, C-92–94
Goupy, Joseph, 35, 36, C-7, 130*n*36
gout, 64
Graham, Miss, 80, C-43
Great Confinement, 95
Greaves, Miss, 80, 89, C-19
Grecian coffee house, C-23, 159*n*21
Griffin, Mr., 31, 77, C-79
Guy, Thomas, 9

Hackney, 9, 43
Hales, Charles, 65, 140*n*35
Hall, John, case book of, 25, 27
hallucinations, 60, 61
Hamilton, Mr., 91, C-6–7
Hampson, Mrs., 54, 66, 70, 110, C-89
Hanbury, Sir Charles, 106
Handasyde, Dr., 63, C-110
Hardinge, George, 101
Harris, Mrs., 31, 67, 69, 77, 80, 87, C-46, C-114

Harris family, 32
Harrison, J. F. C., 89
Haslam, John, 25–26, 91, 148*n*39
Hastings, Warren, 55
Hatton Garden, C-44
Hawkins, Mr., C-59
Heber, Mr., C-124, 173*n*89
Heberden, Dr. William, C-56, 161*n*42
Hendon, C-46
Henry VIII, 7
heredity, 64
heroic medicine, 96, 149*n*18
Hertfordshire, 33, C-89
Highgate, 31, C-118
Hitchin, C-89
Hobbes, Mrs., 59, 81, C-99
Hogarth, William, 37, *38*, 82, 131*n*46
Holborn, C-23
Holford, Mrs., 58, 80, C-37
Holman, Mrs., 67, 80, C-121
Hook, Robert, 8
Hook Norton House, 32
Hooper, Mr., C-109
Hooper, Mrs., 86, C-109
Horace, 36
Horsley, 114, C-65
Horton, C-114
hospitals, London, 7, 9, 41
Howard, Miss, C-31
Hoxton, 9, 42, C-4, C-115
Hudson, Mr., C-67
Hume, Miss, 58, C-13
humoral medicine, 26, 78
Hunter, John, case books of, 25
Huntingdon, Selena Countess of, 49, 50
Huntingdonshire, 33, C-120
hypochondria, 11, 46, 100, 113, C-62
hysteria, 11, 60, 62, 86, 113, C-45, C-71

iatromechanical medicine, 75, 144*n*66
idiocy, 64, 87, C-6, C-61
incontinence, 31, 78, C-11–12, C-27, C-35
India, C-102
Inge, Mr., 31, C-63
Ingleby, David, 5
Ingram, Allan, 91
Ingram, Dale, C-124
Inner Temple, 104–5, 150*n*48
inoculation, 165*n*53
insanity. *See* madness
Inskip, Peter, 43, 104, 155*n*10
Inskip's madhouse, 35, 43, 104, C-7
insomnia, 56, 62
Italian artists, 34, 35

Jackson, Goodwife, 3

Jackson, Mr., C-114
Jacobitism, 82
Jamaica, C-15, C-48, C-49
James, Robert, 101, 153n8
James's Powders, 101, 102, C-5, 153n8
jealousy, 63
Jefferies, Miss, 87, 111, 112, C-4–5
Jefferiss, F. J. G., xi, xii, xv, 16
Jewin Street, C-79
Jewson, Nicholas, 48, 49
Johnson, Samuel, 36, 72
John Street, C-115
Jones, Mr., 113, C-75
Jubilate Agno (Smart), 10
Jütte, Robert, 23

Kensington, 35, C-61
Kent, 33, C-123
Kinder, Mr., 32, C-73, C-74
Kinder, Mrs., 32, 56, 70, C-73, C-74
King's Bench, Court of, 3, C-50, C-54
King's Road, C-115
Kirby, John, 10
Knapstone, Captain, 31, C-106

Lady's Magazine, 72, 73, 74
Lambert, Mrs., 60, 80, C-29
Lane, Joan, 25
Lavater, Johann Casper, 77
Laverstock House, 32
Law, Mrs., C-76
lawyers, 29
Leather Lane, C-99
Lee, Nathaniel, 115
Leicester Lunatic Asylum, 32
Levellers, 84
Lisson Green, C-98
London: City of, 8, 33, 35; economy of, 9
London Wall, 41
Long Acre, C-124
Lovell, Miss, 59, 64, 78, 83, C-21
Loxham, Richard, 18–19, 21, 122n9

MacCune, Mr., 34
MacDonald, Captain, 59, 69, 76, 77, 112, C-68, C-72
MacDonald, Michael, 25, 52, 61, 84, 88, 89, 113
Macham, William, 29, 76, 110–11, C-27, 159n23
Mackenzie, James, xii, xv
Mackenzie, Mr., C-51, C-52, C-53
Mackenzie, Mrs., 77, C-50, C-51, C-52
mad-business. *See* trade in lunacy
mad-doctors, 19; caricatures of, 41, 115; and case histories, 47–48; and definition of madness, 62; as emerging pro-

fession, 6, 11, 42, 115–16, 121n9; and families, 46–48, 115, 135n2; and passions, 76; and patients, 15, 21; as "smiling hyena," 105; and stigma, 30, 42, 47, 105, 106; and therapeutics, 93
madhouses, 6, 9, 10, 32, 42, 43–44, 67, 95, 96; lay vs. medical, 43; and paupers, 10; profits of, 43, 115; and restraint, 99
Madhouses Enquiry (1763), 96
madness: and animality, 79, 87, 98–99; and astrology, 113; and behavior, 58, 66–67, 69; and the body, 63–64, 66, 76–78, 81–82, 87; definition of, 4, 46; demography of, 30; domestic management of, 30, 32, 45, 47, 95, C-88; and dress, 68, C-98; and eating, 79–80, 81, 96–97, 114, C-32, C-57, C-59, C-62, C-66, C-70, C-78, C-105; etiology of, 51–52, 55–56, 63, 108–9; experience of, 15; and eyes, 77, C-45; and heredity, 31, 56, 64, 87, C-4, C-11; and the imagination, 66; and incontinence, C-11; and insensibility, 59, 77, 96, 99, 114, C-11, C-39; and laity, 13, 24, 46; and language, 58–59, 60, 61, C-11–12, C-14, C-35, C-37, C-39, C-42, C-62, C-64, C-71, C-106–8; and literature, 52, 54; and the moon, 52, 113, C-16, C-30, C-42, 137n25; and passions, 55, 56, 69, 71, 76, 109; and psychology, 52, 109, 113; raving, 39, 67, 70; and religion, 81–90, 110; secularization of, 61; and sin, 109; and social class, 21, 28–29, 71; and social control, 33, 115; stereotypes of, 7; and stigma, 42, 46, 47, 112, 137n32; and the supernatural, 109; symptoms of, 21, 30–31, 45–46, 51, 58–59, 61–62, 68–69, 75, 87, 94, 114, 115; and violence, 66–68, 114
Madrid, C-15
Malling, C-123
manacles, 37
mania, 50, 70, 87, 115
Manley, Mrs., 80, 97–98, 111, C-66
Mansion House, 41
masturbation, 21, 56, 113, C-8, 155n11
Matthews, James Tilly, 26, 148n39
Mead, Richard, 32, 52, 96, 104
mechanical restraint, 97, 98, 99, C-105
medical careers: building of, 31–32; and patronage, 48
medical knowledge, 48
medical marketplace, in eighteenth century, 28, 32, 33, 100
medical police, 67

melancholy, 7, 45, 47, 58, 69, 70, 71, 79, 87, 90, 113, 115, C-15, C-30, C-44, C-46, C-55, 143*n*60, 147*n*24. *See also* depression
Mendez, Moses, 37, 131*n*46
mental patients, 14, 24; as cases, 18, 20, 31; and families, 11, 30, 32, 45, 46, 47, 48, 108, 113; and historians, 5; language of, 108–9, 115; and mad-doctors, 5, 15, 32–33, 46, 48, 115–16; marital status of, 30; narratives of, 26, 64–65, 76, 91, 107–8, 115; and secrecy, 20–21, 42; self-diagnosis of, 107–8, 110, 112, 115; social origins of, 28, 29–30, 34; suffering of, 109–10, 111, 113, C-40, C-55; symptoms of, 22, 45, 46, 51, 60, 62, 92, 94, 110, 111, 114, 115
Mercer, Mrs., C-39
merchants, 28, 29
Methodism: and madness, 3, 82, 83, 85, 146*n*10; and satirists, 82
Middlesex, 33
Miles, John, 42, 43
Miles's madhouse, 67, 84, 95–96, 113, C-1, C-2, C-20, C-37, C-38, C-39, C-65, C-67, C-68, C-79, C-89, C-111, C-114
Miller, Justice, C-54
Mitchell, Mr., 68, 98, C-105
Mitford, John, 41
Molyneux, Mr., 56, 80, C-3
Mombray, Miss, 61, C-19
Monro, Edward Thomas, 38, 119*n*1
Monro, Henry, 41, 132*n*48
Monro, James, 6, 8, 14, 17, 31–32, 34, 37, 43, 83, 104, 105, 113, C-25, C-45, C-106, 121*n*10, 131*n*46, 132*n*48, 150*n*49
Monro, John, 7, 11; and art world, 34, 35–40, 42; and Battie, 75, 77, 79, 104, 112, 141*n*41; and Bethlem, 5, 6, 8, 9, 131*n*46; and Brooke House, 43–44; caricatures of, 39–41, 40; and case book, xii–xiv, 13, 15, 16–20, 21–23, 31, 60; case outcomes of, 102; and competitors, 33, 112; and compulsion, 97, 99–100; and confidentiality, 20; corpulence of, 40–41, 40; and the courtroom, 19; and Cruden, 83, 121*n*10; and diagnosis, 46, 47, 48, 50, 58, 60, 61, 62, 63, 64, 66, 68, 77–79, 81, 88, 90–91, 92, 108, 113, 115; and diary, 36; and etiology of madness, 56, 63, 75, 76–77, 87; and expertise, 33, 115, 116; and families, 26, 46, 48, 57, 64, 94, 95, 108, 113, 114, 115; and fees, 105; and Ferrers, 140*n*27; as gentleman, 20, 28, 33, 42, 66; and

Hogarth, 37; library of, 34, 36, 37, 62, 79, 86; and madhouses, 6, 42–43; and management, 93; and James Monro, 101, 102; and nature of clientele, 28, 29, 30, 33; and Oxford University, 34, 36; and patients, 26, 30–32, 42, 45–47, 48, 50–51, 53, 55, 59, 64, 70, 71, 75, 76–77, 79–80, 87, 89, 91, 94, 95, 96, 102, 104, 108, 111, 112, 113, 114, 115; and politics, 82; portrait of, 7, 41, 132*n*48; private practice of, 6, 14, 20, 26, 32, 33, 43, 50–51, 67; professional ties of, 29, 42–43, 103–4; referral networks of, 33–34; religious views of, 82, 83–85, 86, 89; and Royal College of Physicians, 104; and Scottish connections, 34; social status of, 29–30, 43; and therapeutics, 92, 93, 103, 115; and Walpole family, 36
Monro, Thomas (John's son), 26, 41; and artists, 34, 37, 38, 39, 133*n*50
Monro, Thomas (of Magdalen College), 4, 55, 67, 74, 75, 143*n*62, 144*n*68
Monro family, xi; and the arts, 42; and Bethlem, 6, 26, 38, 119*n*1; and mad-business, 6, 31–32, 44, 105
Montague, Lady Mary Wortley, 54
Montague, Mrs. Elizabeth Robinson, 55
Moore, Mr., 31, 60–61, 62, 80, 103, C-40
Moorfields, 8, 41, C-116
Moreati, Mrs. Elizabeth, 34, 58, 114, C-41
Mount Pleasant, 33, C-112
Muggletonians, 84
Murphy, Elaine, 10, 133*n*56
Murphy, Terence, 88

Napier, Richard, 25
nervous disorders, 26, 42, 46, 49, 50, 62, 71–72, 95, 96, 100, 109, 113
Newgate Gaol, 41
Newington family, 32
Newport, Mr., 67, 69, C-81, C-83
Newport market, C-118
New Testament, 86
Newtonian medicine, 26, 56, 96
Nicholson, Margaret, 59
Nicolson, 81

Old Bailey, 29, 109, C-29, C-61
onanism. *See* masturbation
Orford, third Earl of, 28, 106
Ormond Street, C-94
Oxfordshire, 32
Oxford University, 34, 36

Paddington, 43, C-53
Pamela (Richardson), 49

paranoia, 61, 70, 110
Pargeter, William, 25, 29, 47, 52, 77–78, 146*n*10
paupers, madhouses' treatment of, *10*
Peace, Sarah, C-81
Peers, Alderman Richard, 28, 93, 113, C-62, 164*n*50
Perfect, William, 85–86
Peter's Street, C-76
physical examination, 81, 107
physiognomy, 77–78
Pigot, Mrs., C-36
Pilgrim's Progress (Bunyan), 3
Pinel, Philippe, 62
Pitcairn, David, 104
Pitcairn, William, 104
Pitt, William, 40
Plow, Mrs., 63, C-110
Poland Street, C-50
poor. *See* paupers
Pope, Alexander, 71, 82
popery, 85
Porter, Roy, xv–xvi, 23, 24, 25, 26, 100, 107
Potter, George, *10*
Pottinger, Mr., 61, C-108
Preston, Miss, C-99
pride, 61, 75–76
Pringle, Sir John, C-58, C-59, 162*n*44
Printer, Miss, C-78
professional status, 28, 30, 43
Prowsett, Captain, 48, 78, C-75, C-77
psychiatric therapeutics, 5
psychiatry: and case notes, 25; history of, 5, 14–15, 23
puerperal insanity, 70
pulse, C-28, C-35; significance of, 81, 88
Purcell, 46
purging, 92

quacks, 28, 100, 101, 112
Quakerism, 83–84, C-21, C-47
quantification, and eighteenth century, 17
Queen's Square, C-94

rabies, 33, 66
Rake's Progress (Hogarth), 37, *38*
Rakewell, Tom, 37, *38*
Ramsay, Mr., 91, C-111
Ramsgate, 100, C-109, C-123
Ranters, 84
Reading, 43
Red House, *10*, 121*n*10
Reeve, Dr. Thomas, 104, C-85
Reformation, English, 8
regimen, 107
Relhan, Dr., Anthony, C-59, 164*n*47

religious enthusiasm, and madness, 82–86, 89, C-106
Restoration, English, 8, 84, 115
Richardson, Mr., 33, C-112
Richardson, Samuel, 49
Risse, Günther, 23
Robinson, Captain, 64–65, 67, C-48
Robinson, Nicholas, 19, 56, 96
Robinson, Sir George, 28, C-8, 156*n*12
Rosat, Mr., 29, 111, C-119
Rosenberg, Charles, 120*n*4
Rosicrucianism, 86
Rotherhithe, C-91
Rowlandson, Thomas, 39–40, *40, 41, 42*
Rowley, Mr., 64, 67, 69, 79, 114, C-58
Rowley, Sir William, 114, C-58
Royal College of Physicians, 7, 41, 43, 75, 101, 104, 132*n*48
Ryan, Mr., 76, 84, C-65

St. James's Park, C-25
St. Luke's Hospital, 9, 41
St. Thomas's Hospital, 104
satire, Augustan, 71, 75, 86
Savoy Hospital, 65
Sayer, Robert, 36
Schupbach, William, 39–40
Scotland, 34, C-3, C-7
Select Committee on Madhouses (1815), *10*
self-dosing, 100
self-mutilation, 67, C-56
senility, 30
sensationalist theory, 21
sensibility, cult of, 72
Sergison, Mr., 58, 80, C-61
servants, 29
Seymour, Lord Robert, *10*
Shaftesbury, Lord, 9
Shakespeare, William, 36
Sharp, William, *39*
Sheeles, Mrs., C-94
Sherratt, Mr., C-54
Shoreditch, C-17
Shoreland, Mrs., 31, C-39
Showalter, Elaine, 143*n*60
sick role, 23
Sigerist, Henry, 23
slaves, 29, 62, C-1–2
sleep, disturbances of, 80–81, 86–87, 90, 93, 113, 114, C-4, C-10, C-11, C-19, C-28, C-32, C-37, C-40, C-46, C-55, C-57, C-62, C-64, C-70, C-78, C-90, C-116
Smart, Christopher, *10*
Smithfield, 110, C-71
Smollett, Tobias, 52, 86

Snow, John, *10*
Snowhill, C-98
South Sea Bubble, 112
Southwell, Thomas, 104, C-7
Speak, Gill, 110
Spitalfields, C-117
spleen, 11, 46
Spring Vale Asylum, 32
Staffordshire, 32
Stanfield, Mr., 33, 89–90, 110, C-120
Steevens, George, 36
Stevenson, Christine, and asylum architecture, 8
stoicism, 73; criticism of, 74, 143*n*62
Stone, Mrs., 58, 79, 114, C-10
Stothard, Thomas, 39
strait waistcoats, 99
Strange, Sir Robert, 34
Strutt, Joseph, 36
Strutton, Mr., C-43, C-117
Stubbs, Mrs., C-116
suicide, 74, 88, 103; attempted, 65, 67, 70, 71, 72, 73, 87, 91, 111, 114, C-5, C-7, C-39, C-50; as sign of madness, 88
Sussex, 33, C-80
Sutton, Miss, 31, C-64
Suzuki, Akihito, 23
Swift, Jonathan, 82
syphilis, 60

Taylor, Mr., C-91
Theobald, Miss, 32, 68, 69, C-47
Theobald, Mrs., 32, C-47
therapeutics, 13, 49, 50, 92; and the historian, 120*n*4
Ticehurst Asylum, 32
Tonkin, Mr., 56, 77, 85, C-44
trade in lunacy, 9, 11, 14, 15, 26, 30–32, 42, 43, 115; and endogamy, 32
tradesmen, 28, 29, 49
Trecothick, Alderman Barlow, 28, 89, 171*n*84
Trecothick, Mrs., 89, C-115
Tunbridge, C-63
Turkey, 111, C-119
Turner, Trevor, 15, 23
Turner, William Joseph Mallord, 37
Tuten, Bella, 30–31, 79, 114, C-26

Tuthill, George Leman, 119*n*1
Tyson, Edward, 52

Undertaker of the Mind (Andrews and Scull), xi, 28
undertakers, 120*n*9; emergence of trade, 9

Vadall, Mr., 86
Van Hock, Mrs., 31, 64, 111, C-94
vanity, 61, 75
vapors, the, 11, 46, 49
venereal disease, 65, 113, C-2, C-48, C-59, C-124. *See also* syphilis
violence, by patients, 66–67, 114, C-25, C-59, C-60, C-65, C-82–84
vomits, 92

Walker, Mr., 109, C-17
Walker, Mrs., 35, 60, C-7
Walpole, Horace, 54, 137*n*32
Warburton, Thomas, 10, 41, 133*n*56
watercolorists, British School of, 37, 38
Webb, Mrs., 31, C-117
Weindling, Paul, 23
Wesley, John, 3, 82
Westminster, 33, 101, 109, C-18, C-105
Wharton, Lord, 9
Whitbread, Samuel, 29, C-3
Whitby, Mr., 59, 80, C-63
Whitefield, George, 82
Whitehead, Mr., 31, 51, 67, 110, C-56
White House, Bethnal Green, 10, 104, 121*n*10
Wilkes, John, 165*n*50
Williams, Elizabeth, 36
Williams, Mr., C-81, C-85
Willis, Francis, 32
Willis, Thomas, 96
Wilmot, Mrs., C-117
Wilson, Mrs., 67, 70, 110, C-80, C-85
Wiltshire, 32
Winchester Street, C-121
Winter, Mrs., 110, 115, C-68, C-71
women, and madness, 30, 53–55, 59–60, 70–71, 144*n*82; popular depictions of, 72, 73, 74
Worth, Mrs., C-45
Wright, Matthew, 9, 10, 121*n*10, 160*n*30

Text: 10/13 Sabon
Display: Sabon
Compositor: BookMatters, Berkeley
Printer and Binder: Edwards Brothers, Inc.